A Book for Midwives

A manual for traditional birth attendants and community midwives

by Susan Klein

Medical editor: Suellen Miller, CNM, PHD
with Judith Bishop, CNM, MPH
and Marcia Hansen, CNM, MSN

Editor: Sandy Niemann

Blanche with great pleasure + gratitude for your words + your friendship

Charlotte

THE

HESPERIAN

FOUNDATION

1995

D1293749

Each pregnant woman and each birth is unique. Birth attendants have a responsibility to be honest with themselves and the pregnant mother about the limits of their skills. This means: **do only what you know how to do**. Do not try to do things you have not learned about or have not had enough experience doing, so that you do not harm or endanger a mother or her child. At the same time, do not be afraid to learn from this book or from others who have more experience, so that you can improve your knowledge and skills.

The Hesperian Foundation and contributors to *A Book for Midwives* do not assume liability for the use of information contained in this book. This book should not replace properly supervised hands-on training. If you are not sure what to do in an emergency situation, you should try to get advice and help from people with more experience or from local medical and health authorities.

This manual can be improved with your help. We would like to hear about your experiences, traditions, and practices. If you are a midwife, traditional birth attendant, village health worker, doctor, nurse, mother, or anyone with suggestions for ways to make this book better meet the needs of your community, please write to us. Your comments can help make future editions better and more useful. Thank you for your help.

Published by:

The Hesperian Foundation

P.O. Box 1692

Palo Alto, California 94302

U.S.A.

Copyright 1995 by the Hesperian Foundation. All rights reserved.

First published March 1995

Printed in the U.S.A.

Library of Congress Catalog Card Number: 94-07378

ISBN 0-942364-22-8

A Book for Midwives is printed on paper that contains 10% post-consumer waste. Soy-based ink has been used to further reduce the harmful environmental impact of the printing process.

A note about the author

The author, Susan Klein, passed away before this manual was completed. Before Susan died she asked that this book be dedicated to all the women and men who attend women in childbirth. Susan hoped that *A Book for Midwives* would become a tool to assist midwives and traditional birth attendants in making decisions—a tool that provides information and yet respects their ability to make the best decisions for each birth. The Hesperian Foundation hopes that readers and users of this manual will feel Susan's concern and compassion throughout this book and will carry her spirit with them in their work.

Thanks

A Book for Midwives was completed through the cooperative effort of many people. Although Susan Klein passed away before completing the final draft, her vision and spirit guided it through its last stages. In addition, many people contributed their time and expertise. Some provided information on specific topics or birthing practices in different parts of the world. Others helped with illustrations, typed, edited, proofread, or worked on paste-up and correspondence. The Hesperian Foundation is extremely grateful to all those who provided their generous help. We have undoubtedly overlooked some of the contributors and wish to apologize to them. The omission is inadvertent.

The following people were extremely helpful over the course of the book's development:

Samia Altaf, Steve Babb, Naomi Baumslag, Deborah Bickel, Trude Bock, Bill Bower, Jenny Bowers, Kate Bowland, Ann Boyer, Colin Bullough, August Burns, Jennie Corr, Kyle Craven, J.T. Dunn, Maya Escudero, Sylvia Estrada-Claudio, Sadja Greenwood, Caitlin Higginbotham, Kathleen Huggins, Christine Johnson, Mary Johnson, Angela Kamara, Lisa Keller, Raven Lang, Julie Litwin, Ronnie Lovitch, Alan Margolis, Jane Maxwell, Nicky May, Iris Moore, Nimal Perera, David Sanders, Merrie Schaller, Mira Shiva, Judith Standley, Michael Tan, Greg Troll, Gilberte Vansintejan, and David Werner.

The final manuscript was completed during 1994. The following people provided exceptional and dedicated work to prepare it for publication and deserve special thanks:

Project coordinator: Lisa Ziebel
Medical editor: Suellen Miller, with Judith Bishop and Marcia Hansen
Editor: Sandy Niemann
Book design and production: Peter Ivey
Copy editor and proofreader: Susan McCallister
Index: Ty Koontz
Medicines research: Carol Thuman
Medical questions: Davida Coady, Bill Parer, Alan Margolis, Margaret Marshall,
     Robert Keast, Sadja Greenwood, James Green, and Brian Linde
Illustrations: Deb Greene
Editing and production assistance: B.A. Laris, Jane Maxwell, and Lisa de Avila

A number of texts were used in preparing this manuscript. Susan Klein received much of her inspiration from Ina May Gaskin's book, *Spiritual Midwifery*. The following books were also helpful: E. Davis, *A Guide to Midwifery: Heart and Hands*; L. Eloesser, E. J. Galt and I. Hemingway, *Pregnancy, Childbirth and the Newborn: A Manual for Rural Midwives*; G. Gordon, *Training Manual for Traditional Birth Attendants*; M.A. Marshall and S.T. Buffington, *Life-Saving Skills Manual for Midwives*; and M. Myles, *Textbook for Midwives*. (A complete list of references follows the index.)

The costs of developing this book were met by generous grants from the Carnegie Corporation of New York, the Packard Foundation, the Compton Foundation, UNICEF, Oxfam UK, Save the Children Fund, the Swedish International Development Authority (SIDA) and the Danish International Development Agency (DANIDA). We are very grateful to these organizations and to the inividual donors who supported this work.

Contents

SECTION A

Introduction

A Book for Midwives is written for caregivers who are concerned about the health of pregnant women and their babies. It is especially for people who live far from maternity centers or in places where it is difficult for poor people to get medical care. Since it is written in clear, simple language, people with little education can use it to learn more about pregnancy and birth.

In this book we may use the word *midwife* differently than people do in your area. In some parts of the world, only those health workers who have been trained to work in a hospital, maternity center, or clinic are called midwives. In other parts of the world, anyone who gives care at a birth is called a midwife, whether she has received training or not. We will use the word midwife to describe anyone who is the main care giver during pregnancy and birth—and who is not a doctor. This includes:

- *Traditional midwives* who have learned their skills by experience (or from other traditional midwives) and work in the community. They are sometimes called *traditional birth attendants (TBAs)* or *direct entry midwives* (DEMs).

- *Auxiliary midwives* who have had some medical training, and may work in the hospital, maternity center, or in the community.

- *Professional midwives* and *nurse-midwives* who have a lot of medical or nursing training and work in the hospital, maternity center, or in the community.

- Community health workers who sometimes attend births.

- Anyone who happens to find herself (or himself) giving care to a woman during pregnancy and birth.

Just as there are many different kinds of midwives, there are also many different ideas about what midwives can and should do. Some people think that midwives primarily attend births. Others believe that midwives can do much more. In this book, we encourage midwives to do all of the following things:

- help mothers stay healthy during pregnancy

- help mothers have safer labors and births

- give care to new babies

- help mothers and babies through many kinds of emergencies (but get medical help when needed)

- teach women and the community about pregnancy and birth

- be aware of health issues that affect the entire community

- help stop the spread of disease (like AIDS)

The following 2 chapters contain general information that will help midwives who are involved in any of the tasks listed above:

- Words to midwives (chapter 1)

- Tools for safer births (chapter 2)

In this book we have tried to include suggestions from midwives, doctors, and other health workers from all over the world. Some of these suggestions will work in your area, but some of them will not. Many times a midwife is limited by national or local rules or laws; this is called her *"scope of practice."* For example, in some areas a midwife can give injections or perform internal (vaginal) exams, but in other areas a midwife cannot do these things. We encourage all midwives to check the local rules with their local health authorities or health officers, and to discuss their scope of practice with community leaders.

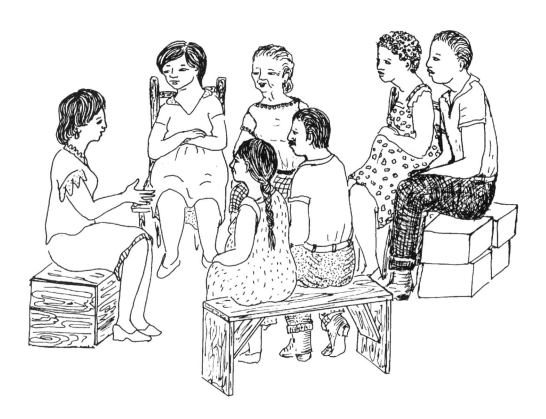

Words to midwives

Chapter 1 contents

Words to midwives

How to be a better midwife

A midwife needs to have many different skills to meet the health needs of women. The following 11 things are needed by all midwives, no matter how much training they have had or where they work. We will remind you of these skills throughout the book and give you ideas about how to use them in specific ways.

1. Help stop the spread of infection and disease

Most diseases and **infections** are caused by **germs** (very small living things that cannot be seen). Germs can be passed from a midwife to a pregnant woman, or from a pregnant woman to a midwife. **The "3 Cleans"**—clean hands, clean birth area, and clean cord cutting—can prevent the spread of germs during childbirth.

In chapter 9, we talk about how to keep things clean and other ways to help stop the spread of infection and disease. **Every midwife should read chapter 9 very carefully before giving care to pregnant women.**

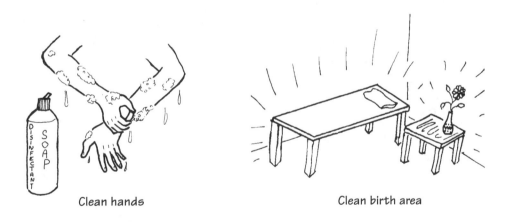

Clean hands

Clean birth area

Clean cord cutting

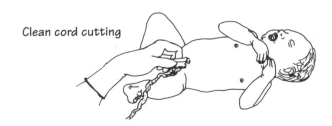

The "3 cleans"

Midwives and AIDS

In some parts of the world, many women giving birth have **AIDS** (Acquired Immune Deficiency Syndrome). AIDS is caused by a small germ *(virus)* called the Human Immune Deficiency Virus *(HIV)*. People who are infected with HIV may look healthy for years before they show signs of AIDS, but they can still spread the disease.

HIV is not easy to get. You cannot get HIV from food, drink, insects, or through the air. HIV is spread when a healthy person is in contact with the blood or other body fluids of a person who is infected with HIV. Some of the most common ways of spreading HIV are: having sex without a **condom** (see p. 347), getting blood from a person with HIV, and using needles or other equipment that have not been treated with heat or **chemicals** to kill ALL of the germs. HIV is also passed from a mother to her unborn child.

Midwives who have cuts or sores on their skin can get HIV when they touch inside a pregnant woman, or when they touch any of the mother's body fluids or anything (like the afterbirth) that has been inside the mother. If a midwife has HIV and has cuts or sores on her hands, she can spread HIV to the mother if she touches the mother inside. For this reason we recommend touching inside the mother **only** when it is necessary to save the mother's life and only when the midwife has gloves or plastic bags on her hands (see p. 160–161).

Midwives can also help stop the spread of HIV in their communities by teaching others how to protect themselves. Midwives can encourage men to wear condoms during sex and discourage practices like circumcision and ear piercing that break the skin and may be done without sterile instruments. Midwives should only use sterile needles when they give *injections* (see p. 157).

2. Be kind and respectful

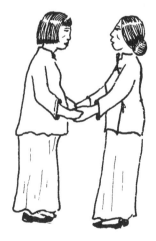

Although much of a midwife's job is to meet the health needs of women, she also must be aware that women have human needs, too. Sometimes the most important thing you can do for someone's health is to listen to them, try to understand them, and let them know you care about them.

This is especially true in pregnancy and birth. Often a kind word, a gentle touch, a massage, or a respectful talk will do more than medicine. When you show a woman care and respect, you help her to respect and care for herself.

3. Learn as much as you can from those who already know

If you are just learning to be a midwife, it is best to train with someone who is already a skilled midwife. Many of the things that you will read about in this book are hard to learn without someone to show you how.

You can try arranging an *apprentice* program with experienced midwives. This means that one or more new midwives or students works with an experienced midwife when she does checkups and attends births. This way you will have attended many births with experienced midwives before becoming the main care giver at a birth.

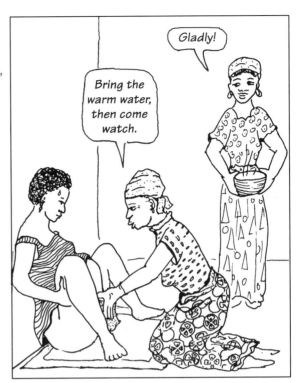

4. Keep learning more

Some midwives think they already know everything there is to know about birth. But they are wrong! There is always more to know.

Use every chance you have to learn. Study whatever books or information you find. Talk to people. Ask questions of doctors, other midwives, health workers, and community elders—anyone who may know something helpful.

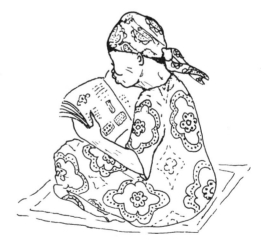

You can also learn from the women you help. Watch and see how well your practices work. Ask new mothers how they felt about their births—what they feel you did well, what you could have done better, and what needs they had that you did not notice.

5. Always ask *why?*

There are 2 kinds of learning: learning what to do and learning why it works.

If you understand why something works, you can avoid many mistakes. You will also be able to figure out the answers to other problems. Here is a true story:

> A group of health workers started attending births in their village. They knew how to deliver a baby, but they did not know how to cut the **cord**. They knew that the midwife had special scissors that were supposed to be safe. But they did not know why they were safe. After the birth they would call the village midwife to cut the cord. The midwife was very greedy, and the mother had to pay her a lot of money.

The reason the midwife's scissors were safe was that she boiled them before she used them! The health workers could have boiled a knife or a razor blade or their own scissors for 20 minutes, and they could have cut the cord safely, too!

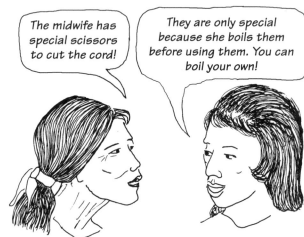

> The midwife has special scissors to cut the cord!

> They are only special because she boils them before using them. You can boil your own!

Try to find the reason for everything you do. But remember—try to find the **real** reason. Sometimes when people do not know, they make up stories and decide they are true. This will not help.

6. Know when to do nothing

If a woman eats a healthy diet, gets enough rest, exercises, and gets checkups, her birth is likely to go well. Although in this book we talk a lot about what to do when things go wrong, it is important to remember that most births are normal.

If you start doing unnecessary things during a normal birth, you can actually cause problems. Instead, honor the natural process of birth. Watch and wait.

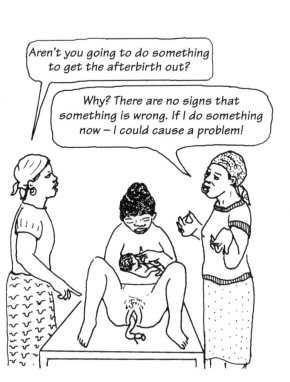

> Aren't you going to do something to get the afterbirth out?

> Why? There are no signs that something is wrong. If I do something now – I could cause a problem!

7. Know when to get help

Even if a midwife is very skilled and keeps learning more, there will be situations in which expert medical help is needed. Knowing when to get medical advice, or when to send a woman to the doctor or hospital, is part of a midwife's skill, too.

Often what you decide to do or not do will depend on how far you are from medical help. For example: If a new mother gets a *fever* with pain in the belly a few days after giving birth, she probably has an infection and needs medicine. If you have no training in giving medicine, the best thing to do is to go to a nearby clinic, doctor, or trained health worker. But if it will take more than one day to get medical help, you may decide to give the medicine to the mother while she travels, so she does not die or get much sicker on the way.

8. Share what you know

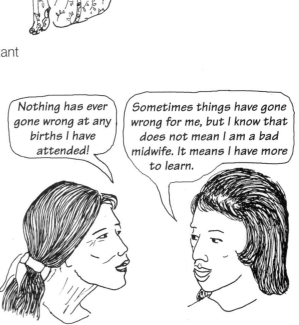

One of the most important things a midwife can do is teach. Midwives can teach pregnant women about how to care for themselves during pregnancy (see chapter 4), and about childbirth (see chapters 8–12). They can also teach the community about women's health needs (see chapters 20–23).

It is also important to share your knowledge with other midwives and health workers. Midwives should learn from and help each other—not guard the secrets of their practices. When midwives meet, it is important to avoid 2 common problems:

- Sometimes midwives start talking about all the bad or frightening experiences they have had. This may frighten new midwives who are just learning.

- Sometimes midwives will not admit they have ever had problems caring for pregnant women. Usually they are not telling the truth, but do not want people to doubt their skills. But you can help others learn if you talk about problems in a helpful way. For example, you can talk about how something could be done better next time.

9. Practice what you teach

The women you care for will pay more attention to what you do than to what you say. As a midwife, it is important to be a good example to the women you help:

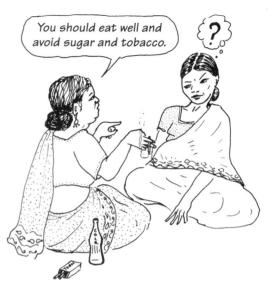

You should eat well and avoid sugar and tobacco.

- Before you tell a woman to eat more green vegetables, make sure you eat them, too.

- Before you tell a woman to get an *injection* against *tetanus*, make sure you have already had an injection.

- Before you tell a woman to **breast feed** her baby, make sure you breast feed your babies, too.

- Before you tell a woman not to smoke, make sure you do not smoke, either.

- Before you teach a woman how to keep clean, make sure your own house and hands are clean.

10. Use local resources in new ways

You may not be able to apply everything in this book to your area. But there are often ways you can use local resources instead. Be creative.

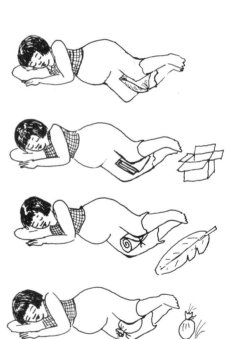

For example: A pregnant woman may have trouble sleeping because her hips hurt. In this book we say that placing a pillow between the knees when the woman is in bed can help her sleep. But what if she has no pillow? She might roll up clothes and use them. Or she can roll up banana leaves, or fold up a cardboard box, or use a bag filled with dry grass.

Think about what goal you are trying to reach. Then invent new ways to reach it.

11. Work for the joy of it

It is important to enjoy what you do. If you do, you will do better work and people will want to follow your example.

Working with the community

The longer a midwife practices, the more she will find that there are many reasons why women have a hard time being healthy. Some of these reasons are poverty, lack of medical care, lack of education, harmful beliefs, and hostile husbands or family members.

A midwife can try to work with individual women to solve these problems. But often these are problems in the community as well. To solve them, the community must be involved. Here are some methods you can use to encourage the community to care about women's health needs:

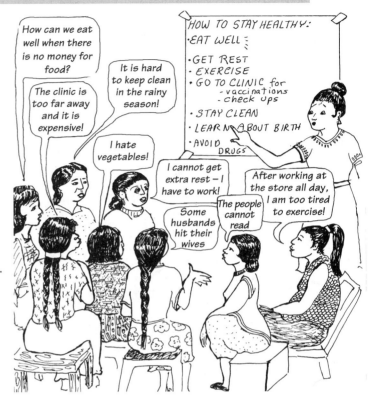

1. Community organizing

Organizing the community means getting people to work together for change. To work together, you will need to find out:

- What do different members of the community think about this problem?

- Who is willing to work on the problem?

- Who can provide money, skills, land, materials, or ideas?

- Who are the people with power or money who might be helpful or difficult?

For example: If the people in your community do not eat well and many women do not get enough iron, the community could:

- Start a community garden where people can work together and share the crops.

- Start a food co-op where people put their money together to buy food in large amounts. Food costs less this way. If the people also share work at a co-op store, the food can be sold even cheaper.

- Start a community education campaign that teaches people to eat better. Teach what to eat and how to make healthy food taste good.

- Start a community project to raise money for iron syrup or iron pills for pregnant women.

2. Teaching

To help women stay healthy you must often teach the community how to stay healthy, too. Here are some general rules for helping others learn:

- If there is more than one person, sit in a circle. The teacher should sit on the same level as the people.

- Share your own experiences freely. Don't set yourself apart. Let people know who you are.

- Listen to people. Learn about their opinions, experiences, needs, questions, and worries. Show respect for them. Talk **with** them, not **at** them.

- Be ready to change the way you teach—and what you teach—as you learn more about the needs of the people.

- Be prepared. Think about what you want to share before you start teaching. If you teach a class, have a plan.

- Use many different methods. People learn better if they see the same thing in different ways, and if they are active in their learning. For example, you could discuss something in a group, act out a play or tell stories about it, or make posters or signs about it.

- Pay attention to how well people are learning, and to what works and does not work. Ask the people you teach to give you ideas and suggestions for being a better teacher.

- Try to make teaching and learning fun.

Sometimes it is also necessary to teach trained health professionals. People can learn a lot from books, but they cannot learn everything. For example: Some women in your area might not go for checkups while they are pregnant because they do not like being scolded by the nurse or doctor. The nurse or doctor must learn that scolding does not make people take better care of themselves. Scolding frightens people away. The nurse or doctor needs to be taught about the needs and feelings of women.

I worried about you when you did not come last month. Was something wrong?

I'm glad she is not yelling at me. Now I can explain that I missed my checkup because my other child was sick.

3. Networking

There may be individuals, local groups, national groups, or even international groups that would like to help your area. Finding out who they are and sharing your needs with them is called **networking**.

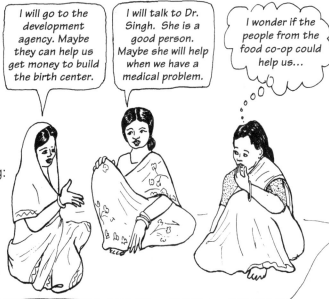

Here are a few examples of networking:

- Finding a doctor who is willing to help when you find problems during pregnancy or birth. This doctor might also teach some skills to local midwives.

- Finding women's organizations in your area. They might be interested in arranging child care when women get medical checkups.

- Finding national or international groups that might be willing to give some money for local projects, like building a birth center. Then a group of people in your area could help build the center.

- Finding male health workers who would be willing to help teach men about women's health needs.

4. Empowering others

Empowering others means helping them make their own decisions and change their lives for the better. When people feel empowered, they have the courage to use their own abilities, and they take pride in the special wisdom and beauty of their culture.

When people are not empowered, they accept unhappiness and abuse. For example: A woman who does not believe that she should be treated with respect will allow others to eat the best food first. She will not look for a way to get her fair share. Or a community that believes that it is not as good as others will accept less land, pay, and power than other groups receive.

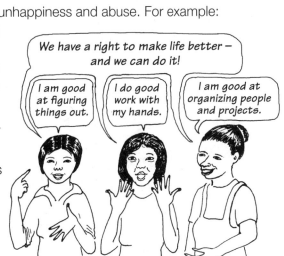

To empower others, a midwife must help them know their own value. If you respect their beliefs and ideas, you teach them that they are intelligent. If you respect their feelings, you teach them that what they feel is important. If you listen to them, you teach them that they have a right to be heard.

5. Talking openly about personal problems

Some problems may seem to be too personal to talk about—especially if they have to do with the family or with sex. But these same problems may affect the whole community. Or they may come from harmful beliefs that the whole community shares.

For example: A man in your community may hit his wife when she is pregnant. This may seem like a problem for that family alone. But is it? Here are some reasons why a man may beat his wife:

- He may think women are property and are owned by men.

- He may feel that the only acceptable emotion is anger. So when he feels sad or helpless, he may hit someone instead.

- He may think he is supposed to hit women (and women may feel they should accept violence from men).

- He may drink too much alcohol, which makes all problems worse.

Many of these reasons come from beliefs that men are taught by their families and by the community. But if people talk about the problem, they may learn the harm that these beliefs cause.

Here is another example: In many parts of the world, people are suffering from AIDS. People can help protect themselves from AIDS by using condoms (see p. 347) during sex. But if people will not talk openly about diseases spread by sexual contact, they cannot learn how to stay healthy.

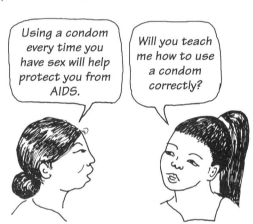

6. Preparing for a life long struggle

Change takes time. Remember that when you work with others to build a stronger community, you do make a difference—even if you do not see change right away. You also encourage others in ways you may not realize.

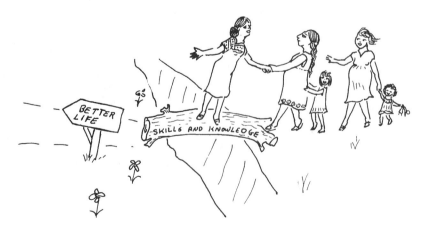

Making the best use of this book

This book can be used in several different ways. Student midwives can study this book before they ever go to a birth. Experienced midwives can use this book to learn new things or to teach others. Practicing midwives can also take this book along when they work with pregnant women. If there is some unusual problem and they are not sure what to do, they can look up the problem in this book.

If you give this book to others:

- Show them the inside of the front cover, which explains how to use the list of contents, the index, the list of medicines, and the vocabulary section.

- Talk with them about how to "read" the pictures (see below). Make sure they understand what they are looking at—especially when the pictures are of things inside the body.

1. How to look things up

See the inside of the front cover of this book to learn how to look things up.

2. How to know what the boxes mean

Throughout this book we use 2 kinds of boxes. The first kind of box has a thick line around it and looks like this:

> **Caution!**

We use this box whenever we want to alert you to something that could be very dangerous. **Read these boxes very carefully.**

The second kind of box looks like this:

> Note:

These boxes contain "notes"—additional information that is helpful for you to know.

3. How to read the pictures

When you use the pictures in this book, be sure to look at the picture **and** the words that go with it. Sometimes the words give you important information about the drawing.

Looking at a part of the body

When we draw a person, we often try to draw the whole body. But if there is not room on the page, we may draw only the part of the body we are talking about. You must use your imagination to fill in the rest of the picture:

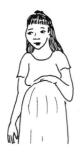

This woman looks like she has no legs, or like her legs are too short.

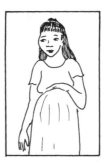

You must imagine that you are looking through a window. The legs are there but you cannot see them. It is as if they are hidden behind a wall.

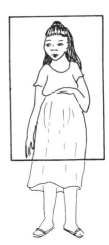

Sometimes we want to show something large and close up, so that you can see it clearly. Again, the rest of the body will not be shown:

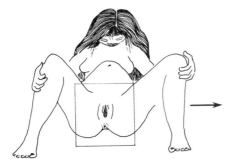

This picture shows the mother pushing the baby out. The baby's head is just inside the vagina. If it is important to see the head and the vagina more clearly...

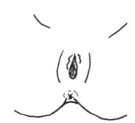

we will make one part of the picture bigger, like this.

Things that are inside the body

Sometimes we want to show things that are hidden inside a woman's body. Some books use drawings that look like the body has been cut open. It is easy to see what is inside her body this way, but the picture is unpleasant to look at.

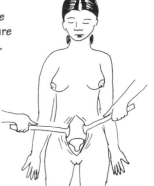

This woman looks as if her belly has been cut open.

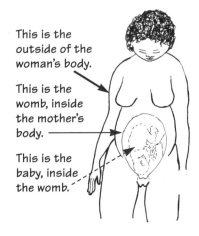

This is the outside of the woman's body.

This is the womb, inside the mother's body.

This is the baby, inside the womb.

This book shows what is inside and what is outside the body by using different kinds of lines. When you see a drawing like the one at left, the thickest, darkest lines show the outside of the body (what you really see when you look at someone). The thinner or broken lines show what is inside (things you cannot see when you look at someone).

Or we may draw the inside of the body as it would look if we could see through the skin:

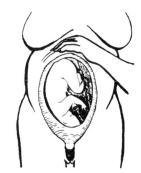

This is a picture of a baby inside the womb. In real life it does not look like this. We have taken away the front of the body and the front of the womb so that you can see inside.

Things inside the body shown by themselves

Sometimes we need to make things inside the body very large. We draw these things without the body around it.

This is a picture of the womb in the belly of a woman who is not pregnant. The womb is small and hard to see.

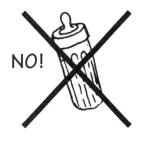

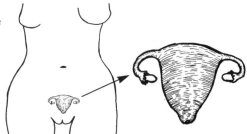

This is a drawing of the same womb. It is larger so you can see it better. We did not draw the body around it.

A sign for *NO!*

In this book, we will use an X over a drawing when we mean **Do not do this!** Often we will add the word **NO!** Or, if something is good, we may add the word **YES!** to that picture.

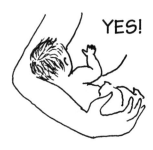

NO!

YES!

4. A note on words

Some common words—especially words for parts of the body and things the body does—are different in different parts of the world. This can be confusing.

We often use common words in this book, especially the first time a word is used. Your area may use different common words. You can write in the words that you and the women you care for will understand.

We also use the medical term for many of these common words. This way you will be better able to talk with medical people and to understand other books.

5. What it means when we suggest getting medical help

As you read this book you will find 3 different kinds of suggestions for getting medical help. It is important to remember what these mean so that you can respond in the appropriate way:

- **Get medical advice.** This means that you need to talk with a doctor or skilled health worker about the problem in order to decide what to do. You should do this as soon as possible, but it is not an emergency.

- **Get medical help.** This means that a woman or her baby needs to see a doctor or skilled health worker. The woman or her baby should be seen as soon as possible, but it is not an emergency.

- **Go to the hospital.** This means that there is an emergency, or that there is likely to be an emergency soon. The woman or her baby should start travelling to the hospital immediately.

6. Some ideas on how to study this book

You can learn the information in this book in many different ways. Here are some suggestions you can adapt to your area:

Study groups

A group of people can meet to study this book. It is a good idea to have a teacher, but you do not need one. If you do not have a teacher:

- People can read one section of the book at a time and then talk about it.

- People can take turns leading the study group.

- Experienced midwives can come and talk about their experiences with the information in different sections.

If you are leading a study group:

- Try to find out what people already know and build on that.

- Encourage them to read each section very carefully. Ask them to keep these questions in mind while they are studying: *What is the most important thing on this page? What are the most important things in this chapter?*

- Help them understand the sections on *Step-by-step thinking* (see p. 29) and *Making decisions: thinking about risks and benefits* (see p. 35). Have them practice using these thinking methods on many kinds of problems.

- Encourage them to pay special attention to the chapters called *Helping pregnant women stay healthy* (see p. 46), *Taking a pregnancy health history* (see p. 74) and *Prenatal checkups* (see p. 96). Talk with them about how care during pregnancy can prevent many problems.

- Ask a lot of questions to get people thinking about what they are learning. Some good questions are: *What do you think about this? Have you ever seen this happen? What did you do? Is this true in our area?*

- Encourage experienced midwives to come to the study group and share their knowledge. They may have useful and important knowledge that is not in this book.

Helping people who cannot read

Some people in your study group may not be able to read well. But they may be very intelligent and have good memories. They can learn a lot by watching, listening, and doing. However, it is impossible to remember everything, especially at first!

When you help someone study this book, go slowly. Study one section at a time. Make sure the person understands that section before you go on to the next one. It sometimes helps to ask people to listen and then explain what they have learned, using their own words. All the methods listed here can be used by both those who cannot read and those who are very educated.

Role playing

You can make learning easier and more fun if you act things out. Here are some examples of things you can try:

- A woman can put a doll under her dress or shirt and pretend to be a pregnant woman. Someone else can practice giving her a checkup. If the pregnant woman has any problems, the person giving the checkup can look it up in this book. (See Appendix B for how to make a doll.)

- The role play group can practice including pregnant women in their own health care. One woman can play the pregnant woman. Another woman can talk with her about ways to get healthy and prevent problems, asking questions to find out what she wants and needs. You can even practice teaching pregnant women to look things up in this book.

There are many other things that can be acted out. Be creative and see what works best in your area.

Working with real pregnant women

It is always best to learn by working with real pregnant women. One of the best ways to do this is to work with more experienced midwives. For example: If you are working with a study group, ask local women to come to it for checkups and advice. Students can watch midwives do these checkups and can also try giving checkups themselves. The teacher or an experienced midwife can make sure that the checkups are done correctly and to help students who have any problems.

7. Adapting this book to local needs

Because this book is written for people everywhere, the information in it is very general. We encourage those who use this book to adapt it to local health needs. Here are a few ways you can do this:

- Write local information next to the words and drawings in this book.

- Write the local brand name, dosage, and price of a medicine in the Green Pages. You can also include local plant medicines.

- Add leaflets or inserts to the books when you give them to other people.

- Use some of the drawings and words from this book, along with your own ideas, to prepare a local manual for midwives.

Note: When adapting this book to local needs, think about a midwife's scope of practice (see p. 2) in your area. For example, in some areas a midwife can give injections or internal (vaginal) exams, but in other areas a midwife cannot do these things. We encourage all midwives to discuss their scope of practice with both health authorities and community leaders.

Anyone has permission to copy or adapt any parts of this book, including pictures, provided the parts copied are distributed free or at cost (not for profit). We would be grateful if you would include a note of credit and send a copy of your book or pamphlet to us at:

The Hesperian Foundation

P.O. Box 1692

Palo Alto, California 94302

U.S.A.

This book is a "work in progress." To make this book better we would like to know how you do things in your area and how we can improve this book. Please send your ideas to us at The Hesperian Foundation.

Tools for safer births

Chapter 2 contents

Tools for
safer births

Traditional and modern medicine

Traditional medicine is based on beliefs that have been passed from midwife to midwife, and from parents to children, for hundreds of years. These beliefs come from knowledge about the body and mind, contact with the spirit world, and from understanding plant medicines. Traditional birth care is often learned from experienced traditional midwives or healers.

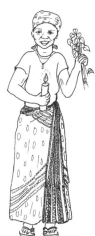

Modern medicine is based on the knowledge of the body and physical world learned through science—a special way of thinking and testing ideas about how things work. Modern birth care is usually learned in schools, in training courses, and from books.

Both traditional and modern medicine are helpful if practiced carefully and correctly. But to use each method well, it is important to remember that both traditional and modern medicine teach:

- helpful methods
- useless methods
- harmful methods

A midwife can help her people use the best of both traditional and modern medicine. She can help her people understand what is helpful about modern medicine, and she can encourage doctors, health workers, and local health departments to study traditional methods.

1. How do you know whether a method is helpful, useless, or harmful?

The only way to know whether a method is helpful, useless, or harmful is to study it carefully.

You can learn how well a particular method works by talking to people who have used it. But remember that some midwives base their methods on experience, while others may simply make something up and decide it is true. If they can make others believe it, their new idea or method will become a tradition—even if it has no real value. This means it is important to ask many different people and then think carefully about what they have said.

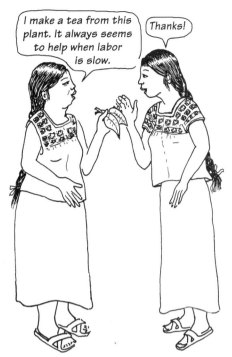

I make a tea from this plant. It always seems to help when labor is slow.

Thanks!

Here are some helpful questions to ask other midwives:

- Why do you use this method?

- When do you use it?

- How do you use it?

- What happens when you use it?

- How often does it help the problem?

- Do things ever go wrong?

Then, when you try different methods yourself, keep your eyes and your mind open. If possible, write down why you used these methods and what happened. You may learn something new.

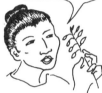

It was a difficult birth. I used this plant to make labor stronger...Then the mother bled a lot.

Hmmm... Maybe the plant medicine caused the bleeding.

If you are still unsure whether a method is useless or harmful, it may help to consider these things:

- The more methods there are to solve any one problem, the less likely it is that any of them will work. This is because when a method does not work well, people keep trying new things. For example: In rural Mexico there are **many** home remedies for *goiter*, **none** of which does any real good. Here are some of them:

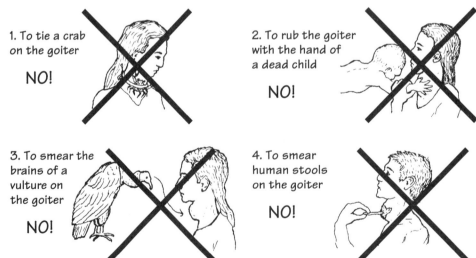

1. To tie a crab on the goiter

NO!

2. To rub the goiter with the hand of a dead child

NO!

3. To smear the brains of a vulture on the goiter

NO!

4. To smear human stools on the goiter

NO!

For prevention and treatment of goiter, use iodized salt (see p. 53).

- Foul or disgusting methods are not likely to help, and often are harmful. They may cause illness or infection. For example:

The idea that leprosy can be cured by a drink made of rotting snakes

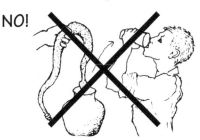

The idea that syphilis can be cured by eating a vulture

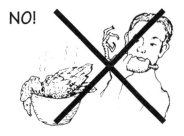

- Methods that use animal or human **stools** do no good, and can cause dangerous infections and illness. For example:

Putting human stools around the eye does not cure blurred vision and can cause infections.

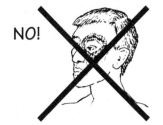

Smearing cow dung on the head to fight ringworm can cause tetanus and other dangerous infections.

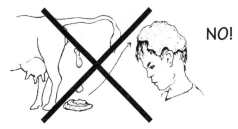

- Methods that deny people food, exercise, or rest usually make them weaker, not stronger.

- Methods that are supposed to work because they look like the problem usually do not work. For example: A red plant will not necessarily stop bleeding.

- Methods that blame people for their problems usually add to their suffering and pain.

It may also help to make a chart of traditional and modern methods used in your area. Here is an example of a chart we made during a midwife training in the Philippines. We all listed common birth care practices. After talking about them, we knew better which were helpful, useless, or harmful.

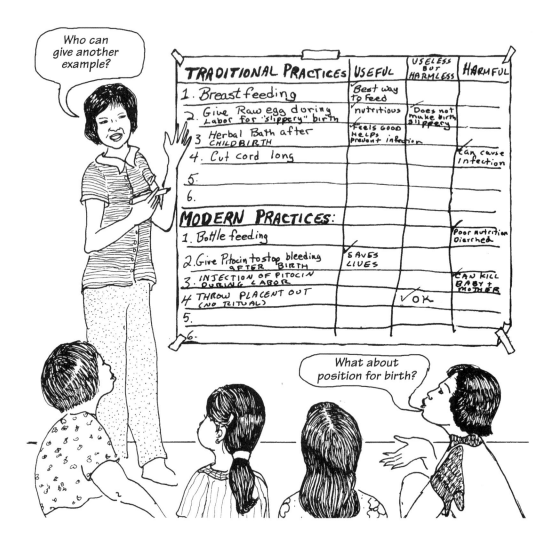

2. Helpful methods

Some traditional methods are helpful because they are based on a healthy, natural way of doing things, or because there are physical powers in the method used. Here are some examples of helpful traditional methods:

- In Guatemala, midwives sometimes cut the cord with a knife that has been heated in a fire. This is a good practice, because heating the knife kills the germs that can cause infection.

- In many cultures, a woman is given 40 days of rest and care after childbirth. This is helpful because it gives the mother time to recover her strength and to care for the baby. (But a mother should not stay in bed all the time. This can make her body weak and cause other problems.)

- In some cultures a woman is given a ritual bath after childbirth. This helps prevent infection.

Some modern methods are helpful because they are based on knowledge about things that cannot be seen (like germs) or on how **chemicals** affect the body: Here are some examples of helpful modern methods:

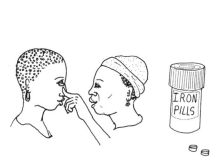

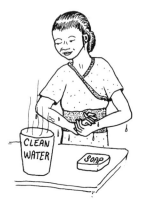

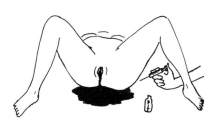

Checking women for anemia and giving iron pills when needed makes the blood strong.

Keeping everything clean at births prevents infections.

Giving medicine _after a birth_ to stop heavy bleeding saves lives.

Helpful methods can also become harmful if used incorrectly. For example, plant or modern medicines used in the wrong amount can be very dangerous. Remember: Never use a medicine simply because someone told you about it. Know the correct amount to use, and the correct time and way to use it.

3. Useless methods

Useless methods are methods that are neither helpful or harmful in themselves. But they can become helpful or harmful, depending on how they are used:

- If a woman strongly believes in a method or finds it comforting, it may be helpful by lessening her fear and worry. For example: In the Philippines, midwives sometimes have a pregnant woman eat a raw egg during *labor*. They believe this will help the baby slip out easily. But since the egg goes into the stomach, and the stomach is separate from the womb where the baby is, an egg cannot really help the baby slip out. However, if the mother believes that the egg will help her, she may relax and have an easier labor.

- If using a method means not using another, more helpful method, the useless method may not only be useless but harmful. For example: In parts of Africa, women tie a string around their waist to prevent pregnancy. This does no harm, but it does not prevent pregnancy (see chapter 22). If a woman does this instead of using a *family planning* method that works, she will probably get pregnant.

> **Caution!** Do not use a useless method **instead of** a helpful method. It is usually OK to use both.

4. Harmful methods

Some methods are harmful even if a woman believes in them very strongly or if a midwife has been told by others that they work.

Here are some examples of harmful traditional methods:

- Pushing on the *womb* to help a labor go faster. This can cause the mother's womb to tear.

- Putting plant medicines inside the *vagina* during labor. This can cause a serious infection.

Here are some examples of harmful modern methods:

- Giving an injection of *oxytocin* (see p. 460–461) before the birth. This can kill the mother and the baby.

NO!

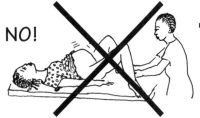

NO!

- Making a woman lie on her back to deliver. This can slow—or even prevent—the birth.

- Feeding a baby with a bottle. This can lead to illness and loose stools *(diarrhea)*.

NO!

> **Caution!** If you think a method might be harmful, do not use it!

Step-by-step thinking

Step-by-step thinking is the kind of thinking that trained people use when they are trying to figure out the answer to a problem. Step-by-step thinking helps you use both modern and traditional medicine in the right way.

Step-by-step thinking has 9 steps:

1. Notice that there is a problem.

2. Start with doubt. This means admitting that you do not know what the answer is—yet.

3. Think about all the possible causes of the problem and answers to the problem. If there is time, ask other people for their ideas.

4. Look for clues that can tell you which causes and answers are most likely:

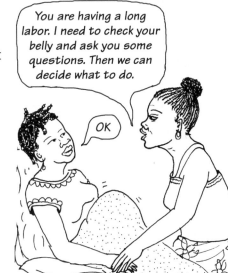

> *You are having a long labor. I need to check your belly and ask you some questions. Then we can decide what to do.*

> OK

- notice everything you can about the problem

- examine what you find

- ask questions

- make tests if needed

5. Eliminate the unlikely answers.

6. Decide which answer is probably the right one (make a guess).

7. Try out the answer.

8. Look for results.

9. If the answer does not work, start all over again.

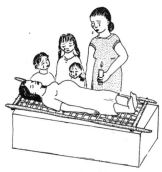

This midwife was afraid to admit that she was unsure. She gave the first medicine she could think of.

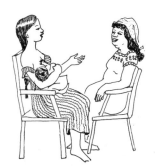

This midwife thought carefully about the problem and considered all of the possibilities.

Remember: In step-by-step thinking, admitting that you do not know yet is a strength, not a weakness.

All of us use step-by-step thinking often, even when we do not realize it. Here is an example:

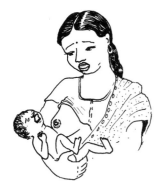

Indira was breast feeding her first baby. Suddenly, the baby started to cry. Indira wondered what could be wrong. She began to think:

"He might still be hungry, but then why did he not keep breast feeding?" She got worried, "Maybe I don't have enough milk." But when she squeezed her nipple, milk squirted out.

She thought about other possibilities. He could not be lonely, since she was still holding him. She kissed his forehead with her lips to feel for fever, but he felt cool.

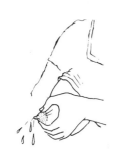

She held him gently and watched him closely. She noticed that he would pull his knees up when he cried. "Well," she thought, "He just ate, and my mother says that sometimes babies get gas while eating. Pulling the knees up like that might mean that his belly hurts." So she decided to try burping him. She laid him on his belly across her knees and patted his back.

Soon he had a huge burp, and stopped crying. When she put him back to the breast, he nursed happily until he was full. She had found the answer. From then on, she burped him often to prevent gas from becoming painful again.

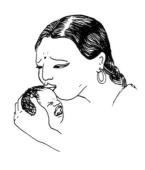

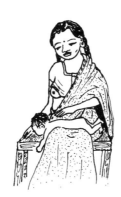

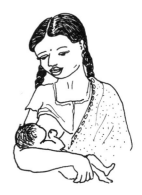

If Indira had simply decided that the baby was crying because she did not have enough milk, she would have been wrong. She could have made serious mistakes. She might have started giving the baby a bottle for no good reason. The baby would still have had the gas in his belly. She might have lost her milk from not nursing, and the baby might have become ill from bottle feeding. So it is a good thing that she decided to test her idea by squeezing the nipple. It is also good that she took the time to think about other possibilities, and watched her baby for more clues.

Here is another story:

When Elena was 5 months pregnant, she came to see the midwife for the first time. She complained that she was always feeling tired and weak.

"Hmmm…" said her midwife, Celeste. "I wonder what the problem is. You do look tired. You may be working too hard, or you may have an illness, or you may have thin, pale blood or be malnourished in some other way— or you could just be upset about something. How are things in your life in general?" As she asked this, Celeste noticed that Elena looked calm and content, and that her clothes were clean, but ragged. She wondered if Elena could afford to eat well.

"Well, I don't think I am upset about anything," said Elena. "My husband is very good to me and I am glad to be pregnant. And I am not working any more than I usually do."

"Do you have any signs of illness?" asked Celeste, "Like a fever, headache, cough, loose stools, bleeding, or unusual pain?"

"No," said Elena, "Just the ordinary small aches and pains of pregnancy. Nothing unusual."

"Well, tell me about your diet," said the midwife. " Are you getting lots of protein and iron foods?"

"Protein is like meat and beans, right?" asked Elena. "Yes, I think so. I eat maize (corn) and beans every day, and sometimes an egg or some chicken, too."

"That's wonderful!" said Celeste, "What about iron foods like liver or red meat, leafy green vegetables, and yams?"

"Well… once in a while," said Elena. "I had some green vegetables last week. And some red meat the week before. I mostly eat maize and beans. Mostly maize, actually. Meat is so expensive."

"Beans do have some iron," responded Celeste, " and so do eggs, but sometimes not enough just by themselves. Let me see your fingernails—and the insides of your eyelids and lips. How pale they are! It is very likely that you are not getting enough iron in your diet. You may be anemic."

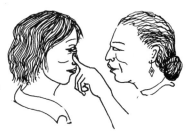

Celeste then gave Elena some ideas on how to add more iron foods to her diet. "You must eat some strong iron foods with every meal. Leafy, dark green vegetables and yams are not expensive, and organ meats like liver and heart are sometimes cheaper than other kinds. I also want you to put a clean piece of iron (like an iron nail) in the pot when you cook beans, and add tomatoes if you can. This will probably help you feel less tired, and you should start feeling better. Can you do that?"

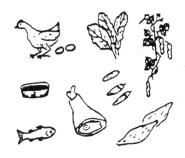

"I think so," said Elena.

"Good!" said Celeste, "but I'd like to hear from you in 3 or 4 weeks just to make sure that these things are working. Also, if you start to feel worse, please let me know right away! There is always a chance that there is some other problem."

If there had been a clinic nearby, Celeste could have sent Elena there for a blood test, to see if she really had too little iron in her blood. But the clinic was quite far away. She also knew that iron medicine (such as iron pills or iron syrup) could help, but that it was very difficult to get in her village. Celeste decided that if the change in diet did not help, or if Elena felt worse, she would take her to the clinic a few hours away for a checkup, and to get whatever medicine was needed.

Here is a chart that shows how both Indira and Celeste used step-by-step thinking:

The steps	Indira's story	Celeste's story
1. Notice that there is a problem.	Indira noticed that her baby got upset when she started to breast feed.	Celeste noticed that Elena was unusually tired and weak.
2. Start with doubt.	Indira wondered: "why?"	Celeste wondered: "why?"
3. Think about all the possibilities.	Indira thought: "Is he hungry? Do I have enough milk? Is he lonely? Does he have a fever? Does his belly hurt from gas?"	Celeste thought: "Is she unhappy at home? Is she bleeding? Is she sick? Does she have diarrhea or fever? Is she working too hard? Is she eating enough?"
4. Look for clues.	Indira noticed that the baby was not trying to breast feed anymore. She squeezed her nipple to check for milk and felt his forehead for fever. She noticed he was pulling his knees up.	Celeste asked about Elena's family life, work, and diet. She asked about signs of illness and diarrhea. She noticed Elena's clothes and mood. Celeste checked Elena's fingernails, lips, and eyelids for signs of anemia.
5. Eliminate unlikely answers.	Indira thought: "He is not lonely because I am holding him. I have plenty of milk. There is no fever."	Celeste thought: "She looks and sounds happy. She works no more than usual. She has no signs of illness, diarrhea, or bleeding."
6. Decide what the answer probably is.	Indira decided: "It is probably gas in his belly."	Celeste decided: "It is probably anemia caused by a poor diet."
7. Try out the answer.	Indira burped the baby.	Celeste gave good diet advice.
8. Look for results.	Indira put the baby to the breast after burping and saw that the baby was now happy.	Celeste asked Elena to come back in 3 to 4 weeks to see if she is feeling better.
9. If there are no results, start all over again.		If Elena does not feel better, Celeste will take her to the clinic to get help.

Intuition

Intuition is knowledge that comes through feelings. It is an important kind of knowledge—as long as you remember that it is not always right. When you get a feeling that something is right or wrong, it is a good idea to also test it against the physical world.

This true story was told to a group of community midwives by a hospital nurse. The community midwives had insisted that intuition could be useful. At first the nurse said intuition was not important. Then she remembered something that made her change her mind:

"I was in the hospital," the nurse said, "taking care of a woman in labor. Every $1/2$ hour I would listen to the baby's heartbeat, and it was always fine. Suddenly, I got the feeling that something was wrong. It was not time to listen again. But I listened anyway—just to make sure."

It is not really time yet, but I want to listen to the baby again anyway...

"Well," the midwives asked, "what happened?"

"I was right," she said. "I could tell from the baby's heartbeat that the baby was in trouble! During a contraction it got much too slow, and it stayed slow afterwards. We rushed the mother into surgery and delivered the baby by operation. The doctor found that the cord was down in front of the head and was getting squeezed against the mother's bones."

The baby's heartbeat is too slow. It needs help!

"You see," the midwives said, "if you had not listened to your intuition, the baby might have died!" And it was true.

Intuition **can** save lives. But notice that this nurse also checked the *physical signs* (the baby's *heartbeat*) to see if something was wrong. If the baby's heartbeat had been fine, she would have continued to watch and wait. This would have been the right thing to do.

Other people use intuition in harmful ways. For example: If a midwife has a feeling that everything is going well at a birth, she may ignore signs that there are problems. Or if a midwife has a feeling that something is wrong but does not check whether she is right, she may interfere with an otherwise normal birth. So it is always important to check intuition against the physical world—even if you believe that the feeling comes from the spirit world.

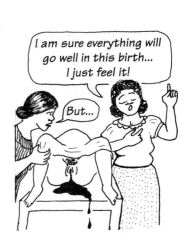

This midwife used intuition in a harmful way.

Creativity

Creativity is the ability to make something new out of materials and information you already have. A creative midwife is one who can think of new and better ways to handle problems when the old ways do not work.

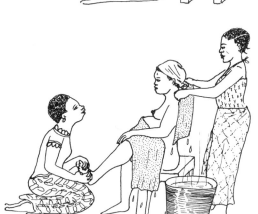

The following is based on a true story:

> Sophie was having trouble pushing her baby out. She was tired from her long labor. She also seemed tense. Since Sophie had lost her last baby when she was 6 months pregnant, the midwife wondered if Sophie's fear of losing this baby was slowing the birth.
>
> The midwife tried all the usual methods to help Sophie push, but nothing worked. There were no other signs that some-thing was wrong. The baby's heartbeat was still normal. Because the midwife knew the baby was probably OK, she felt it was probably time to try something new.
>
> She had Sophie take off all her clothes and sit on a comfortable wooden stool. She wrapped Sophie in warm, wet cloths while her helper massaged Sophie's feet. The midwife said, "When you get a contraction, just push right where you are." The warm, wet cloths and massage relaxed and refreshed Sophie. She was soon able to give birth.

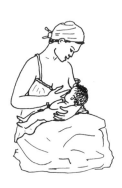

In this story, the midwife's intuition told her that Sophie was tense. Her knowledge of the labor and birth told her that Sophie and the baby were probably OK. The midwife's solution was creative. It had not been done before in her area, but it worked!

It is important to be careful when you are trying something new, especially if there are other problems with a birth. In Sophie's case, the creative solution was a good one because there were no other problems. But if Sophie's baby had been butt down **(breech)**, or if Sophie had been bleeding a lot, it would have been better to get medical help right away.

Making decisions: thinking about risks and benefits

Any time you make a decision, you must consider the risks and benefits. A *risk* is the harm that something may cause. A **benefit** is the good that something will cause. The best choice is to do something that has the biggest benefit and the least risk. If the risk is greater than the benefit, it is not worth doing. But often the answer is not simple.

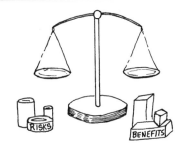

Note: A risk does not mean that something bad will happen. It only means that something bad is more likely to happen.

Here is a story about risks and benefits:

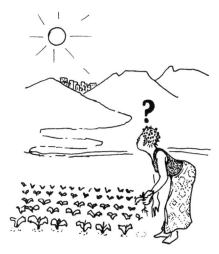

Akua makes money for her family by growing vegetables. Usually, she takes the vegetables to a nearby town on market day to sell them. She knows that people will buy them there. Recently, a friend told her that she can get much more money for her vegetables in the big city, which is farther away. The problem is that there are robbers in the hills around the city, and once in a while they attack people on their way back from the market. Akua has to decide if the benefit of making more money in the city is worth the effort of travel and the risk of being robbed on the way home.

What do you think she should do? To decide, you will need to weigh the risks and benefits.

Risks and benefits in pregnancy and birth

Before you decide to do anything that interferes with pregnancy and birth, ask yourself these questions:

- What are the benefits of doing it? Is there a very good reason to do it?

- What are the risks of doing it? How likely is it that something bad will happen? If something does go wrong, how bad will it be?

- Will it be expensive? Will it be painful? Will it take a long time?

- Is there something else that will work as well and is safer?

Here are 3 examples of weighing risks and benefits in pregnancy and birth:

Deciding on a birth by operation (cesarean section)

A **cesarean section** is always a risk for the mother and baby. The doctor has to give the mother medicine to prevent pain, and then has to cut her belly open to take the baby out. There is a small risk that the medicine will make the mother sick, or that she will bleed a lot or get an infection from the cut in her belly. In a good hospital these problems do not happen very often, but they do happen.

This is why it is not a good idea to do a cesarean section without a good reason. But if there is a serious problem (such as the baby being too big to fit through the mother's pelvic bones), a cesarean section can save the mother's and baby's life. The risk of problems caused by the operation is small, but the benefit of saving the life of the mother and baby is very great.

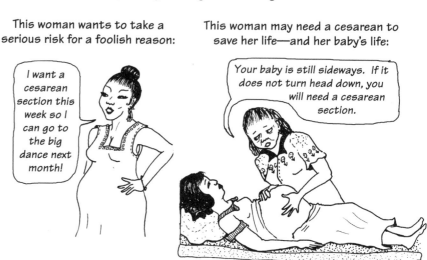

Removing the placenta by hand

Removing the placenta by hand

Removing the **placenta** by hand is very dangerous to do. There is so much risk that you would almost never do it. But in an extreme emergency, the risk of not doing it is even greater. For example:

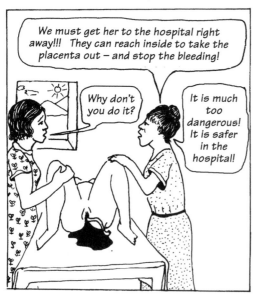

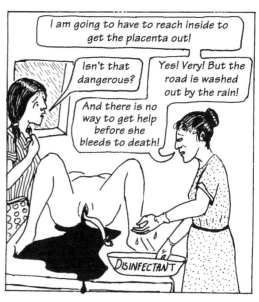

Giving medicine to hurry a labor

Giving medicine to hurry a labor is never worth the risk! This is why:

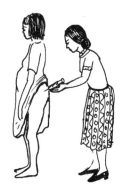

Giving an injection
to hurry labor

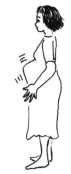

often makes labor
stronger and faster.

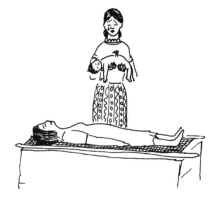

But there is a real risk of harming the
baby, or making the mother bleed inside.
The mother and baby could die.

SECTION B

Prenatal care

Introduction

The *prenatal* (before birth) period starts when a woman gets pregnant and ends when she gives birth. If a woman gets good prenatal care, she is more likely to have a safer, healthier pregnancy and birth.

It is best if a midwife can give 2 kinds of prenatal care: 1) she can teach a woman about how to have a healthier pregnancy (for example, how she can eat a healthy diet and avoid harmful things during pregnancy), and 2) she can give a woman regular *prenatal checkups* (also called *ante-natal checkups* or *ante-partum checkups*). During these checkups a midwife can talk with a woman about any questions or problems she may have, teach a woman about how to have a healthier pregnancy, and check a woman's body for *signs* that the pregnancy is going well *(healthy signs)* and signs that something may be wrong *(risk signs)*.

Every pregnant woman should begin having prenatal checkups as soon as she thinks she might be pregnant. Check with your local health department to find out the number of prenatal checkups they recommend. Here is one common prenatal schedule for healthy women:

Prenatal checkup schedule

when a woman thinks she is pregnant .....first prenatal checkup

first 5 months of pregnancy ....1 prenatal checkup every other month

months 6, 7, 8 of pregnancy ....1 prenatal checkup every month

month 9 of pregnancy ....1 prenatal checkup every week

You may need to see a woman who has risk signs more frequently. It will depend on what her risk sign is and what is considered good care where you live.

You can give prenatal checkups anywhere. We recommend that you give the prenatal checkups yourself—even if the woman is also getting checkups at a clinic. Giving the checkups yourself will help you know the woman and her pregnancy better. You may also find a problem or solution that the doctor or clinic has missed.

The following chapters will help teach you how to give good prenatal care:

- A woman's body during pregnancy (chapter 3)

- Helping pregnant women stay healthy (chapter 4)

- Helping pregnant women with common complaints (chapter 5)

- Taking a pregnancy health history (chapter 6)

- Prenatal checkups (chapter 7)

Think ahead: Arrange for emergencies!

No matter how well you take care of a woman during pregnancy, there is always a chance that something will go wrong. With good care and good habits this is not likely to happen, but it is still possible.

During the prenatal period it is very important to:

- Arrange emergency transportation to a hospital or clinic—just in case it is needed. There should be a car or truck with a full tank of gas available for the whole last month of the pregnancy. If there is no car or truck, see if there is a donkey (or horse) and cart, a blanket and pole to use as a stretcher, people to carry the woman, or some other kind of transportation.

- Arrange someplace to go for help. It is a good idea to talk with individual doctors, and with local clinics or hospitals, in case you need to call on them in an emergency. It is best to find out what their policies and procedures are **before** the birth, so that you do not have to find out in the middle of an emergency.

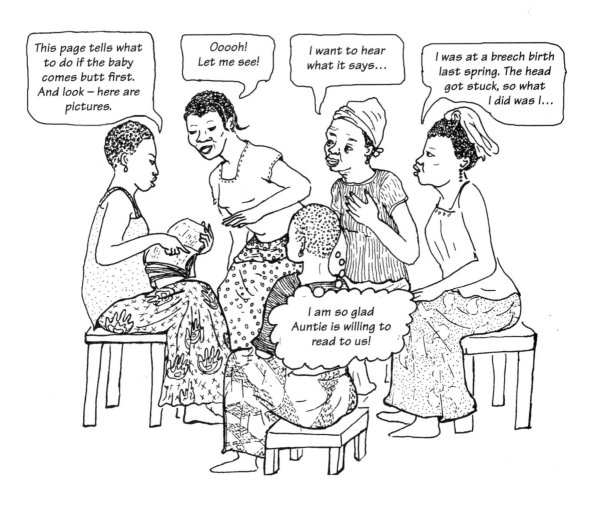

A woman's body during pregnancy

Chapter 3 contents

A woman's body during pregnancy

How things look on the outside

This is how a woman's *genitals* look on the outside:

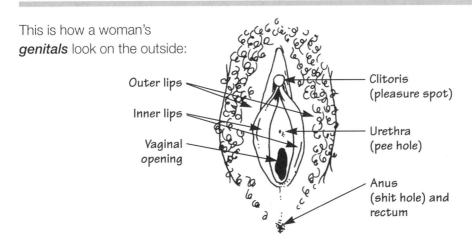

Outer lips

Inner lips

Vaginal opening

Clitoris (pleasure spot)

Urethra (pee hole)

Anus (shit hole) and rectum

How things look on the inside

These are the inside parts of a woman's body that are important to know about during pregnancy and birth.

1. The pelvic bones

The *pelvic bones* are inside the belly. A woman can feel them by putting her hands on her hips like this:

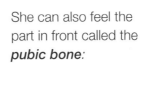

Pelvic bones

She can also feel the part in front called the *pubic bone:*

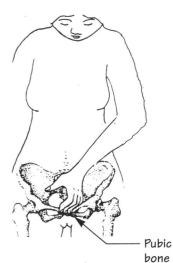

Pubic bone

The pelvic bones are like a bowl with a hole in the bottom. During childbirth the baby must pass through the hole to get out:

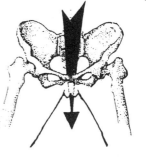

2. The womb

The **womb** is a bag of strong muscle. It lies inside the belly between the pelvic bones. When a woman is not pregnant, she cannot usually feel her womb from the outside.

If you looked inside the mother's belly, the womb would look like this:

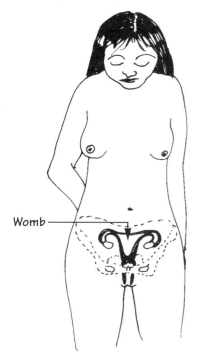

Womb

Two tubes come from the top of the womb and connect to the egg sacks or **ovaries**. The bottom of the womb is called the **cervix**. It has a small hole in it, which is usually plugged with **mucus** (a thick, sticky material). The cervix attaches to the **vagina**, a small tunnel that leads to the outside of the woman's body. Both the cervix and the vagina are made of muscle.

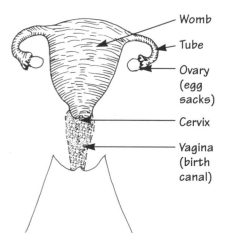

Womb

Tube

Ovary (egg sacks)

Cervix

Vagina (birth canal)

A woman can touch her own cervix by putting 2 very clean fingers into the vagina, and then reaching up and forward. The cervix feels round, hard, and smooth—with a small bump (the hole) in the middle.

How women get pregnant

A woman's body makes an egg that travels through one of the tubes into the womb. The father's body makes a seed (**sperm**). When he and a woman have sex, the man enters the woman's vagina. His seed travels up into the womb and meets the woman's egg. The egg and seed together form a baby that grows inside the womb.

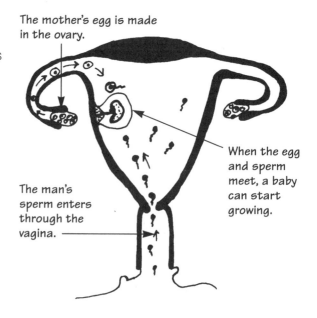

The mother's egg is made in the ovary.

When the egg and sperm meet, a baby can start growing.

The man's sperm enters through the vagina.

How a baby grows

1. If you could see inside the womb, you would find the baby floating in a bag of water. The baby is connected to the mother by a **cord** and the *afterbirth (placenta)*.

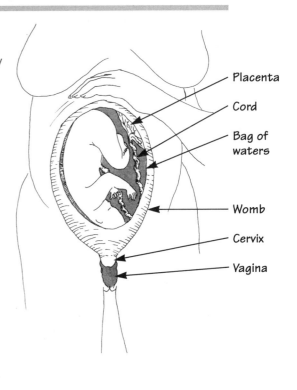

Placenta

Cord

Bag of waters

Womb

Cervix

Vagina

2. The baby grows by getting air and food from the mother, like this:

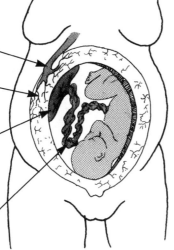

The mother's blood gets air from her lungs and food from her stomach and brings it to the womb.

The mother's blood gives air and food to the baby's blood in the placenta.

Then the baby's blood takes the air and food to the baby through the cord.

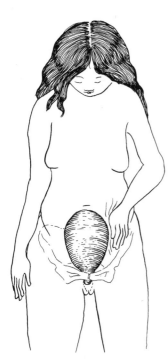

3. As the baby gets bigger, the mother can start to feel her womb by putting her hand on her belly. This woman is about 5 months pregnant.

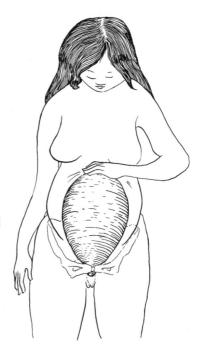

4. When a woman is about 9 months pregnant, she can feel the top of her womb just below her ribs.

Helping pregnant women stay healthy

Chapter 4 contents

Helping pregnant women stay healthy

There are some very important things a woman can do to stay healthy during pregnancy. It is good to talk with a woman about these helpful things as soon as you learn she is pregnant. The earlier she practices healthy habits, the healthier she and her baby will be at the birth.

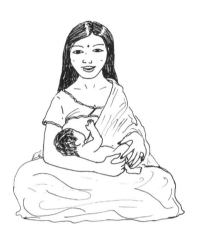

This woman ate well, kept clean, and avoided harmful things while pregnant and breastfeeding.

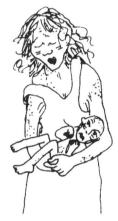

This woman did not.

Eating well to stay healthy

The best way the mother can stay healthy is to eat enough food and the right kind of food:

- Eating well gives a woman strength to work, resist illness, and stay healthy.

- Eating well protects a woman's teeth and bones.

- Eating well makes the baby grow stronger in the womb.

- Eating well helps prevent heavy bleeding during birth.

- Eating well helps a mother recover her strength quickly after birth.

- Eating well helps a mother resist infections after birth.

- Eating well helps a mother produce plenty of milk for breast feeding.

To find out whether a woman is eating well, ask her what she usually eats, like this: *What did you eat yesterday? The day before? The day before that?* The answers to these questions will give you better information than if you ask questions that she can answer with a *yes* or *no.* Some women will answer *yes* to a question because they think it is what you want to hear—even if it is not true.

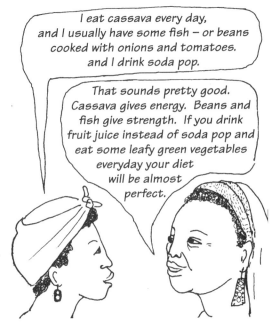

I eat cassava every day, and I usually have some fish – or beans cooked with onions and tomatoes. and I drink soda pop.

That sounds pretty good. Cassava gives energy. Beans and fish give strength. If you drink fruit juice instead of soda pop and eat some leafy green vegetables everyday your diet will be almost perfect.

After she tells you about her diet, first tell her what is good about what she eats. Then, if needed, make suggestions that she will like and can afford for making her diet better. The sections below contain some of the most important things a woman can do to eat well.

1. Eat 4 kinds of food at every meal

To stay healthy, pregnant women (just like everyone else) need to eat 4 kinds of food at every meal: *main foods, grow foods, glow foods,* and *go foods.*

Main foods

In most parts of the world, people eat one **main food** at every meal. This may be a grain like rice, maize (corn), millet, or wheat; a starchy root like cassava or potato; or a starchy fruit like breadfruit or banana. The main food usually gives at least $1/2$ of all the **nutrition** people need.

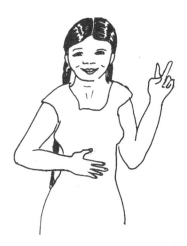

Generally, main foods are more nutritious when they have not been refined (processed to take out the color). Taking out the color takes out healthy things, too. For example, white bread and white rice are not as healthy as brown bread and brown rice.

Main foods are a good, low-cost, healthy source of energy. But they will not give a woman complete nutrition. She must also eat other things.

Grow foods (proteins)

Grow foods contain **protein**, which helps build muscles and bones that make the body strong. Everyone needs protein to be healthy. Babies and children also need protein to grow. Proteins are found in **legumes** (beans, peas, and lentils), and in nuts and seeds. Proteins are also found in animal products like meat, cheese, fish, insects, eggs, and milk. (If you do not eat animal products, the other protein foods are just as good. See p. 50, 55–56.)

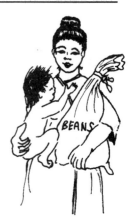

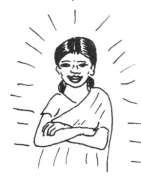

Glow foods (vitamins and minerals)

Glow foods contain **vitamins** and **minerals,** which help the body resist disease and recover after illness or injury. Vitamins and minerals are found in fruits and vegetables. In addition to the vitamins and minerals needed for general health, women need larger amounts of certain minerals during pregnancy (see p. 51–53).

Note: If a mother eats well, she can get all the vitamins and minerals she needs from food. It is always better to get vitamins and minerals from real food than to buy vitamin pills, injections, syrups, or tonics. But there are exceptions to this rule. For example: A woman who has **anemia** (pale blood) should take iron and folic acid in pills or some other medicine form (see p. 51). Or a mother with certain illnesses or severe **malnutrition** may need other kinds of injections. These women should get medical help.

Go foods (sugars and fats)

Go foods contain **sugars** and **fats,** which give energy. Sugars and fats also help the body store energy to use later, when it is needed. Sugars are found in fruits, sugar (white, brown, and raw), and honey. Fats are found in animal meat, nuts, eggs, seeds, vegetable oil, butter, ghee, and lard.

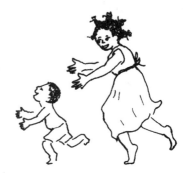

Note: It is best to get sugar from fruits, which have vitamins and minerals as well as energy. Using a lot of sugar on your food, or eating a lot of foods made from sugar (like candy or soda pop) can be expensive and bad for the teeth. Foods made from sugar do not contain any vitamins or minerals.

Too much fat (especially animal fat) is not good for the heart and blood. But it is good to eat a little bit.

A woman does not need to eat all the foods listed below to be healthy. She can see what foods from each of the 4 groups are available in her area and try to use some food from each group when she prepares meals:

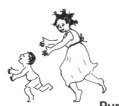

GO FOODS
(energy helpers)

Examples:

Pure fat: Ghee, butter, vegetable oil, lard

Fat-rich foods: Cheese, fatty meat, coconut

Nuts: Cashews, almonds, ground nuts

Oil seeds: sesame, sunflower

Sweet foods: Fruits, sugar, sugarcane, molasses, honey, jaggery

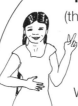

MAIN FOODS
(the center of the meal)

Examples:

Cereals and grains:
Wheat, Millet, Rice, Maize,
Sorghum

Starchy roots: Taro,
Cassava, Potato

Starchy fruits: Banana,
Breadfruit, Plantain

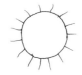

GLOW FOODS
(vitamins and minerals or
protective helpers)

Examples:

Vegetables: Dark green leafy
plants, tomatoes, carrots,
sweet potatoes, peppers,
pumpkin, leeks, turnips, kale,
avocado, eggplant

Fruit: Melons, oranges,
papaya, mango, banana,
pineapple, grapefruit

Pregnant and
breast feeding
women need extra
grow and glow
foods and 3
important minerals:
calcium, iron,
iodine.

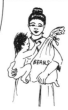

GROW FOODS
(proteins or
body-building helpers)

Examples:

Legumes: Beans, peas, lentils

Nuts: Cashews, almonds,
ground nuts

Oil Seeds: Sesame, sunflower

Animal products:
Milk, cheese, yogurt, meat,
fish, chicken, small animals,
insects

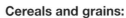

2. Eat 3 important minerals every day

Pregnant and breast feeding women need larger amounts of 3 important minerals—
iron, calcium, and **iodine**—than other people do. Pregnant women should try to get
some of these minerals every day because the baby needs these minerals to grow and
be healthy. The pregnant woman needs enough for the baby to take and still have
enough left to stay healthy herself.

Iron

Iron helps make blood healthy and helps prevent **anemia** (thin, pale blood) (see p. 110).
A pregnant woman needs to get a lot of iron so that the growing baby can form healthy
blood and store iron for the first few months after birth.

It is best for a woman to eat iron foods along with fruits or tomatoes. This way the body
uses more of the iron in the food.

These foods contain a lot of iron:

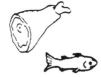

meat (especially liver
and other organ meats)

fish

chicken

eggs

These foods also have some iron:

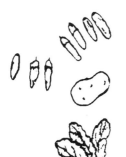

beans	brussel sprouts
peas	cabbage
potatoes	cauliflower
lentils	turnips
sunflower seeds	strawberries
dark green leafy vegetables	pineapples
yams	dried fruit (especially dates, apricots, raisins)
seaweed	
broccoli	blackstrap molasses

It is possible to get even more iron by cooking foods in certain ways.
If a woman cooks food in iron pots and adds tomatoes, lime juice, or
lemon juice to the food while it is cooking, iron will go from the pots
into the food. Or she can put a clean piece of iron—like an iron nail or
horseshoe—in the pot when she cooks beans or other foods. (Make
sure that the nails are pure iron, not a mixture of iron and other
metals.) Or she can put a clean piece of pure iron in a little lemon juice
for a few hours, make lemonade with the juice, and drink it.

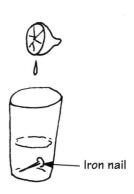

Iron nail

But even when a pregnant woman eats iron foods and uses these methods every day, it is still difficult for her to get enough iron from food. She should also take iron pills or iron syrup, if possible. These medicines may be called ferrous sulfate, ferrous gluconate, ferrous fumerate, or other names. In addition, she should take a substance called folic acid (folicin, or folate) to avoid or treat anemia.

In many areas the Department of Health or health system will have iron and folic acid pills for pregnant women. Sometimes these are two separate pills; sometimes they come in one pill (iron and folic acid). To prevent anemia a woman should have at least 60 mg of iron and 1 mg of folic acid every day. If a woman is already anemic or if she becomes anemic, she should take 2 iron pills and one folic acid pill a day. Warn the woman that the iron may make it hard to move her bowels (constipation) and her stools (shit) may turn black. This is normal. If she does not get better she may need medical help (see p. 110–111).

> **Caution!** Too much ferrous sulfate is poisonous. Tell women to take only the dose you give them and to keep their pills away from children.

Calcium

Calcium makes bones and teeth strong. A growing baby needs a lot of calcium to make its new bones, especially in the last few months of pregnancy. When a pregnant woman eats calcium, it goes first to the baby to help it grow. So if the mother does not eat enough calcium, her bones and teeth will become weak.

These foods contain a lot of calcium:

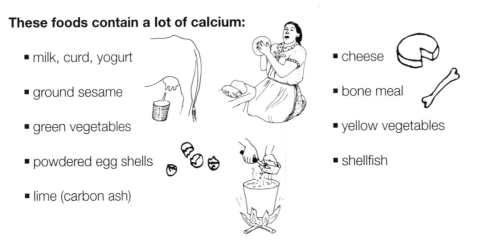

- milk, curd, yogurt
- ground sesame
- green vegetables
- powdered egg shells
- lime (carbon ash)

- cheese
- bone meal
- yellow vegetables
- shellfish

A pregnant woman can increase the amount of calcium she gets from food in several ways. She can soak a bone or some egg shells in vinegar or lemon juice for a few hours, and then use that vinegar or lemon juice in soup or other food. Or she can add a little lemon juice, vinegar, or tomato to the water when cooking bones for soup. She can grind up egg shells into a powder and mix it with food.

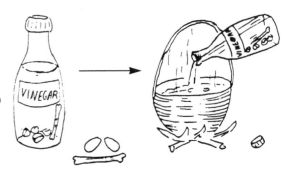

She can also soak maize (corn) in lime, making it richer in calcium. If a pregnant woman cannot get enough calcium from food, she can take calcium pills.

Once calcium is in a woman's body, sunshine will help her body use the calcium better. She should try to be in the sun at least 15 minutes every day. (Remember that it is not enough to just be outdoors. The sun's rays must touch the skin.)

Iodine

Iodine in the diet helps prevent a swelling on the throat called **goiter** and other problems in adults. In children, iodine prevents mental slowness (**cretinism**).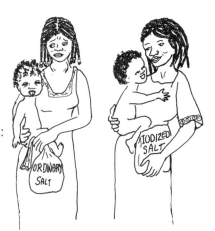

The easiest way to get enough iodine is to use iodized salt instead of regular salt. Or women can eat some of these foods:

- fresh or dried shellfish (like shrimp)
- fresh or dried saltwater fish
- fresh or dried freshwater fish

If iodized salt or these foods are hard to get, or if there is goiter or cretinism in your area, it might be wise to have people drink a special iodine preparation. Check with the local ministry of health to see if they have a program giving iodized oil by mouth or by injection. When taken by mouth, people need iodized oil once a year. When given by injection, people need one injection of iodized oil every 4 years. Smaller amounts of iodine preparation are used for babies and small children.

If there is no ministry of health program, people can make an iodine solution at home with Lugol's iodine (an antiseptic that is often available at the local dispensary, pharmacy, clinic, or hospital). It contains 6 milliliters (ml) of iodine per drop. Here is how to make an iodine solution to drink:

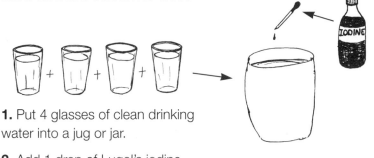

1. Put 4 glasses of clean drinking water into a jug or jar.

2. Add 1 drop of Lugol's iodine.

3. Everyone over 7 years old should drink 1 glass of this iodine solution every week of their life. This is especially important for pregnant women and children.

Note: Do **not** give more than this amount. Iodine is important, but too much iodine can cause problems.

3. Learn which ideas about diet are harmful

In many parts of the world, certain customs about women and food are harmful rather than helpful. Some of these harmful ideas affect young girls; others affect pregnant women and mothers.

Feeding girls less food than boys

Sometimes young girls are not fed as well as young boys. Some people believe that boys need more food because they must work when they grow up. But these people are wrong! Girls need just as much good food as boys do—in order to grow well and do their own work. When young girls do not eat well, their bones may not grow right. This can cause serious problems when they try to give birth.

Feeding the family first

It is often the custom for a woman to feed her family first. She eats only what is left and often does not get as much food as the rest of the family. This is never healthy. But when a woman is pregnant, or has just had a baby, it can be very dangerous. The whole family should understand that eating well during pregnancy and breast feeding is important. They should encourage the woman to eat well.

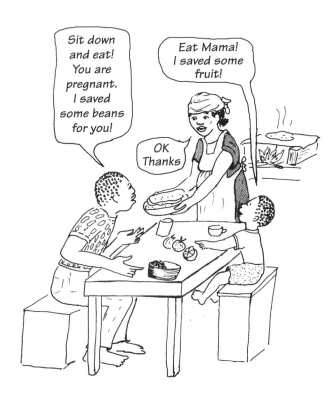

If the family does not help, we encourage the woman to do what she must to get enough food. She may need to eat while cooking, or hide food and eat it when her husband is out of the house.

Sometimes no one in the family is eating well. The family may be too poor or may have other problems. The best solution is to find a way for everyone to eat better.

Avoiding foods during pregnancy and breast feeding

In some areas, people believe that pregnant women or new mothers should avoid certain foods—like beans, eggs, chicken, milk products, meat, fish, fruits, or vegetables. But a pregnant or breast feeding woman needs all these foods. Avoiding them can cause weakness, illness, and even death.

Finding creative answers

If a woman has any of these harmful beliefs, it is still important to respect her feelings. Try to find ways to work with these beliefs, not against them. This example is based on a true story:

> Maria is a midwife in Guatemala. She and her people believe that some foods are hot foods and some are cold foods. They believe pregnant women should not eat cold foods.
>
> Maria and her people believe beans and eggs are cold foods (even when they are cooked). But Maria also knows that beans and eggs are good, cheap ways for pregnant women to get the protein and iron they need.
>
> Maria has a problem. She wants pregnant women to eat well. But they will not eat cold foods. Also, Maria is not sure that cold foods are good for pregnant women. Her solution is simple but very smart. She tells women to eat beans and eggs, but to always add a little hot pepper or other hot food spice to the beans or eggs. This way they will not be cold foods any more.
>
> Maria has found a creative answer to a problem. She has found a way for her people to eat better and respect their traditional ways.

4. Buy better foods for less money

Most people eat more plant foods (like grains, fruits, and vegetables) than animal foods (like meat, fish, milk products, or eggs). They do this because plant foods cost less than animal foods.

If custom allows, it is wise to eat a little animal food with most meals because animal foods mix with plant foods to give more protein, vitamins, and minerals. But people can also be strong and healthy by eating just plant foods, if they are careful to eat different kinds of plant foods at the same meal. For example, it is better to eat beans and maize together than to eat either of these foods alone. Adding other vegetables and fruits at the same meal is even better.

Another way to get more nutrition from plant foods is to cook vegetables in a small amount of water. Take the vegetables off the fire when they are finished cooking. Drink the water you cooked the foods in, or use it in soup.

Use a small amount of water to cook vegetables.

Here are some ways to get both animal and plant foods at low cost:

Eggs and chicken

Eggs are a good source of protein, iron, and vitamin A. In many places, eggs are one of the best and least expensive forms of animal protein. Babies also can eat them as they get older, along with breast milk.

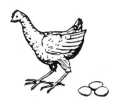

Chicken is a good form of animal protein that often costs less than other meat, especially if the family raises its own chickens.

Liver, heart, kidney, and blood (organ meats)

These foods all have a lot of protein, vitamins, and iron. They sometimes cost less than other meats. Make sure these foods come from healthy animals.

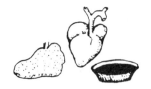

Fish

Fish contains as much protein as meat but often costs less.

Beans, peas, lentils, and other legumes

Legumes are good, cheap ways to get protein, vitamins, and minerals. They will have even more vitamins if they are sprouted first: rinse them with water 2 times per day for 3 days and keep them covered. Eat the legumes when sprouts appear. Baby food can also be made from legumes—cook them well, peel off their skins, and mash them.

Legumes even make your soil richer when you grow them. Other crops will then grow better in this rich soil.

Dark green leafy vegetables

These vegetables have a lot of vitamin A, some iron and calcium, and a small amount of protein. Dark green leafy vegetables usually have more nutrition than light green leafy vegetables.

The leaves of some kinds of sweet potatoes, beans, peas, pumpkins, squash, and certain kinds of yams and baobab are also very nutritious. For babies, the leaves can be dried and powdered, then mixed with baby food.

Cassava leaves

The leaves of a cassava plant have more protein and vitamins than the root. Eat the leaves with the root to get more nutrition. The young leaves are best.

Dried maize

Maize contains protein and vitamins. Soaking maize in lime (calcium ash) before cooking makes the maize richer in calcium. Soaking also makes it easier for your body to use the nutrition in the maize.

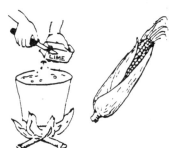

Wild fruits and berries

These are a good source of vitamin C and natural sugars. But be careful not to eat fruits and berries that may be poisonous or dangerous in pregnancy.

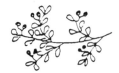

More ways to stay healthy in pregnancy

When you meet with the mother, also encourage her to:

1. Keep her body clean

Keeping the body clean helps prevent infections. If possible, the mother should wash her body with clean water every day. She should also wash the outside of her genitals gently with clean water.

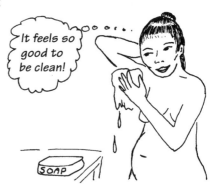

It feels so good to be clean!

SOAP

2. Take care of her teeth

Some places have a saying *Have a baby, lose a tooth.* But a woman can protect her teeth by eating calcium foods and avoiding sweets. She should also clean her teeth carefully after every meal with a soft brush, tooth stick, or finger wrapped with a piece of rough cloth. Toothpaste is good but not necessary; salt, charcoal, or even plain water will work. Clean the surface of all teeth (front and back), between the teeth, and under the gums.

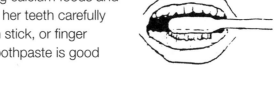

If possible, every mother should visit a dentist or dental worker at least one time during pregnancy.

To make a toothbrush:

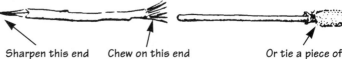

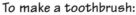

Sharpen this end to clean between the teeth.

Chew on this end and use the fibers as a brush.

Or tie a piece of rough cloth on the end of a stick.

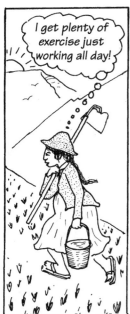

I get plenty of exercise just working all day!

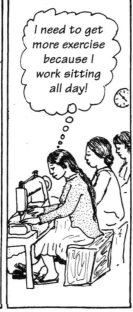

I need to get more exercise because I work sitting all day!

3. Exercise

Exercise makes a woman's body stronger. During pregnancy, exercise helps her body get ready for the hard work of labor and birth. Exercise can also make her feel happier and more full of energy.

In many places, women get all the exercise they need by hauling water, working in the fields, milling grain, chasing after children, and walking up and down hills. But women who work sitting or standing (for example, in offices, stores, or factories), or who work in their own homes, usually need more exercise. They can take long walks, dance, do some physical work, or find some other form of lively exercise.

4. Get sleep, rest, and relaxation

Sleep, rest, and relaxation are very important for pregnant and breast feeding women. These things help women stay strong and resist illness. They also help prevent *miscarriages*, high blood pressure, sick babies, and other problems.

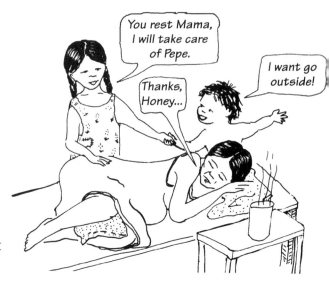

Many women carry a double burden of work. They work all day in fields, factories, gardens, or stores helping to feed and support their families. They might also haul water, prepare food, get fuel, mill grain, clean and repair clothes, clean the house, and take care of their families. And they go through the work of pregnancy and birth.

Many women feel guilty when they stop work to rest. You may need to reassure a woman that it is good to take a few minutes every 1 or 2 hours to sit, rest, and put her feet up. Also, try to help a pregnant woman's family understand why it is important for her to rest and sleep well.

5. Schedule regular prenatal checkups

When a woman gets a prenatal checkup, the nurse, midwife, or doctor makes sure that her pregnancy is normal. If they find problems, they can often do something right away to correct the problem or to keep it from getting worse.

We recommend that you give prenatal checkups to every pregnant woman whom you plan to help in labor and birth. Check with your local health authorities for a schedule of how often to see each woman. She should also get prenatal checkups from a doctor or professional midwife if possible. Sometimes public hospitals or clinics offer these checkups.

6. Enjoy the pregnancy

If women have enough good food, rest, and emotional support, and if they are not worried about how to feed and care for their new baby, pregnancy can be a peaceful, enjoyable part of life. Some women are easily upset during pregnancy, but others feel unusually strong, healthy, and happy.

Many cultures have rituals and practices that honor a pregnant woman. People help her with her work, bring her special foods, give her massages and gifts, and take care of her special needs. Customs like these are very good. They help a woman to get the food and rest she needs. They give her emotional strength. They also help her feel good about herself and her pregnancy.

Things to avoid during pregnancy and breast feeding

Some things are very harmful during pregnancy and should be avoided. The following things will cause the most harm during the first 3 months (when the baby is growing very quickly). But it is best to avoid these things all during pregnancy and breast feeding. Encourage a pregnant woman to:

1. Stay away from anyone with measles

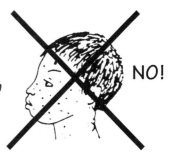

It is usually best for a pregnant woman to avoid being near any people who are ill. But it is extremely important for a pregnant woman to stay away from anyone with measles, especially **German measles** (rubella). If a woman gets German measles during the first 3 months of pregnancy, the baby can be stillborn or born deaf or with a heart problem.

If a woman has already had German measles, she is not likely to get them again. But, to be sure, she should avoid anyone who has them.

Note: The German measles **vaccine** should not be given to a pregnant woman because it could damage the baby inside. It can be given after birth.

2. Avoid taking medicines

When a woman takes medicine, the medicine first gets into her blood and then gets into the baby's blood. Medicines that are helpful to grown women, and even to children, can hurt a baby who is still inside the mother. These harmful medicines include cough syrups and pain relievers, home remedies (like strong plant medicines), and modern medicines (like antibiotics). Some of these medicines can cause the baby to be born deformed or mentally slow.

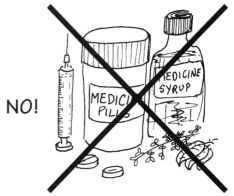

A pregnant woman should avoid taking medicines whenever possible. If she is ill, or thinks she needs medicine, it is very important to find out whether a particular medicine is safe for her baby. For example, it is probably OK for a pregnant woman to take acetaminophen or paracetamol once in a while.

Other medicine should be taken only when there is a good reason. A good reason is when the risk of **not** taking the medicine is greater than the risk of taking it. If you think a pregnant woman needs medicine, get medical advice from someone who knows which medicines are safe for her baby.

3. Avoid smoking, drinking alcohol, or using drugs

Cigarette smoke, alcohol, and drugs are all harmful to the mother **and** to her baby. All these things get into the mother's blood first, then into the baby's blood.

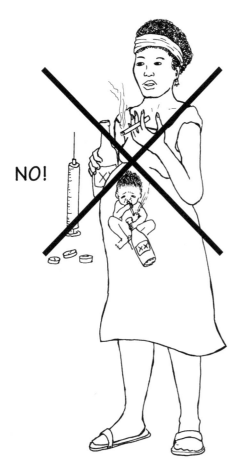

NO!

- **When a pregnant woman smokes, her baby smokes with her!** When a woman smokes, her blood vessels get smaller. This is harmful for her, but it also makes it hard for her blood to carry food and air to the baby in her womb. The baby starves and cannot grow properly. It might even become ill and die.

- **When a pregnant woman drinks, her baby drinks with her!** Alcohol can cause a baby to be deformed, with a head that is too small for its body. The baby might be mentally slow. Also, women who drink a lot of alcohol may not eat as well as they should. This can lead to health problems for her and her baby.

- **When a pregnant woman takes drugs, her baby takes them, too!** Drugs like opium, heroin, cocaine, and barbiturates are very dangerous. If a pregnant woman uses them, her baby can be born dead or sick. Or it might be born addicted to the drug and suffer greatly after its birth.

Smoking, drinking alcohol, and using drugs are difficult habits to stop. Some women will be able to slow or stop their harmful habits when they understand the dangers. Some women will not be able to do so. If the baby is not growing well during the last months of pregnancy, it will probably need special care after birth. It is probably best for it to be born at a hospital or clinic. The mother may need special care, too.

Like many things, smoking, drinking alcohol, and using drugs are social and economic problems. People need to learn how dangerous these habits are. They also need hope for the future and a sense of their own value, so they will not need to do these harmful things.

4. Stay away from strong fumes or poisonous chemicals

Many **chemicals** have great benefits. Some help farmers to grow and store more food. Some are used to make products that make life easier. But many of these chemicals are also poisons and can cause serious health problems. Some poisonous chemicals can cause **infertility**, illness, and death in both men and women. In pregnant women, poisonous chemicals can also cause miscarriage, or a dead or deformed baby.

Poisonous chemicals include:

- pesticides (chemicals that kill insects)

- herbicides (chemicals that kill weeds)

- factory chemicals

- anything that is poisonous or has strong fumes

Everyone should avoid poisonous chemicals whenever possible. A pregnant woman should have **no contact** with them. She should not work with chemicals, she should not breathe chemical fumes or dust, and she should not cook or store food in containers that once had chemicals inside. Small, dangerous amounts of the chemical can remain in the container, even after washing.

Also, if someone in the family works with chemicals, they should remember these rules:

- Do not breathe chemical dust or fumes (wearing a mask may help).

- Avoid getting chemicals on the skin. Wear gloves whenever possible.

- Wash carefully and change clothes after working with chemicals, **before** entering the house. Do not let a pregnant woman wash the clothes.

- Never use more of a chemical than is absolutely needed.

- Keep chemicals away from food and places where food is stored.

- Wash foods that have been sprayed with pesticides or herbicides before eating.

- Keep chemicals where children cannot reach them.

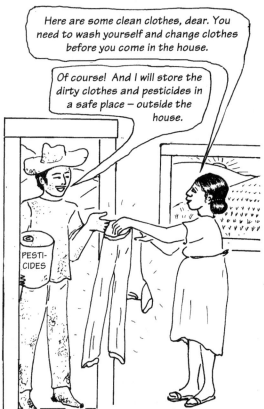

Here are some clean clothes, dear. You need to wash yourself and change clothes before you come in the house.

Of course! And I will store the dirty clothes and pesticides in a safe place – outside the house.

PESTI-CIDES

Caution! Factories should not dump poisonous chemicals into the air or drinking water, or onto the land. They should not store poisonous chemicals near places where people eat, work, grow food, play, or live.

Helping pregnant women with common complaints

Chapter 5 contents

Helping pregnant women with common complaints

Common complaints are the things that many pregnant women complain about. These complaints are bothersome, but they are usually not serious.

In this chapter we describe these complaints and how to help pregnant women who have them. We also talk about how to tell when a complaint may be a sign of risk.

Complaints about feelings and emotions

1. Sudden crying or laughing, extreme sadness (depression), anger, and irritability

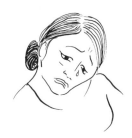

Pregnancy sometimes makes women very emotional. They may laugh or cry for no reason; some women will cry even when they are happy. Or women may feel depressed, angry, or irritable.

It is important that everyone knows that pregnancy can cause strong emotions. Odd laughing or crying, or other extreme emotions, are normal. They should pass quickly. But do not ignore a woman's feelings simply because she is pregnant; her feelings are still real.

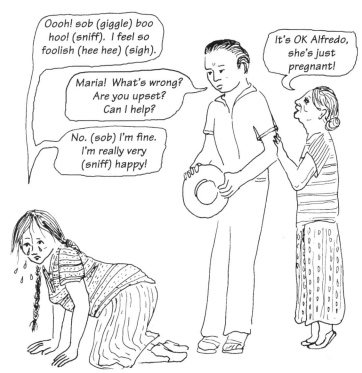

2. Worry and fear

Some women worry when they are pregnant, especially about the baby's health or about giving birth. A pregnant woman may also become very worried about other problems in her life.

These fears are normal. They do **not** mean that something bad will happen. This woman will need emotional support. But she may also need help with real problems.

3. Strange dreams and nightmares

Many pregnant women have strong, vivid dreams. They can be beautiful, meaningful, frightening, or just strange.

A nightmare does not mean that something bad will happen. If a woman is worried about nightmares, it may help her not to eat before going to sleep. It also may help her to talk to a caring person about her dreams, and about her hopes, fears, and feelings.

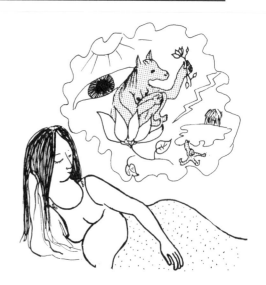

4. Feelings about sex

Some women do not want much sex when they are pregnant. Others find that they want sex more than usual. Both feelings are normal. Both having sex and not having sex are OK for the woman and her baby.

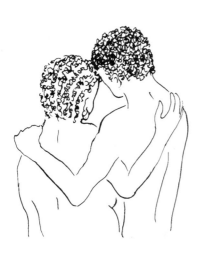

If a woman is having sex, it is important that anything put inside her body is clean (to avoid infection). This includes the man's sex organ (penis) and his hands. If the man is having sex with **anyone** other than his wife, he should always use a condom during sex (with his wife and with someone else) to help prevent infections, AIDS, and other illnesses.

If sex is uncomfortable, a woman and her partner can try different positions for love making. It may feel better with the woman on top, or in a sitting or standing position. If their needs are different, perhaps they can do something that makes both of them happy. There may be other ways to be close and please each other.

Note: Pregnant women may want to avoid sex in the last 3 to 6 weeks of pregnancy. This may help prevent infection and keep the bag of waters from breaking early.

If a woman has had miscarriages, it might be good to avoid sex in the first 3 months. If she has had early labors in other pregnancies, it might be good for her to avoid sex after the 6th month.

Complaints about body changes

1. The mask of pregnancy

The **mask of pregnancy** is a name for the dark-colored areas that appear on the face, breasts, and belly of some pregnant women.

This mask is not harmful. Usually most of the color goes away after the birth. If a woman wishes to avoid dark areas on her face, it may help to wear a hat when she goes out in the sun.

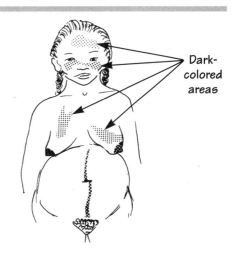

Dark-colored areas

2. Purple spots on the skin

Purple spots come from small groups of veins under the skin. Some people call these spots **spiders.** They usually happen when blood vessels swell. They are not harmful and usually go away after the birth.

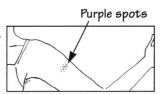

Purple spots

3. Swollen, leaking breasts

A woman's breasts get bigger during pregnancy because they are getting ready to make milk for the baby. Sometimes the breasts are also sore.

During the last months of pregnancy, a clear, yellowish fluid may leak out of the nipples. This is called **colostrum.** This fluid is normal. Women should dry their nipples often and keep them clean to protect them from infection.

A woman who is already breast feeding a baby when she gets pregnant may continue to make milk. If so, she can continue breast feeding. But it will be **very** important for her to eat plenty of good food (see p. 47–56).

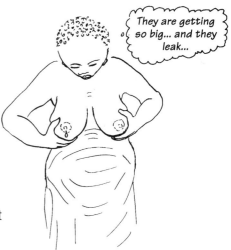

They are getting so big... and they leak...

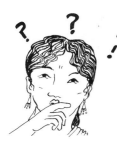

4. Forgetfulness

Some women forget things when they are pregnant. For most women, this is not a big problem. But some may worry if they do not know it is normal. It usually stops after the birth.

Complaints about eating and sleeping

1. Upset stomach (nausea) and dislike of some foods

Many women have **nausea** in the first months of pregnancy. Sometimes it is called **morning sickness**. If the nausea is mild, encourage the mother to try any of these remedies:

- Eating a few crackers, dry bread, dry tortillas, dry chapatis, or other grain food before she gets up in the morning.

- Eating small meals instead of 2 or 3 larger ones, and taking small sips of liquid often.

   - Drinking a cup of ginger tea or cinnamon tea 2 or 3 times per day, before meals. To make ginger tea, put $^1/_2$ to 1 teaspoon of ground ginger root in a cup of boiled water. To make cinnamon tea, put $^1/_2$ to 1 teaspoon of grated cinnamon in a cup of boiled water.

   - Taking vitamin B–6 capsules. We recommend the 50 mg size. Take one capsule, 2 times per day. (Do not take more.)

A mother can also ask traditional healers about other plant medicines or remedies that will help morning sickness.

Although there is no food that should be avoided during pregnancy, a pregnant woman may find that she suddenly dislikes a food that she usually likes. It is OK not to eat that food, and she will probably begin to like it again after the birth. But she should be careful that the rest of her diet contains a lot of nutritious food (see p. 47–56).

2. Food cravings

A food craving is a strong desire to eat a certain food, or even things that are not food at all—like dirt, chalk, or clay.

If a woman gets a craving for good, nutritious foods (like beans, eggs, fruits, and vegetables), it is OK for her to eat as much as she wants. But she should not eat a lot of "junk foods" (like candy, soda, or packaged snacks).

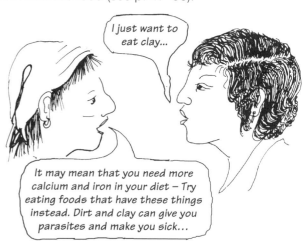

I just want to eat clay...

It may mean that you need more calcium and iron in your diet – Try eating foods that have these things instead. Dirt and clay can give you parasites and make you sick...

If a woman gets a craving for things like dirt or clay, she should be warned **not** to eat them. They may poison her and her baby. They may also give her **parasites** that can make her sick. Encourage her to eat high calcium and high iron foods instead (see p. 51–53).

3. Burning or pain in the stomach or between the breasts

A burning or pain in the stomach or between the breasts is called *indigestion* or *heartburn*. This happens because the growing baby crowds the mother's stomach and pushes it higher than usual. This is not dangerous and usually goes away after the birth.

Here are some things a woman can try to make herself more comfortable:

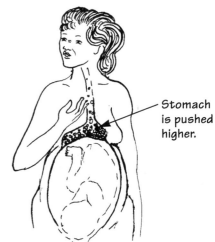

Stomach is pushed higher.

- Eat smaller meals more often.

- Eat papaya with each meal.

- Eat foods and liquids separately.

- Drink more milk.

- Avoid spicy or greasy foods.

- Avoid coffee and cigarettes.

- Sleep with her head higher than her stomach.

- Wear loose clothing.

- Take antacids (see p. 461) that are low in salt and contain no aspirin.

Also, traditional midwives or healers may know of local plant medicines or other remedies that may help.

4. Sleepiness

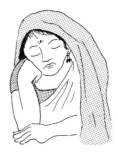

Some pregnant women feel sleepy much of the day. This is most common during the first 3 months.

It is best for a woman who feels sleepy to get plenty of rest. If the woman also feels weak, she may have other problems—like an infection (see p. 115), depression (p. 63), or anemia (p. 110–111).

5. Difficulty sleeping

If a woman cannot sleep because she is uncomfortable at night, it may help if:

- she lies on her side with something comfortable—like a pillow or rolled up banana leaves—between her knees and at her lower back.

- her husband, children, or family talks quietly with her before bed to help her relax.

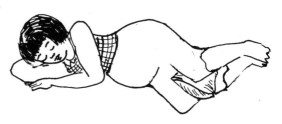

- someone gives her a massage.

- she drinks warm milk or hot soup before trying to sleep.

Complaints about physical aches and pains

1. Baby's kicks hurt the mother, or the baby stops kicking

Most of the baby's movements feel good. But sometimes babies kick very hard or always in the same place. And sometimes the baby's head may bounce against the mother's back or bladder when she walks during the last weeks of pregnancy. These movements may make the mother sore or uncomfortable, but they are not harmful.

The mother is usually feeling regular kicks every day by the 6th or 7th month. If the baby stops kicking for a few hours, it is OK. But if the mother feels no movement for more than a day and a night, there may be a problem. The mother should get medical advice immediately.

2. Sudden pain in the side of the lower belly

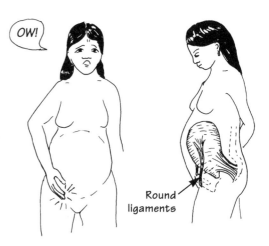

The womb is held in place by *ligaments.* Ligaments are like strong ropes that attach the womb to the mother's bones.

Round ligaments hold the bottom of the womb in place. A sudden movement will sometimes cause a sharp pain in these ligaments. This may be very painful, but it is **not** dangerous. The pain will stop in a few minutes. It may help to stroke the belly very gently, or to put a warm cloth on it.

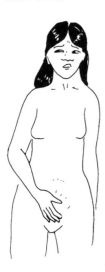

3. Cramps in early pregnancy

It is normal to have **mild** cramps (like easy monthly bleeding cramps) from time to time during the first 3 months of pregnancy. These cramps happen because the womb is growing.

But if the cramps are regular (come and go evenly) or constant (do not come and go but are always there), are very strong or painful, or if the woman also has *spotting* or bleeding, these are risk signs. See p. 100. The woman may need medical help immediately.

4. Aches and pains in the joints

A pregnant woman's body gets soft and loose so the baby can get bigger, and so she can give birth more easily. Sometimes her joints also get loose and uncomfortable, especially the hips. This is not dangerous. It will get better after the birth.

It is also common to have other small aches and pains during pregnancy. But if you see any of the following risk signs, you should get medical advice: red, swollen joints; severe pain; signs of anemia with joint pain; or weakness.

5. Back pain

Many women get back pain. The weight of the baby, the womb, and the waters puts a strain on the woman's bones and muscles. Hard work can also cause back pain. Most kinds of back pain are normal. (See p. 101–102 for the kinds of back pain that may cause problems.)

Encourage husbands, children, friends, or family members to massage the mother's back. This will not only feel wonderful, but will be a great help. Warm cloths or hot water bottles on her back may also feel good. Her family can also help by doing some of the heavy work (carrying small children, washing clothes, farming, and milling grain) for her.

A woman can also do an exercise—called the **angry cat exercise**—to reduce lower back pain. She should do this exercise several times in a row, 2 times per day, and whenever her back hurts her.

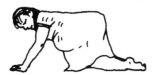 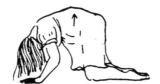 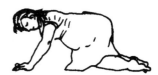

| Start on hands and knees with back flat. | Push the lower back up. | Return to flat back... repeat. |

6. Leg cramps

Many women get foot or leg cramps—especially at night, or when they stretch and point their toes.

Here are some suggestions you can give the mother. If her foot or leg is cramping, she can flex her foot (point it upward) to stop the pain, and then gently stroke her leg to help it relax (do not stroke hard!).

Point the toe up,   not down.   Then stroke the leg.

To prevent more cramps, it will help if she remembers not to point her toes (even when stretching), and to eat more calcium foods or take calcium pills.

7. Swollen feet

Swelling of the feet is very common, especially in the afternoon or in hot weather. Swelling of the feet is usually OK, but it is a risk sign if the feet are already swollen when the mother wakes up in the morning, if the swelling is severe or comes on suddenly, or if there is *pitting edema* (see p. 113). Swelling of the hands and face is also a risk sign (see p. 112).

It may help the mother if she puts her feet up for a few minutes at least 2 to 3 times a day, eats less salt, and drinks more water or fruit juices.

8. Difficulty getting up and down

It is usually best if a pregnant woman does not lie flat on her back. The weight of the womb presses on the big blood vessels that bring food and air to the baby. If the mother wants to be on her back, she should put something behind her back, so she is not lying completely flat. She may also be more comfortable if she puts something under her knees or puts her feet up.

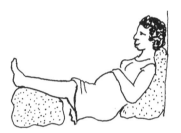

When the mother is on her back, she should be careful about how she sits up. She should not sit up like this:

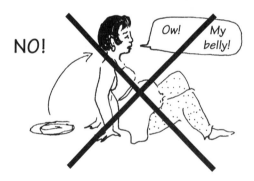

Instead, she should roll to the side and push herself up with her hands, like this:

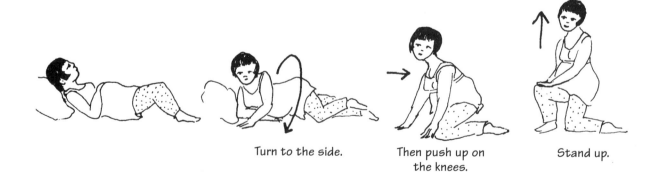

Turn to the side.   Then push up on the knees.   Stand up.

9. Difficulty moving the bowels (constipation)

Some pregnant women have a hard time moving the **bowels** (passing waste, shitting stools). This is called **constipation**.

It may help if the mother:

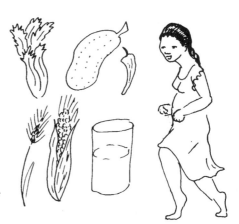

- Eats more vegetables and fruits.

- Eats whole grains (brown rice and whole wheat instead of white rice or white flour).

- Drinks more water.

- Gets more exercise.

Home or plant remedies that soften the stools or make them slippery (like those remedies made from psillium seed or certain fruits or fiber plants) may also help.

> **Caution!** Pregnant women should not take modern medicines called *laxatives* or *purgatives* for constipation. These work by making the bowels tighten or contract. They may cause labor to start too soon. Some can harm the baby inside. Pregnant women should also not wash out the bowels with water (**enema**). This could start labor too soon.

10. Swollen veins (varicose veins)

Swollen blue veins that often appear in the legs or on the woman's genitals are called **varicose veins**. Sometimes these veins hurt. If the swollen veins are in the legs, it may help to have the mother put her feet up often. Strong stockings or Ace bandages (tight, elastic bandages) may also help. If the swollen veins are around the genitals, they can cause bleeding problems if they tear during delivery.

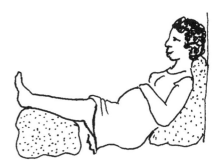

11. Piles (hemorrhoids)

Hemorrhoids are a type of swollen veins around the **anus.** They may burn, hurt, or itch. Sometimes they bleed when the woman moves her bowels, especially if she is constipated.

Sitting in a cool bath can help. Some women say it helps to soak a clove of garlic in vegetable oil and then insert it all the way inside the anus. The mother should also try to avoid getting constipated. If you have heard of other remedies, ask a doctor or experienced health worker whether they are safe. Some remedies are dangerous for pregnant women and may hurt the baby inside.

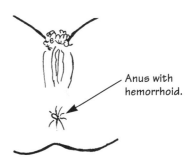

Anus with hemorrhoid.

12. Need to pee (urinate) often

Needing to urinate often is normal, especially in the first and last months of pregnancy. This happens because the growing womb presses against the **bladder** and leaves less room for the bladder to hold urine. It is so common that there is an old joke among midwives: *If a man cannot find his pregnant wife, he should wait near the place where she urinates. If she is not there, she will be soon!*

If urinating hurts, itches, or burns, the woman may have a bladder infection (see p. 115) or a vaginal infection (see p. 362–365).

13. Wetness from the vagina (discharge)

Discharge is the wetness all women have, all month long, from the vagina. It is one way that the body washes itself from the inside. Pregnant women often have a lot of discharge, especially towards the end of pregnancy. It may be clear or somewhat yellow. This is normal.

If there is discharge with itching, burning, or a bad smell around the vagina, the woman may have a vaginal infection (see p. 362–365). If possible, get medical help.

If the discharge is white and lumpy with itching and burning, she may have a **yeast infection**. Yeast infections are common in pregnancy. They are uncomfortable but not dangerous. The medical remedies (clortrimozole, miconazole, and nystatin) work well and are safe in pregnancy if you can get them. (See p. 365 for more information about yeast infections.)

14. Headaches

Headaches are common in pregnancy but are usually harmless. It may help if the mother rests and relaxes more, drinks more juice or water, and gently massages her temples. It is OK for a woman to take 2 acetaminophen or paracetamol tablets with water once in a while.

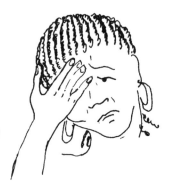

Some women have **migraine headaches**. These are strong headaches, often on the side of the head. The woman may see spots and feel nauseated. Bright light or sunshine can make them worse.

Migraines may get worse in pregnancy, but migraine medicine (ergotamine) is very dangerous in pregnancy. It can cause labor to start too soon; it may also harm the baby. It is better for a pregnant woman with migraines to take acetaminophen or paracetamol tablets, and rest in a dark room. It is also a good idea to get medical advice.

If a woman has headaches with swelling, dizziness, or high blood pressure, this is a risk sign (see p. 112–113).

15. Shortness of breath

Many women get short of breath once in a while, especially late in pregnancy. This is because the growing baby crowds the mother's lungs and she has less room to breathe. Reassure her that this is normal.

But if a mother is also weak and tired, or if she is short of breath **all of the time**, she should be checked for signs of heart problems, anemia (see p. 110–111), poor diet (see p. 111), infection (see p. 115, 362–364, 372, 87), and depression (see p. 63). Get medical advice if you think she may have any of these problems.

16. Feeling hot or sweating a lot

This is very common, and as long as there are no other signs of risk (such as infection, see p. 115, 362–364, 372, 87), the woman should not worry. She can dress in cool clothes, bathe frequently, and drink plenty of fluids.

Taking a pregnancy health history

Chapter 6 contents

Taking a pregnancy health history

The first prenatal checkup has 2 parts:

1. taking a pregnancy health history

2. the regular prenatal checkup

This chapter covers part 1: 14 questions that make up a pregnancy health history. These questions will be asked only at the first prenatal visit. The next chapter covers part 2—the regular prenatal checkup—which will be given at each prenatal visit, including the first visit.

Taking a pregnancy health history will help you learn about a woman's general health, her past health, and her past pregnancies and births. This information will help you make a plan and give advice to make this pregnancy and birth as safe as possible.

The first prenatal checkup is also a time for a pregnant woman to become comfortable talking with you. If she feels shy talking about her body or about sex, it may be difficult for her to tell you things that you need to know about her health. Try to help her feel comfortable by listening carefully to her, answering her questions, and treating her with respect. Try to be relaxed and practical.

It is a good idea to write down all the things you learn about each pregnant woman. This information may be needed later in the pregnancy, or during labor and birth.

14 questions in a pregnancy health history

1. Does she have signs of pregnancy?

There are 2 kinds of signs of pregnancy: **probable signs** (those signs that mean the woman is probably pregnant but could mean something else) and **sure signs** (those signs that mean the woman is definitely pregnant).

Probable signs of pregnancy

Since each of these signs could be caused by something other than pregnancy, we have given other possible causes for you to think about.

1. The woman's monthly bleeding stops. This is often the first sign of pregnancy.

Other possible causes of this sign are malnutrition, emotional troubles, or "change of life" *(menopause)*.

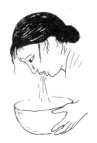

2. The woman feels like she wants to vomit (nausea). Most women have nausea in the morning (morning sickness), but some women may feel this way all day. Nausea is common during the first 3 months of pregnancy.

Other possible causes of this sign are illness or parasites (see p. 98).

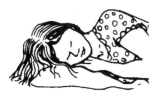

3. The woman feels tired and sleepy. This should go away after 3 or 4 months of pregnancy.

Other possible causes of this sign are anemia (see p. 110), other kinds of malnutrition, emotional troubles, or too much work.

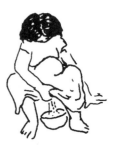

4. The woman needs to urinate (pee) often. This is most common during the first 3 and the last 3 months of pregnancy.

Other possible causes of this sign are bladder infection (see p. 115), tension, or blood sugar disease (diabetes) (see p. 88).

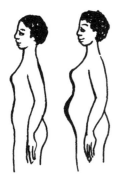

5. The woman's belly grows. The baby and womb are growing, especially after the first 3 months.

Other possible causes of this sign are that the woman is getting fat or has a growth in her belly.

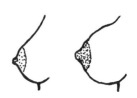

6. The woman's breasts get bigger. A pregnant woman's breasts get bigger to prepare to make milk for the baby.

Other possible causes of this sign are upcoming monthly bleeding or other changes during the monthly cycle.

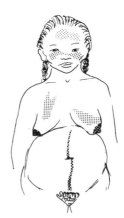

7. The woman has a dark line on her belly, dark nipples, or dark patches of skin on her belly or face. Most women's nipples get darker when they are pregnant. The dark line may appear by the 3rd month; the dark patches may appear by the 5th month. These things usually go away after the birth.

8. The woman feels light baby movements. Early movements (in the first 4 months) are very light.

Another possible cause of this sign is gas.

Sure signs of pregnancy

Each of these signs could only be caused by pregnancy:

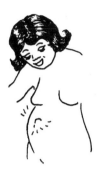

1. The woman feels strong baby movements inside. Most women begin to feel the baby move by the time they are 5 or 6 months pregnant. Some women feel it sooner.

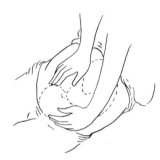

2. The baby can be felt inside the womb. By the 6th or 7th month, a skilled person can usually find the baby's head, neck, back, arms, and legs by feeling the mother's belly. The baby will be harder to feel if the woman is very fat.

3. The baby's heartbeat can be heard. By the 7th month, a skilled person can usually hear the baby's heartbeat when she puts her ear on the woman's belly. At the 5th or 6th month, the heartbeat can sometimes be heard with special equipment, like a *stethoscope* or *fetoscope* (see p. 127). The heartbeat will be harder to hear if the woman is very fat.

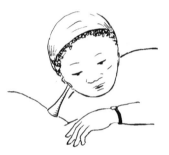

4. A medical pregnancy test says the woman is pregnant. This test is done in a laboratory with a little of the woman's urine or blood. This test is expensive and is usually not necessary. But it can be useful, for example, if a woman needs to know if she is pregnant before taking a medicine that might harm a baby inside her.

2. How pregnant is she now? When is the baby due?

You will need to find out how many months pregnant the woman is at the time of her first checkup and the probable date of the birth (the **due date**). It is normal for the baby to be born as much as 3 weeks earlier or 2 weeks later than the due date.

There are 2 ways to figure out how pregnant the woman is now and her due date. 1) You can use the date of her last monthly bleeding, or 2) you can measure the size of her womb.

Using the last monthly bleeding

If a woman bleeds regularly every 4 weeks, she will get pregnant about 2 weeks after her last monthly bleeding. This makes it easy to figure out when she got pregnant.

To find out if you can use this method for this pregnancy, you must first ask the mother 3 questions:

> **1.** Has your monthly bleeding been mostly regular, once every 4 weeks (or every month or one time between 2 full moons)?
>
> **2.** Was your last monthly bleeding normal for you (or was it unusually light or heavy)?
>
> **3.** Do you remember the date of the first day of your last monthly bleeding?

If the mother answers *no* to any of these 3 questions, you should not use this method as your only method. You cannot be certain this method will give you a correct due date.

If she answers *yes* to all 3 questions, you can figure out the due date and how pregnant the woman is at this visit. Remember that a pregnancy lasts about 9 calendar months or 10 lunar months from the last monthly bleeding.

Using a calendar

1. To figure out the due date, take the first day of the last monthly bleeding and count backwards 3 months. Then add 7 days. Be careful to count the right number of months. Use your fingers or write it down to make it easier.

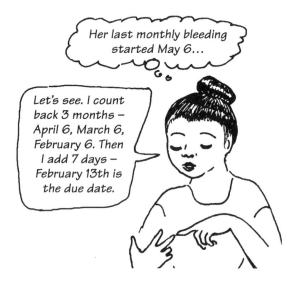

Her last monthly bleeding started May 6...

Let's see. I count back 3 months – April 6, March 6, February 6. Then I add 7 days – February 13th is the due date.

2. To figure out how pregnant the woman is now, take the first day of the last monthly bleeding and count the number of months that have passed between that day and the first visit.

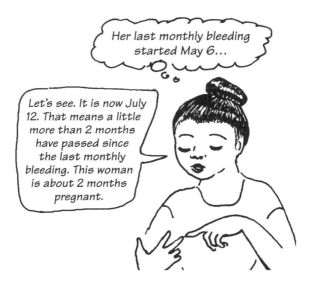

Without using a calendar

If you do not use calendars, you can find the due date by using the moon. If a woman's monthly bleeding is usually about one moon (4 weeks) apart, the baby is due exactly 10 moons after the first day of her last monthly bleeding. If a woman's monthly bleeding starts on a quarter moon, the baby is due 10 quarter moons later. If her bleeding started on a new moon, the baby is due 10 new moons later, and so on.

For example:

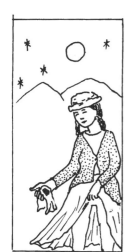

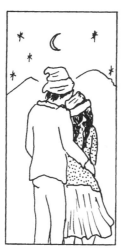

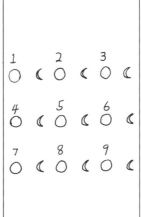

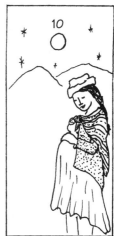

If her bleeding started on the full moon,

she probably got pregnant on the new moon.

The baby is always due 10 months after the first day of her last monthly bleeding –

in this case, 10 full moons after the first day of her last monthly bleeding.

Measuring the woman's womb

Feeling the size of the woman's womb is another method to use if:

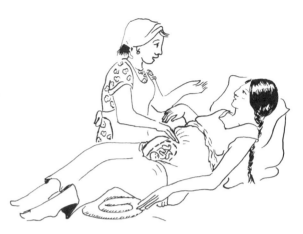

- the woman does not remember when her last monthly bleeding started.

- the last monthly bleeding was unusually light or heavy.

- her monthly bleeding is not regular.

- the woman was breast feeding and not bleeding regularly when she got pregnant.

Since you will be measuring the woman's womb as a regular part of a prenatal checkup, this is explained in the next chapter (see p. 117–119). You can wait to figure out the due date until you examine the woman's body. You will also see if the size of the womb matches the due date that you figured out from the last monthly bleeding.

3. How old is she?

Women who are between 18 and 35 usually have the fewest problems giving birth.

Less risk	More risk
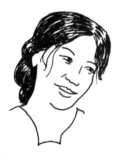	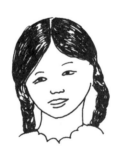 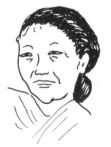
The woman is between 18 and 35.	The woman is younger than 18 or older than 35.

If a woman is younger than 18 years, her hips may not be fully grown. This can make birth more difficult. If a woman is more than 35 years old, her body may be tired and less flexible. She may suffer more from working too hard, stress, and illness. If the woman is more than 40 years old, there is more chance that the baby will be mentally slow.

If a woman is younger than 18 or older than 35, it is best for her to give birth in or near a hospital or maternity center, especially if she seems tired or if she is not as strong and healthy as a young woman. The older a woman is, the more important it is for her to be near medical help. These women may also need special advice, care, and support during pregnancy.

4. How many children has she had?

Women who have had 1 or 2 babies, whose last baby was born at least 2 years ago, and whose children are alive and healthy usually have the fewest problems giving birth.

Other women may have more problems. First births are often more difficult than later births. It is safest for a woman giving birth for the first time to give birth in or near a hospital. If she is not in a hospital, watch carefully for risk signs and have transportation available for emergencies.

A woman who has given birth to 5 or more babies is more likely to have some of the following problems:

- a labor that stops before the birth
- a long labor
- a **torn womb** (after a long, hard labor)
- a fallen womb **(prolapsed uterus)**
- a baby in a difficult position for birth
- heavy bleeding after birth

For these reasons, it is safer for a woman who has had 5 or more births to give birth in or near a hospital or maternity center. The more children she has, the more important it is for her to have medical help.

Less risk   More risk

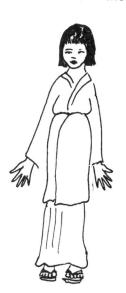

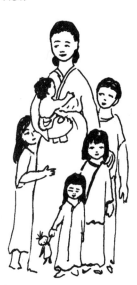

I have one child.   This is my first baby.   I have 5 children.

5. Has she had any miscarriages or abortions?

Miscarriage

A *miscarriage* (also called a *spontaneous abortion*) is when a baby is born before the woman is 6 months pregnant, while the baby is still too small to live outside the mother. If a miscarriage happens very early in pregnancy, the mother may only notice strong pains and a little more bleeding than her usual monthly bleeding. The baby she loses may be too small to be seen. After 3 months of pregnancy, the mother may have real labor pains during a miscarriage. The baby may be born alive but die in a few hours.

Many women have had 1 or 2 miscarriages in their lives. But if a woman has had 3 or more miscarriages in a row, she has a greater risk of another miscarriage. Try to get medical advice.

If a woman had very heavy bleeding or an infection of the womb after a past miscarriage, get medical advice. She may have the same problem after this birth. It may be best for this baby to be born in a hospital or maternity center.

Abortion

When a woman chooses to end a pregnancy before the baby can live outside the mother, it is called an *induced abortion.* In this book we simply use the word *abortion*.

There are several kinds of medical abortions. The most common kind is done by scraping inside the womb. This is called a *D and C* (*D*ilation and *C*urettage). If a woman has had only 1 or 2 of these abortions, and they were done in a hospital or clinic by a trained person, there should not be a problem. But if a woman has had 3 or more abortions, or even 1 abortion done by an unskilled person, it is probably safest for her to deliver her baby in or near a hospital or maternity center. This is because an abortion can sometimes leave small scars inside the mother's womb. In rare cases, the scars left by several of these abortions can cause the placenta to get stuck inside the mother after the birth.

If a woman had very heavy bleeding or infection of the womb after an abortion, get medical advice. She may have the same problem after this birth. It may be best for this baby to be born in a hospital.

> **Caution!** Abortions done at home or by untrained people are very dangerous! They often cause heavy scarring, serious bleeding, and infections of the womb.

Also, remember that a woman who has had an abortion or miscarriage may need extra emotional support when she becomes pregnant again.

6. Has she had any problems with past pregnancies or births?

If a woman has had problems with past pregnancies or births, she may have problems with this birth, too. The risk is greatest if the woman's most recent pregnancy or birth was difficult.

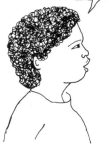

I bled a lot with both children. I was very weak for many days after the birth.

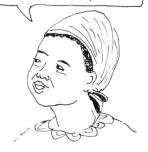

If you bled at past births, you are more likely to bleed at this one. It would be safer to have your next baby in a hospital.

Ask the mother to tell you the story of each of her past pregnancies and births. Let her tell you everything: the good **and** the bad. Then ask the following questions to learn more about problems in past pregnancies and how you can help during this pregnancy. (Many of these questions are explained more fully in other parts of this book. Turn to the page number listed to learn more about the problem.) Write down what you learn.

Questions to ask about past pregnancies

Was she anemic (see p. 110)?

If she was *anemic* in a past pregnancy, find out if she is anemic now and whether she is eating well (see chapter 4). If she is anemic now or not eating well, she is more likely to have many problems during this pregnancy and birth.

Did she have high blood pressure (see p. 107, 109)?

If she had *high blood pressure* in a past pregnancy, she is more likely to get it again. Try to make sure it is checked regularly during this pregnancy, even if the woman has to travel to a clinic to have it done. See p. 108 for how to check blood pressure.

Did she have swelling or pre-eclampsia (see p. 112)?

If a woman had *pre-eclampsia* in a past pregnancy, check her blood pressure and other signs of pre-eclampsia regularly in this pregnancy.

Did she have a bladder or kidney infection (see p. 115)?

If she had either of these infections in a past pregnancy, it is more likely to happen again. Teach the mother the early signs of bladder and kidney infection. Encourage her to get help right away if any signs appear. She should also drink lots of liquids and keep her genitals very clean. If possible, get medical advice now.

Does she have diabetes (blood sugar disease) (see p. 88)?

If she had *diabetes* in a past pregnancy, she is more likely to get it again. Get medical advice. If possible, she should be tested by a doctor or health worker.

Did she have a very long labor (longer than 24 hours for a first baby, or longer than 12 hours for other babies)? Did she have a long pushing stage (more than 2 hours)?

Ask her if this long labor caused problems for her or her baby. If that birth was normal and the baby was OK, then it will probably not be a problem with this birth. If that birth was not normal, ask her why the labor was long. Did she have anemia? An illness? Small bones? A big baby? Was the baby in a difficult position? Was she very afraid? Depending on what you find out, you may need to get medical advice.

Did she have a very short labor (less than 2 hours)?

If the mother had a very short labor in the past, make sure she and her family know what to do if you do not get there in time. You may want to spend some time teaching the family how to deliver a baby and how to handle emergencies, like heavy bleeding. See chapters 20 and 13.

Did she have an early birth (see p. 233)?

If she had a baby born more than 5 weeks early, ask her if she has signs of vaginal infection (see p. 362–365). If possible, have a doctor check her cervix at the 6th or 7th month of pregnancy, to see if it is starting to open too early. Be ready in case this baby is early, too.

Did she have a baby that was less than 2.5 kilograms or 5 pounds?

Find out if the baby was born more than 3 weeks before the due date. If the baby came on time, find out whether the mother had high blood pressure, anemia, or pre-eclampsia. Also ask if she had enough to eat, or if she smoked cigarettes or used drugs. Check carefully to see if this baby is growing normally. Make arrangements for medical care if you think this baby may be very small, too.

Did she have a baby that was over 4 kilograms or 9 pounds?

Find out whether the birth was difficult. Look for signs of diabetes (see p. 88). Check carefully to see if this baby seems big, too. If possible, get medical advice and have the mother checked for diabetes.

Did she have fits (convulsions)?

If she had **convulsions** in a past pregnancy or birth, get medical help **now**! She should have medical care during all her pregnancies and should always give birth in a hospital.

Did she have heavy bleeding before or after the birth (see p. 100–101)?

If she bled a lot in a past pregnancy or birth, it is more likely to happen again. Check for signs of anemia. If possible, she should have her babies in the hospital from now on.

Did she have any problems with the placenta?

If the placenta did not come out easily in a past birth, it is more likely to happen again. Get medical advice.

Did she have a fever or infection of the womb during or after birth (see p. 298)?

Find out if her bag of waters broke before or early in labor, and whether she had a lot of vaginal checkups. This birth may be fine, but there is more risk of infection than for other women. Be sure to check her for signs of vaginal infection (see p. 362–365) and get medical advice.

Was she very sad (depressed) after the birth?

If a woman became depressed after a past birth, there is a chance that it may happen again. Be prepared to help if this happens (see p. 301).

Did the baby get sick or die—before, during, or after the birth?

Find out if the baby was normal or had defects. If her first baby was healthy, but later babies died, she may need a special blood test. Be sure to check the mother for high blood pressure (see p. 107–109), diabetes (see p. 88), anemia (see p. 110–111), malnutrition (see chapter 4), and illness. Get medical advice.

Did her baby have birth defects (see p. 294–295)?

Some **birth defects** run in the family. Ask about the type of birth defect and if anyone else in her or her husband's family has that birth defect. If so, get medical advice.

7. Has she had a cesarean section (birth by operation)?

In a cesarean section the doctor cuts open the woman's belly and womb to get the baby out. After the baby is out, the doctor sews the womb and belly closed. This leaves one scar on the womb and a second scar on the belly. Sometimes a cesarean section is done because the baby is too big to fit through the mother's pelvic bones. Sometimes it is done because there is some reason the baby must get out of the mother quickly.

When the mother has another baby, there is a very small chance that the scar on the womb will tear open during labor. If this happens, she can bleed inside and die. It is safest for a woman with a past cesarean section to give birth in a hospital. She may not need to have an operation with this baby, but she should be in a hospital in case of problems. If a woman understands the risks but does not want to give birth in a hospital, she should give birth near a hospital. Before the birth, arrange to have hospital care in case there are any problems during the labor.

If any of the following are true, this woman should definitely go to the hospital for the birth:

- The scar on the womb is up and down. Unfortunately, you cannot tell anything about the scar on the womb by looking at the belly. The scar on the belly can be one way, and the scar on the womb inside can be another. You can only find out by checking the medical records at the hospital or by asking the doctor who did the operation.

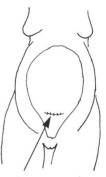

This scar is more likely to open up in labor.

This scar is less likely to open up in labor.

- She had a cesarean section because the baby could not fit through her pelvic bones.

- The cesarean section was less than 2 years ago.

- This baby is big or in a difficult birth position.

- There are any other risk signs with this pregnancy.

8. Is she healthy?

Pregnancy and birth can be more dangerous if a woman is ill. If a pregnant woman has any of the following problems **now**, she should get medical help to plan for her needs during pregnancy and decide if she should deliver in a hospital.

- diabetes
- AIDS
- bladder or kidney infection
- fever over 40°C or 104°F for more than 2 days
- liver disease (**hepatitis**, especially hepatitis B)
- convulsions
- high blood pressure
- heart problems
- untreated **tuberculosis**
- deformity of the hips or lower back

If a woman has **ever** had any of the following problems, she should see a doctor or experienced health worker during her pregnancy—to find out whether she still has a problem:

- hepatitis
- bladder or kidney infections
- frequent fevers
- tuberculosis

Malaria

Malaria is an infection of the blood that causes chills and high fever. Malaria is spread by mosquitoes. Women are more likely to get malaria when they are pregnant. Malaria can cause a miscarriage, early birth, small baby, or *still birth* (baby is born dead).

If you live in an area where there is a lot of malaria, it may be best for all pregnant women to take medicine to prevent malaria. The World Health Organization recommends 2 tablets of 250 mg chloroquine phosphate every week throughout pregnancy. Check with your local health ministry to see if this is recommended in your area.

If a woman already has malaria, she should take tablets of 250 mg chloroquine phosphate on the following schedule:

- Day 1: 4 tablets to start, then 2 tablets 6 hours later
- Day 2: 2 tablets
- Day 3: 2 tablets

If the medicine does not work, the woman should get medical advice.

If a woman has fever over 40°C or 104°F for 2 days or longer, or if she has sleepiness, convulsions, dark urine, or unconsciousness (coma), she should get medical help.

9. Does she have signs of diabetes?

When a woman gets *diabetes*, her body cannot use the sugar in her blood. A woman cannot get diabetes from another person, but sometimes it runs in families. Sometimes women get diabetes only when they are pregnant. They do not have it before, and it goes away after the birth.

Diabetes can make a woman very sick and childbirth more dangerous. Her baby may have birth defects, be very big, or it may become very ill and die after the birth.

Risk signs

If a woman has some of the following risk signs, there is a chance that she has diabetes. A woman does not need all of these signs to have diabetes. But the more signs a woman has, the more likely it is that she has diabetes.

- She is fat.
- She had diabetes with a past pregnancy.
- One or more past babies was born very big (more than 4 kilograms or 9 pounds), ill, or died at birth—and no one knows why.
- Her womb is bigger than you would expect for her months of pregnancy.
- She is thirsty all of the time.
- She is over 35 years old.
- Her wounds heal slowly.
- She has to urinate (pee) more than other pregnant women.

You can also ask your local health department if they have recommendations for how to recognize diabetes.

What to do

Sometimes diabetes can be controlled by a good diet, rest, and exercise. Sometimes medicine is needed to prevent serious problems.

If a woman has had diabetes in the past, get medical advice **now**. Proper medical care during pregnancy can prevent many problems.

If you suspect that a woman may have had diabetes in a past pregnancy, she should have a medical test. The best time of this test is at about 6 months or 24 weeks.

If a woman has diabetes now, she should get medical help **now**. She should plan to have her baby in a hospital. If no medical help is available, she should follow a good diet (see chapter 4); avoid sweets; and eat small, frequent meals. You should get medical advice on how to help her to have a healthy baby.

10. Has she had tetanus injections? If so, when was her last injection?

Tetanus (lockjaw) results when a germ that lives in stools of animals or people enters the body through a wound. A mother can get tetanus if someone puts something that is not sterile into her womb or vagina during or after childbirth (while she is still bleeding). A baby can get tetanus when its cord is cut with something that is not sterile.

All babies and women of childbearing age should get injections *(vaccinations)* to prevent tetanus. The World Health Organization recommends the following injection schedule:

- injection #1: at first contact
- injection #2: 1 month after injection #1
- injection #3: 6 months after injection #2
- injection #4: 1 year after injection #3
- injection #5: 1 year after injection #4

In addition, every pregnant woman should be vaccinated at the first prenatal visit of **each** pregnancy (in case this may be her only visit). Check with your local health authorities for where she can get these injections or if you can give them to her.

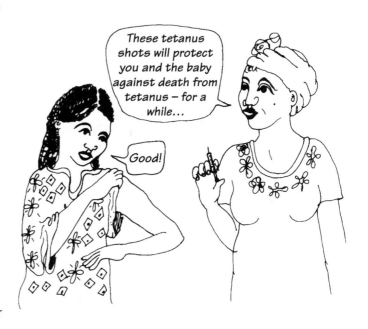

If a pregnant woman has not been properly vaccinated (following the schedule above) or has not had a vaccination for more than 10 years, give her an injection at the first prenatal visit. Give her a second injection 1–2 months later. If she has never been vaccinated, give a third injection 6 months after the second if possible.

Vaccinations during pregnancy will also help protect the baby from tetanus during the first few weeks after birth. The baby must be vaccinated after birth so that the protection will continue (see p. 229).

11. Has any medicine ever given her problems?

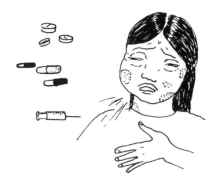

If any medicine has ever given a woman a problem (like a rash, swelling, or difficulty breathing), **do not give her that medicine**. She may be *allergic* to it. If she takes the medicine again at any time during the rest of her life, she might have a very serious problem or even die.

It is a good idea to write down the medicine and talk with a doctor or skilled health worker about it. Make sure everyone who might give the woman medicine knows about the problem. Explain to the woman that she must never use the medicine again, and that she should always tell her doctors or health workers about the problem.

Note: Some kinds of medicines come in "families." For example, penicillin and ampicillin are in the same family. This is why their names are similar. If a woman is allergic to one member of a family of medicines, she is probably allergic to the other members of that family.

But a woman who is allergic to one medicine or family of medicines should not fear all medicines. Other medicines are as safe for her as for anyone else.

12. Is she taking any medicines now?

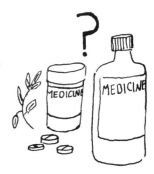

It is best for a woman to avoid all modern medicines and plant medicines during pregnancy. There are many medicines that can harm the baby inside the womb.

If a woman needs to take a medicine, see the Green Pages to find out whether that medicine is listed as **safe** in pregnancy. If the medicine is not listed, the pregnant woman should get medical advice.

13. Does she have any special concerns about this birth?

When you ask this question, give her time to think. It is probably also a good idea to ask the question again at each prenatal visit. If you listen carefully, you may even find answers to this question when you are talking about other things.

14. Does she have any special problems or needs?

Here are some things you may want to find out about:

Physical needs

Money

Does she (or a friend or family member) have enough money to pay for the following:

- healthy food
- supplies
- injections and medicines
- a doctor or hospital care
- transportation

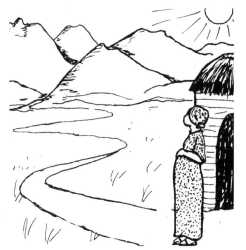

Distance from care

- Will she be able to come to her prenatal checkups? Can you go to her?
- If she lives far away, can you teach her to do some of the prenatal checkup herself?
- How far is the maternity center, clinic, or hospital? Does she need to stay somewhere else to be closer to medical help?
- Is there a telephone or radio she can use in an emergency?

Transportation

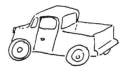

- Does she need help getting to her prenatal checkups or to the hospital in an emergency?
- Is there a car, truck, jeep, horse, bicycle cart, or push cart she can use? If these are not available, 2 wooden poles and a blanket carried between 2 people can be used for emergency transportation.

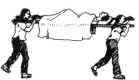

Her work

- How much work does she do at home and outside her home?
- Can she get enough rest during pregnancy?
- Does her work expose her to dangers—like poisons or chemicals (see p. 61). Can she be protected from work dangers?

Living conditions

- Is her house very crowded? Is the area around her house crowded or dirty?
- Is there clean water available?
- Does anyone in her house have a serious disease that she can get too (**contagious** disease)?

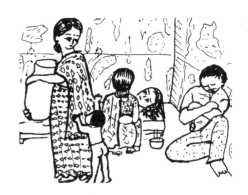

Family and community

Husband or partner

- Is the woman married?
- Is her husband often away from home?
- Does he get drunk?
- Does he treat her well?
- If he does not treat her well, is there someone he respects in the community who could help him understand her needs?
- Does he have sex with other people?
- Does he allow her to do what she needs to do to keep her pregnancy healthy?

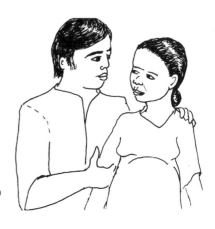

Family and community

- Does her family understand her needs?
- Are there people in her family and community who can help her with this pregnancy and make sure she eats well, rests, and has someone to talk to?
- Who else can help (the clinic, local organizations, a landlord, a government program)?
- Can she borrow what she needs for the birth (clean sheets and **disinfectant**)?
- Is there someone to deliver messages in an emergency?

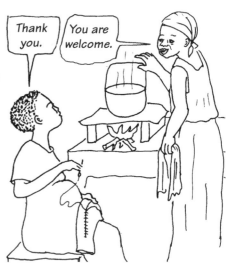

Beliefs and customs

- Does she have traditional beliefs or customs that are helpful or harmful (see p. 23–28)?

- If she has harmful beliefs, can you find ways to help her and still be respectful?

Special groups

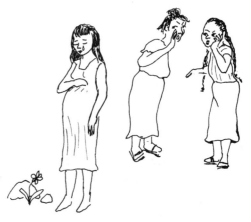

Single mothers

In some communities people are unkind to single mothers who have no husband or partner to help them. But we believe that single mothers and their babies deserve as much caring and kindness as anyone; often they need even more. Never reject them. Do what you can to help these women get the help they need.

Very young mothers and disabled mothers

Very young mothers and disabled or mentally slow mothers may need more help and support than other women during and after pregnancy. If the woman's family cannot help her, perhaps some friendly, experienced women in the community can help her.

Try to help these women learn to take care of themselves and their babies. If you do everything for them, they will not learn. Help them only when they need help.

Women who have been raped (forced to have sex)

Some women or girls become pregnant from a rape. It is important to remember that **rape is not the woman's fault**. She is not dirty or polluted. No one should make her feel guilty or ashamed. Instead, she needs special care, love, and support to heal. She may need to be tested for AIDS and other diseases that can be spread by sex.

If she is thinking about having an abortion to end the pregnancy, try to help her think clearly about how she feels and what she really wants to do. Make sure she gets good medical care.

Sometimes a woman who has been raped fears being touched. She may not want anyone to touch her body during the prenatal checkups or during childbirth. Try to help her feel safe and relaxed. Wait until she is ready before you touch her. Go slowly when you examine her. Explain what you are doing.

Sometimes a woman who is pregnant from a rape will have trouble caring for the child. If this happens, try to help her understand that the child had no part in the rape. It may help her to talk with someone about her feelings.

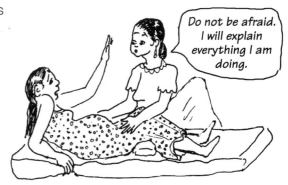

Do not be afraid. I will explain everything I am doing.

Women who have been beaten

In some parts of the word, people think it is acceptable for a man to beat his wife. Wife beating often starts or gets worse when a woman becomes pregnant. Other men do not beat their wives but may torment them emotionally by insulting them.

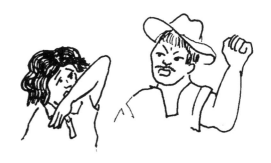

A woman may not admit that her husband beats her. She may feel ashamed or afraid to talk about it. If you see frequent bruises, burns, or broken bones, it may be a sign of wife beating.

Note: **It is never acceptable to beat a woman!** Beatings can lead to injury and sometimes even death. Beatings can also harm an unborn baby. We urge all health workers and community organizers to work together to stop wife beating in their communities.

Prostitutes

Prostitutes, like all women, deserve good care in pregnancy. Give her the same care you would give anyone else.

A woman who works as a prostitute may be exposed to many diseases. It is a good idea for her to go to a clinic for a complete checkup, and for medical tests to see if she has AIDS or other sexually transmitted diseases (see chapter 23).

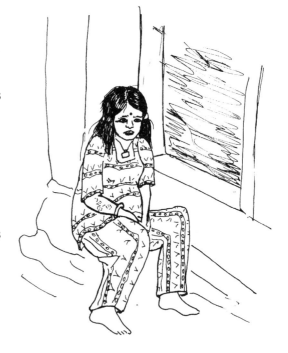

When her belly begins to grow, she may not be able to continue working as a prostitute. She may lose her home. She may not have enough money for food or health care. People may be unkind to her. Try to help her get what she needs. Do not judge her.

After asking the questions in this chapter, it is time to give the woman her first regular prenatal checkup. It is best to give this checkup on the same day. The next chapter will tell you how to do it. (Since you have just been talking with the mother, you can skip p. 97–102. Turn to p. 103, the section called **Check the mother's body**, to begin the regular checkup).

Prenatal checkups

Chapter 7 contents

Prenatal checkups

The regular prenatal checkup has 3 main parts: talking with the mother, checking the mother's body, and checking the baby. It is a good idea to write down what you learn about the mother and baby during each visit (see the sample chart at the end of this chapter).

In each part of the checkup, we have listed healthy signs and risk signs. If you find a risk sign, be sure to follow the instructions under the *What to do if you find risk signs* section. The woman may need medical help, or you may be able to take care of her yourself.

Caution! At each regular checkup, remind the woman of the following risk signs of pregnancy. If they occur between visits, she must contact you at once or seek medical help. If she has these signs, check the page number of the sign for what you can do.

1. Bleeding from the vagina (see p. 100).
2. Swelling of the face and hands (see p. 112).
3. Headache, dizziness, or blurred vision (see p. 112).

Talk with the mother

It is usually best to start the checkup with friendly talking. Ask the mother how she has been feeling and how her pregnancy is going. See if she has any complaints or questions.

1. Observe her general health

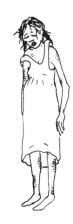

Healthy signs: *Mother looks, sounds, and feels healthy and happy.*

Risk signs: *Mother looks, sounds, or feels unhealthy or unhappy.*

While you are talking with the mother, try to notice everything about her general health. For example:

- Does she seem happy—or is she irritable and depressed?
- Does she have plenty of energy—or is she tired and ill?
- Does she move easily—or is she stiff and slow?
- Does she seem to think and talk clearly—or is she confused?
- Does she have clear skin—or does she have sores and rashes?

What to do if you find risk signs

If the mother's general health seems poor, or if she does not look right, try to give her special attention—even if nothing in particular seems wrong. If she seems unhealthy, encourage her to seek medical help.

2. Ask if she has any nausea or vomiting

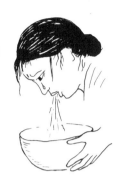

Healthy signs: Mother has no nausea or vomiting, or mild nausea in the first 3 to 4 months.

Risk signs:

- *Mother has severe vomiting or vomiting after the 4th month.*

- *Mother is unable to keep water in her stomach.*

- *Mother can only urinate (pee) a little bit (or stops urinating), or urine is very dark.*

- *Mother gains less than 1 kilo (2 pounds) per month.*

Many woman have nausea in the first 3 or 4 months of pregnancy. This is not usually serious. But if a woman vomits a lot, feels too sick to eat or can't keep down fluids, it is a risk sign. She and her baby may become malnourished. The nausea may also be a sign that something else is wrong.

What to do if you find risk signs

If the nausea is mild and in early pregnancy, see p. 66 for some helpful remedies to give the mother. If these remedies do not work, or if vomiting is severe or continues after the 4th month, get medical advice. There are modern medicines that help calm the stomach so she can eat.

If the mother has diarrhea (loose stools) or other signs of illness along with vomiting, get medical advice. She should be checked for infection, ulcers (sores in the stomach), **parasites** (tiny animals living in people's intestines and causing disease) or a **molar pregnancy** (a tumor growing in the womb instead of a baby, see p. 121).

If the mother has parasites but they are not causing too many problems, she should probably wait until after the birth to take medicine. Some medicines for parasites may harm the baby, especially during the first 3 months. Check with local health authorities about what medicines to use, or get medical help. If illness from parasites is severe and the woman is not gaining weight normally, or has other signs of illness, get medical advice.

If the mother is unable to keep fluids down and stops urinating, get medical help immediately. She will need **intravenous fluids** (fluids given in the veins, which are also called **IV fluids**) (see p. 414–415) and medicine. If you are trained in starting IV fluids, start them while you are travelling to get medical help.

Note: If other people in the area also have trouble with nausea, vomiting, or diarrhea, there may be a problem with the local water supply. It will not help to give the mother medicines for parasites if she will just get them again from bad water. To make the water good for drinking, she should boil or filter it first.

Perhaps the community can work together to build a clean water system. Or you may find other solutions to the problem.

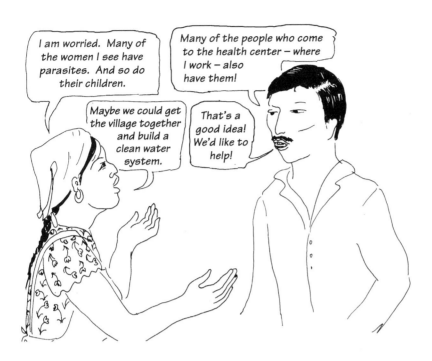

3. Ask if she feels weak

Healthy sign: Mother has plenty of energy.

Risk sign: Mother feels weak or tired all of the time, especially after the 4th month.

A pregnant woman should have plenty of energy, although she may be very sleepy in the first 3 months and in the last 4 to 5 weeks of pregnancy.

If a woman is weak for a long time, she may be suffering from one or more of the following:

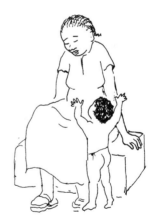

- malnutrition (see chapter 4)

- anemia (see p. 110–111)

- too much work

- illness

- depression

- heart trouble (see p. 102, 107)

What to do if you find risk signs

It is important to check for these problems because a weak mother is more likely to have problems in labor and birth. She may have a long, difficult labor, and bleed heavily or get an infection after the birth. Her baby is more likely to be sick. If you are worried about the mother, ask her to see a health worker for a checkup.

4. Ask if she has spotting or bleeding from the vagina

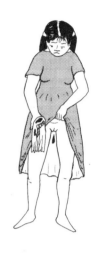

Healthy signs:

- *No bleeding during pregnancy, or very light bleeding without cramps during the first months when the mother's monthly bleeding would have occurred.*

- *Pink or blood-tinged mucus 2 to 3 days before labor begins. This mucus is called* **show**.

Risk signs:

- *Bleeding like a period at any time during pregnancy.*

- *Bleeding with cramps during the first 6 months. There is a risk of miscarriage or natural abortion.*

- *Bleeding with constant pain at any time during pregnancy.*

- *Bleeding with no pain, especially in the second half of pregnancy.*

What to do if you find risk signs

Light bleeding during the first 6 months

If the mother has light bleeding with cramps, she may be starting a miscarriage (spontaneous abortion). If the bleeding is light *(spotting)* and she is in the first 3 months, the risk is low. If the bleeding is like a monthly bleeding or heavier, if the mother is more than 3 months pregnant, or if there is severe pain or a bad smell from her vagina, it is best to get medical advice. Do not put anything in a woman's vagina if she is having a miscarriage.

Bleeding with constant pain at any time during pregnancy

Bleeding with constant pain during the first 3 months may be a sign that the baby is growing in the wrong place. Usually the baby grows in the womb, where it belongs. But in rare cases, it may start to grow in a small tube that is off to the side of the womb. This is called a **tubal pregnancy**.

At first the tube stretches. But as the baby grows, the mother may feel a sore lump on her side, or pain on her side. Then, sometime before she is 3 months pregnant, the tube breaks and bleeds. This is very dangerous. The mother can bleed to death inside her belly.
Go to the hospital immediately!
Watch for *signs of shock* and treat for **shock** (see p. 243).

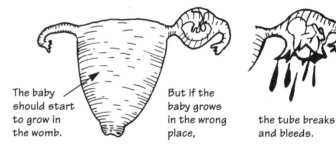

The baby should start to grow in the womb.

But if the baby grows in the wrong place,

the tube breaks and bleeds.

Tubal pregnancy

Bleeding with constant pain during the **last** few months of pregnancy may mean the placenta has come off the wall of the womb. This is called a **detached placenta**, or **abruption** of the placenta. The mother may be bleeding heavily inside. Some of this blood may come out, but it may not. A womb full of blood may feel hard. This is very dangerous. The mother and baby may die. **Go to the hospital immediately!** Watch for signs of shock and treat for shock (see p. 243).

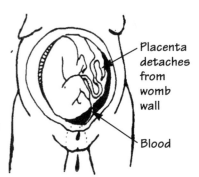

Placenta detaches from womb wall

Blood

Bleeding with no pain, especially in the last half of pregnancy

Bleeding without pain may mean the placenta is covering the cervix instead of being near the top of the womb (where it should be). This is called **placenta previa**. When the cervix starts to open toward the end of pregnancy, the bottom of the placenta is not protected. It is like a raw wound. The mother's blood flows through the placenta and out the vagina. This is very dangerous. The mother and baby may die. **Go to the hospital immediately!** Watch for signs of shock and treat for shock (see p. 243).

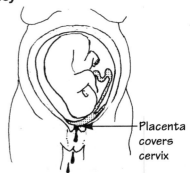

Placenta covers cervix

> **Caution!** Never put your hands inside the vagina when there is bleeding. You could poke a hole in the placenta and make bleeding much worse. You could kill the mother.

5. Ask if she has any unusual pain in the belly, back, or leg

Healthy sign: *No pain in the belly, back or legs.*

Pregnant women often have aches and pains that are normal. These pains are probably OK:

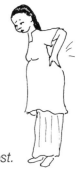

- *Mild, irregular cramps high in the belly or all over the belly (also called* **practice contractions**; *see p. 137).*

- *Womb feels tight, then relaxes.*

- *Sudden, sharp pains low in the front but to the side that last a few minutes and then go away.*

- *Lower back pain that feels better with rest, massage, or exercise.*

- *Sharp pain in the buttocks that runs down the leg and feels better with rest.*

Risk signs:

- *Cramps or pains that get stronger and come more often.*

- *Constant pain in the belly.*

- *Pain in the lower belly that goes through the sides into the back, or back pain that does not get better with rest, massage, or exercise.*

What to do if you find risk signs

If the mother has any of the following pains, there may be a problem. Turn to the page number listed for more information:

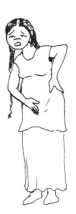

- Cramps or belly pains in the first 3 months that get stronger or come more often may mean that a miscarriage is starting. See p. 82, 100.

- Strong, constant belly or side pain in the first 3 months may mean that this is a tubal pregnancy. See p. 100.

- Constant belly pain in late pregnancy may mean the placenta is coming off the womb wall. See p. 101.

- Constant pain in the lower belly that goes through the sides into the back, or back pain that does not get better with rest, massage, or exercise, may be caused by a bladder or kidney infection. See p. 115.

Note: Just like anyone else, a pregnant woman can get an ordinary illness that makes her belly hurt. The illness could be caused by appendicitis (an infection of part of the *intestines*—with fever, pain on the right side of the belly, and lack of appetite), parasites (with nausea or diarrhea), or ulcers (sometimes with vomiting and black, tarry stools). Get medical advice if you think the mother may have one of these illnesses.

6. Ask if she has shortness of breath

Healthy signs: *No shortness of breath, or mild shortness of breath late in pregnancy.*

Risk sign: *A lot of shortness of breath, especially with other signs of illness.*

Many women get a little shortness of breath when they are 8 or 9 months pregnant. Sometimes it is hard for them to take deep breaths because the baby is in the way. Breathing may get easier when the baby drops lower in the belly shortly before labor begins (see p. 137).

If the mother has trouble breathing all the time, she may have:

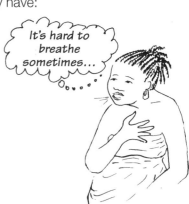

It's hard to breathe sometimes...

- allergies

- anemia (see p. 110)

- heart problems

- tuberculosis (a *contagious* lung disease)

- *asthma*

- lung infection

What to do if you find risk signs

If the mother has trouble breathing all of the time, or if you think she may have any of the problems listed above, get medical advice.

Check the mother's body

1. Weigh the mother

Healthy sign: *Mother slowly and steadily gains between 9 and 18 kilograms (20 to 40 pounds) during pregnancy. This is the same as $1/4$ to $1/2$ kilogram ($1/2$ to 1 pound) per week or 1 to 2 kilograms (2 to 4 pounds) each month. Most of the weight is gained in the second half of pregnancy.*

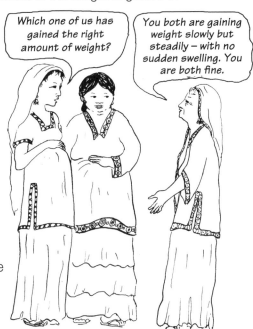

Which one of us has gained the right amount of weight?

You both are gaining weight slowly but steadily – with no sudden swelling. You are both fine.

Risk signs:

- *Mother is very thin or does not gain at least 9 kilograms (20 pounds) during pregnancy.*

- *Mother is very fat or gains more than 19 kilograms (42 pounds) during pregnancy.*

- *Mother gains weight suddenly—more than 1.4 kilograms (3 pounds) in 1 week or $3^{1}/_{2}$ kilograms (8 pounds) in 1 month, especially in the last 2 months of pregnancy.*

Most of the weight a mother gains during pregnancy is from her baby, the placenta, and the bag of waters. The mother also puts on some fat. This is usually good.

If you have a scale, weigh the mother at each visit. If possible, always use the same scale. If you do not have a scale, try to estimate her weight. Keep a record of her weight at each visit.

What to do if you find risk signs

Mother is very thin or does not gain enough weight

If the mother is very thin, or does not gain enough weight, try to figure out what may be causing the problem. Ask the mother about:

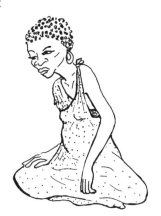

- her diet (see p. 48)

- nausea and vomiting (see p. 98)

- signs of parasites (see p. 98)

- special needs (see p. 91)

- drug use (see p. 60)

- AIDS (see p. 369)

If none of these things seem to be causing the problem, she may have a serious problem. Get medical advice.

Mother is very fat or gains too much weight

Some fat on a woman's body is healthy and good. But extremely fat women may have more problems in childbirth. Here are some of the problems that being very fat can cause:

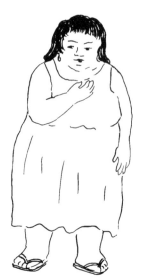

- The mother may feel weak and have less energy.

- The mother may have diabetes (see p. 88).

- The midwife may have trouble finding the position of the baby, the size of the womb, and the baby's heartbeat.

- The mother may have trouble pushing the baby out.

- The baby may get very big and be hard to deliver.

- The midwife may have a hard time massaging the womb if the mother bleeds a lot after birth.

If a woman is eating a good diet in normal amounts, she may be naturally fat. This is OK. But if a woman has too much fat and sugar in her diet, or if she eats more than most women do, encourage her to eat small amounts of better quality foods (see chapter 4). A woman should **not** try to lose weight while she is pregnant.

Encourage all fat women to get vigorous exercise—like walking, dancing, physical work, or other lively activities.

Mother gains weight suddenly

If a mother gains weight suddenly near the end of her pregnancy, it may be a sign of *twins* (see p. 131) or pre-eclampsia (see p. 112).

2. Feel her skin to see if she is hot-to-touch or take her temperature

Healthy sign: *Temperature is 37° centigrade (C) or 98.6° Fahrenheit (F). Woman feels cool.*

Risk sign: *Temperature is above 37.2°C or 99°F. This is a **fever**. Woman feels hot-to-touch.*

How to take the temperature

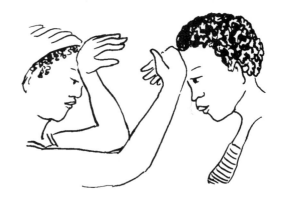

Put the back of one hand on the woman's forehead, and the other on your own, or that of another healthy person. Or kiss the woman's forehead with your lips, which are very sensitive to temperature. If the woman has a fever, you should be able to feel a difference between her skin and that of a healthy person.

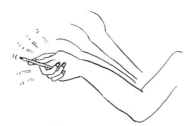

If you have a thermometer, clean it well with alcohol (or soap and clean water). Shake with a snap of the wrist until the thermometer reads less than 36°C or 95°F.

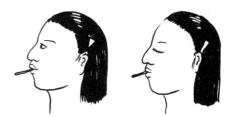

Put the thermometer under the tongue and leave it there for 3 or 4 minutes.

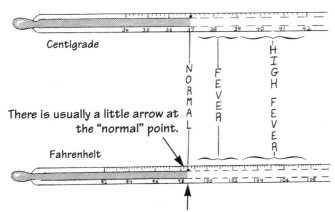

Centigrade

There is usually a little arrow at the "normal" point.

NORMAL   FEVER   HIGH FEVER

Fahrenheit

Take the thermometer out and turn it until you see the silver line. The point where the silver stops marks the temperature.

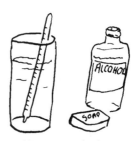

Always wash the thermometer with alcohol, or soap and clean water, after you use it. Do not use hot water. It can break the thermometer!

What to do if you find risk signs

A fever is a sign of infection (harmful germs entering the body and causing illness). Some kinds of infection, like malaria, are more dangerous in pregnancy than at other times (see p. 87). If the mother has a fever it could mean an infection anywhere in the body. Is there a flu or sickness in the community? Is she at risk for malaria? Does she have other signs of infection (see p. 115, 163)?

A high fever (38°C or 100.4°F) needs to be treated to bring it down. Give the woman paracetamol (acetaminophen) 500 mg by mouth every 4 hours and have her drink lots of fluids. If the fever does not come down in 8 hours, get medical help.

3. Take the mother's pulse

Healthy sign: *Pulse is about 60–80 beats per minute when the mother is resting.*

Risk sign: *Pulse is 100 beats per minute or more when the mother is resting.*

The **pulse** tells you how fast the heart is beating. Different pulses are normal for different people.

How to take the pulse

1. Make sure the mother is resting and relaxed.

2. Find the pulse.

3. Count the number of beats per minute:

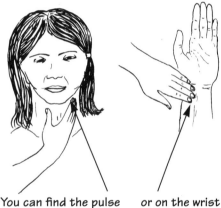

You can find the pulse on the side of the throat, under the jaw, **or on the wrist below the thumb.**

- If you have a watch with a second hand, count the number of beats in the mother's pulse for one minute. Write the number down. (At first it may be best to have someone watch the clock for you and tell you when a minute has passed. Many people find it hard to count accurately while looking at a watch. They tend to count one pulse beat per second, even if this is wrong.)

- If you do not have a watch with a second hand, take the pulse anyway. You can learn to tell if it is slow, normal, or fast compared to your own pulse, and to other women. Or you can make a homemade timer to use instead of a watch (see p. 427).

What to do if you find a risk sign

If the mother's pulse is 100 beats per minute or more, she may have one or more of the following problems:

- tension, fear, or worry from special problems (see p. 91–92)
- heavy bleeding (see p. 100–101)
- anemia (see p. 110)
- illness or fever (see p. 105, 115, 363)
- *thyroid* problems
- heart trouble
- drug use (for example: cocaine, diet pills, heroin, or morphine)

If you suspect any of these problems, turn to the page number listed for more information. If there is no page number listed, or if you do not know what is causing the fast pulse, get medical advice.

4. Take her blood pressure

Healthy sign: *Blood pressure stays between 90/60 and 140/90 and does not go up much during pregnancy.*

Risk sign: *High blood pressure.*

The mother has high blood pressure if either of these is true:

- *The top number is over 140, or goes up 30 or more points during pregnancy.*
- *The bottom number is over 90, or goes up 15 or more points during pregnancy.*

Blood pressure is a measure of how hard the blood presses on the inside of the blood vessels (**veins** and **arteries**). **High blood pressure** usually means that the blood has to press harder to get through tight or shrunken blood vessels.

High blood pressure can cause many problems during pregnancy. It is hard for the blood to bring food to the baby. The baby grows slowly because it is starving. Sometimes high blood pressure can cause the mother to have kidney problems, bleeding in the womb before birth, bleeding in the brain, or convulsions. High blood pressure can even kill the mother.

How to take blood pressure

Anyone who knows how to count can learn to take blood pressure. There are several types of blood pressure equipment. Some have a tall gauge that looks like a thermometer. Others have a round dial. Blood pressure equipment usually comes with a **stethoscope**. (See p. 429 for how to make a homemade stethoscope.)

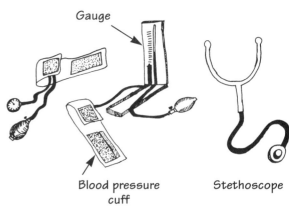

Gauge

Blood pressure
cuff

Stethoscope

To take the mother's blood pressure, first tell her what you are going to do, so she will not be afraid.

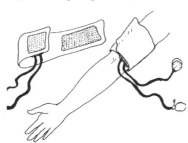

Fasten the cuff around the
bare upper arm.

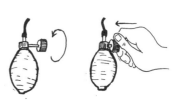

Close the valve on the rubber bulb
by turning the screw to the right.
The valve will get shorter.

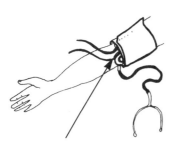

Feel for a pulse just below the elbow,
on the inside of the arm. Put the
stethoscope over the pulse.

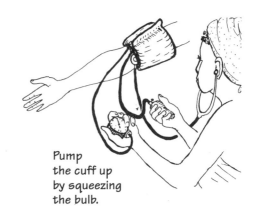

Pump
the cuff up
by squeezing
the bulb.

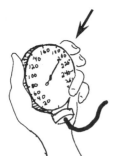

As you pump, the needle
will move. When it reaches
200, stop pumping.

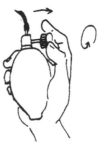

Then release the valve a
little so that the air leaks
out slowly.

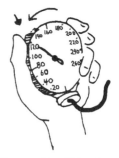

The needle will begin to go
back down. (If the valve is
closed, it will stay at 200.)

As the air leaks out, you will start to hear the mother's pulse through your stethoscope. Notice where the needle or mercury is when you start to hear the pulse (this will be the top number) and when the pulse disappears or gets very soft (this will be the bottom number).

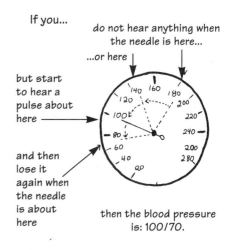

If you...
do not hear anything when the needle is here...
...or here
but start to hear a pulse about here →
and then lose it again when the needle is about here
then the blood pressure is: 100/70.

Sept 13	100/60
Oct 12	110/62
Nov 15	90/58
Dec 10	112/60
Jan 12	110/70

This woman's blood pressure goes up and down a little from month to month. This is normal.

Take the mother's blood pressure at each visit. Write it down on a chart or on one piece of paper, so you can look for changes over time. It is OK if the blood pressure goes up 20 points or less in the top number and 14 points or less in the bottom number from month to month.

What to do if you find risk signs

If the mother has high blood pressure the first time you take it, have her lie on her left side. Talk with her in a friendly way to help her relax (feeling tense can cause blood pressure to go up). In 10 to 30 minutes, take her blood pressure again:

- If the blood pressure goes down to a normal level, things are probably OK. If possible, have the mother come back in a few days so you can take her blood pressure again. Be sure to take her blood pressure at each visit.

- If the blood pressure does not go down, there may be a problem. To find out, take her blood pressure at least 3 times in the next week (or every day for 3 days). If the blood pressure stays high, get medical advice. Teach the mother the danger signs of pre-eclampsia and check to see if she has any of those signs (see p. 112). It will probably be safest for her to give birth in a hospital.

- If the top number of the blood pressure is over 160, **or** if the bottom number is over 100, get medical help now. She must go to the hospital for treatment. In some cases, she may need to stay at the hospital until she has the baby.

Home care for high blood pressure (for blood pressures between 140/90 and 158/98)

If the mother cannot see a doctor or if the doctor advises her to rest at home, she should:

- Rest in bed as much as possible. It is best if she rests on her left side. If she cannot stay in bed, she should rest as much as she can during the day, even if this is only for a few minutes every 1 to 2 hours. The mother can practice relaxing and feeling peaceful during these rest periods. The higher the blood pressure, the more important it is to rest. It is especially important to rest in the last 3 months of pregnancy.

- Eat a good diet—with protein, fruits, vegetables, and high iron and calcium foods (see p. 50).

- Drink a lot of liquid—6 to 8 glasses or more a day.

- Avoid very salty foods.

5. Check for signs of anemia

Healthy signs:

- *pink inside of eyelids*

- *pink gums*

- *pink fingernails*

- *general good health and a lot of energy*

- *normal pulse*

- *normal breathing*

Risk signs:

- *pale inside of eyelids*

- *pale gums*

- *white fingernails*

- *weakness*

- *fast pulse (over 80 beats per minute)*

- *fast breathing*

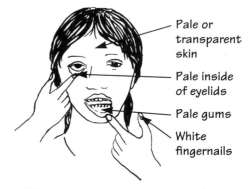

Pale or transparent skin

Pale inside of eyelids

Pale gums

White fingernails

Weakness, fast pulse, fast breathing

When someone has anemia, it means their blood is thin or pale—usually because there is not enough iron in the diet (see p. 51–52). Iron makes the blood red. It helps the blood carry oxygen (from the air) to all parts of the body. (Some kinds of anemia are caused by illness, not lack of iron, but these kinds are less common.)

Many pregnant women have anemia, especially in poor communities. Women with anemia have less strength for childbirth and are more likely to bleed heavily, become ill after childbirth, or even die.

What to do if you find risk signs

Ordinary anemia can usually be cured at home by eating foods high in iron and vitamin C (for example, citrus fruits and tomatoes), and by taking iron medicine. Turn to p. 51–52 to learn about several ways to prevent or cure anemia. After using these methods, the mother should be checked again in about 4 weeks. If she is not getting better, get medical advice. She may have an illness, or she may just need stronger medicine.

If a woman is very anemic by the 9th month of pregnancy, she should plan to have her baby in the hospital.

> **Caution!** The risk signs listed above usually mean anemia, but they may also mean that a woman is losing blood. If the signs of anemia begin suddenly, it is even more likely that the mother is bleeding inside. See p. 243.

6. Check for signs of poor nutrition or lack of iodine

Healthy signs:

- *general good health and a lot of energy*

- *clear skin*

Risk signs:

For general poor nutrition:

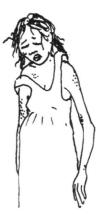

- *poor appetite or weight gain*

- *weakness and general ill health*

- *sores, rashes, or other skin problems*

- *sore or bleeding gums*

- *stomach problems or diarrhea*

- *burning or numbness of the feet*

For lack of iodine:

- *goiter (swelling in the front of the throat)*

- *cretinism (short, deaf, or mentally slow children)*

What to do if you find risk signs

The best way to prevent or cure poor nutrition is to help people eat well. Find out what the mother has been eating. Study chapter 4 to find ways to help her eat better. Remember: Never use vitamin pills, tonics, or injections instead of a good diet!

If you are worried that she may have a hard birth because of poor nutrition, get medical advice. This is especially important if you do not have enough time or resources to help her get well before the birth.

If a pregnant woman has goiter, or if she or other women in the community have cretin children, she probably does not have enough iodine in her diet. See p. 53 for ways to get more iodine.

Goiter

7. Check for signs of pre-eclampsia *(toxemia* of pregnancy)

Healthy signs

- *no swelling (a little swelling in the ankles is OK)*
- *normal blood pressure*
- *no headaches, dizziness, or blurred or double vision*

Risk signs

If the mother has any of these risk signs, she may be developing pre-eclampsia:

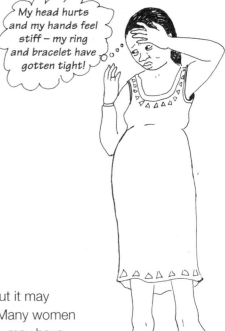

My head hurts and my hands feel stiff – my ring and bracelet have gotten tight!

- *high blood pressure*
- *swelling of the face or hands*
- *rapid weight gain*

If the mother has high blood pressure, and one or more of the following signs, she has pre-eclampsia:

- *headaches*
- *blurred or double vision*
- *dizziness*
- *any swelling (a little swelling in the ankles is OK)*

We do not know exactly what causes **pre-eclampsia**, but it may be due to the mother's body reacting to the pregnancy. Many women with pre-eclampsia often feel fine during pregnancy. They may have quick, easy labors. But other women with pre-eclampsia will have serious problems—like premature birth, convulsions during labor, severe bleeding after childbirth, or even death.

Checking for pre-eclampsia

1. Take the woman's blood pressure (see p. 108). High blood pressure is always a risk sign. If it is combined with any other risk signs listed here, the risk is even greater.

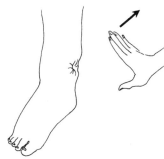

2. Check for swelling. Swelling is sometimes called water weight, water retention, or edema.

Some swelling in pregnancy is normal. If the woman has swollen ankles in the afternoon or in hot weather, this is OK. Swollen ankles are risk signs if they are already swollen

High blood pressure

when the mother wakes up in the morning, if the swelling is severe or comes on suddenly, if there is *pitting edema* (see below), or if there are also other risk signs.

Here are some ways to check for swelling:

- Look at the mother and see if her face or fingers look puffy or swollen. Ask her if she has had to take off her rings or bracelets because they were too tight.

- Weigh the mother to check for sudden weight gain of more than 3.5 kilograms or 8 pounds in one month. This is a sign of general swelling.

- Make the pitting edema test:

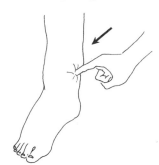

Press her ankle here with your finger, then take your finger away.

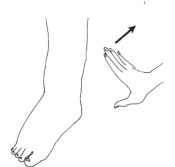

If the skin bounces back quickly, it is not serious swelling.

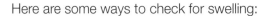

If your finger leaves a pit or dent that stays for a while, it is "pitting edema" or serious swelling.

3. Ask the mother if she has had headaches, dizziness, or trouble seeing. It is OK to have a headache or a little dizziness occasionally. But if these things happen often, or if they are severe, or if she has more than one of these problems, it is a risk sign. If she has any of these problems combined with swelling or high blood pressure, the risk is even greater.

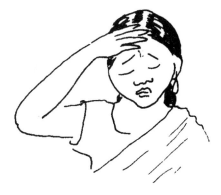

4. If possible, check for protein in the urine. There are 2 methods of checking for protein in the urine.

In the first method, use small plastic strips called **Uristicks**, **Albusticks** or **Labsticks** to check for protein. These sticks are sometimes available from a local health officer or a pharmacy. The strips have different color squares that will turn from yellow to dark green. Ask the mother to urinate on the stick, and then compare the color of the squares with the color chart on the bottle. If the square turns dark green, there is protein in the urine.

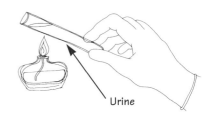

Dark green means protein

In the second method, heat the mother's urine to check for protein. Ask the mother to wash her genitals well and then urinate into a clean container. Then the midwife pours the urine into a test tube to within $2\frac{1}{2}$ centimeters or one inch of the top of the tube. Heat the upper part of the tube over a small burner, low flame, or candle until the urine boils. (Keep turning the test tube or the glass will break.) If the urine is clear, there is no protein in the urine. If the urine becomes cloudy and white, add a few drops of 2% acetic acid. If the cloudiness goes away there is no protein in the urine. If it stays cloudy or gets more white, there is protein in the urine. When a women has pre-eclampsia, the urine may become very cloudy, white, and thick.

Urine

Heating urine to test for protein

What to do if you find risk signs

If a mother has any risk signs get medical help (even if the birth is several months away). It may be safer for the mother to give birth in a hospital. If you must do the birth at home, be prepared for problems. Read the section on home care for high blood pressure (see p. 246), and the sections on bleeding (see p. 243–244), convulsions (p. 247), and small babies (p. 269, 292) in the chapters on labor and birth.

If the mother is told to rest at home:

- Encourage her to lie on her left side as much as possible.

- Encourage her to eat less salt. Salt holds water in the tissues or flesh. She should not add salt to her food, but she can eat a little salt that is already in food.

- Encourage her to eat a lot of protein-rich foods (see p. 49–50, 55–56).

- Encourage her to drink at least 2 liters (about 2 quarts) of water each day. If she works a lot or if it is very hot, she should drink even more. Water washes her system out and helps get rid of the swelling.

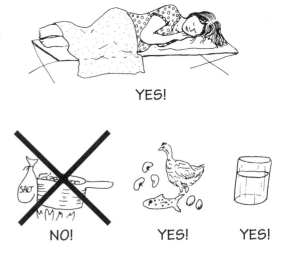

YES!

NO!   YES!   YES!

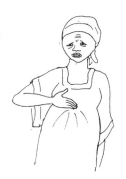

Watch for danger signs that the mother may have a convulsion:

- Severe, new headache with blurred vision.

- Sudden, steady, severe pain in the pit of the stomach, just below the high point between the ribs. It may feel like indigestion. Sometimes it feels like the pain goes through the stomach to the back. Often there are headaches, trouble seeing, or dizziness at the same time as the stomach pain—but not always.

If you think the pain may be caused by indigestion, you can give an antacid (see p. 461). If the pain does not get better in 20 minutes, it is a danger sign.

- Over-active reflexes. Do the **foot-reflex test** to check for over-active reflexes:

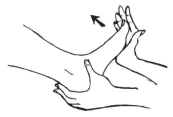

Hold the foot like this. Give a sharp push, then let go.

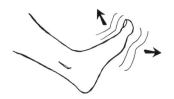

If the foot jerks 2 times or more, it is a danger sign.

If the mother has **any** of these danger signs and her blood pressure is over 140/90 (or the top number has gone up 30 points, or the bottom number has gone up 15 points), **she should be taken to the hospital immediately!** On the way, have her lie on her left side. Someone should go with her in case she has a convulsion (see p. 247).

8. Check for signs of urine, bladder, or kidney infection

Healthy signs:

- *no pain, itching, or burning when urinating*

- *urinates often*

Signs of infection:

- *constant feeling of needing to urinate, even after having just urinated*

- *itching or burning when urinating*

- *pain low down in front*

- *pain that goes from the lower belly around the side to the lower back*

- *pain in the lower back (especially on the sides)*

- *hot-to-touch, or temperature above 37.2°C or 99°F*

- *cloudy or bloody urine*

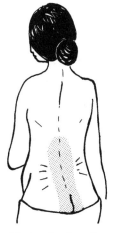

Back pain along the spine is quite common. It can often be helped by massage, exercise, and hot compresses.

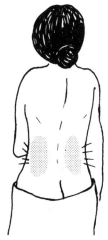

Pain along the sides of the back may be normal, or it may be a sign of kidney infection.

The kidneys, kidney tubes, bladder, and urine tube are all connected and work together to get rid of body wastes. First the kidneys clean the blood and put waste into the urine. Then the urine goes down the kidney tubes to the bladder. The urine sits in the bladder until you decide to urinate.

Infections of the urine, bladder, or kidneys begin when harmful germs enter a woman's body. In pregnancy, a woman is more likely to get these infections than at other times.

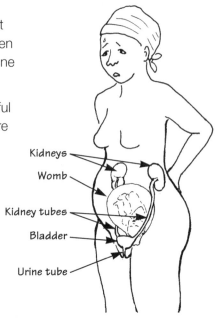

Kidneys

Womb

Kidney tubes

Bladder

Urine tube

These infections often start at the opening where the urine comes out of the body. This opening may itch or burn when the woman urinates. Then the infection travels up the tube to the bladder and causes pain in the lower belly. There may also be fever and back pain, the woman may feel she has to urinate all the time, or there may be blood in the urine. The infection in the bladder can then travel up the kidney tubes to the kidneys. The mother may feel pain going from the front through her sides to her lower back.

If you treat urine or bladder infections immediately, you may be able to prevent the germs from traveling to the kidneys. Bladder infections can also cause early labor if not treated right away.

Note: Itching or burning during urination may also mean that the woman has an infection of the vagina instead. This is usually not as dangerous as a bladder infection, but it should be treated. Sometimes it is a sign of a serious sexually transmitted disease (see chapter 23).

What to do if you find signs of urine, bladder, or kidney infection

- Give the mother **antibiotics** right away. Give ampicillin or amoxicillin 500 mg by mouth 4 times per day for 7 days. (If the mother is allergic to penicillin, give sulfa 500 mg by mouth 4 to 5 times a day for 7 days.) Do not wait until she is so sick that it is an emergency. The longer you wait, the harder the infection may be to cure. If she is not better in 2 days, get medical help.

- Encourage the mother to drink one glass of liquid every hour while she is awake. Liquids help wash infection out of her body. Fruit juices are especially good to drink. There may also be local plant medicines that fight infection or make people urinate a lot.

- If the infection is cured before labor begins, and if everything else is normal, the mother can stay home to have her baby. If the infection is not cured, it is safer for her to have her baby in the hospital.

- Make sure the mother knows how to wipe or wash her genitals from front to back to prevent bladder infections from happening again. The woman's husband should also keep his genitals and hands clean so that he does not get germs on her genitals. This might give her an infection.

Check the baby

1. Measure the mother's womb

Healthy signs:

- *The top of the womb matches the due date the first time you check.*

- *Womb grows about 2 finger widths a month.*

Risk signs:

- *The top of the womb does not match the due date the first time you check.*

- *Womb grows more or less than 2 finger widths a month.*

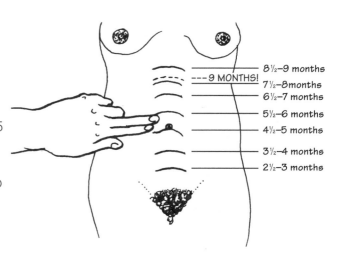

8½–9 months

9 MONTHS!

7½–8months

6½–7 months

5½–6 months

4½–5 months

3½–4 months

2½–3 months

As the baby grows, the top of the womb moves up in the mother's belly. The top of the womb usually grows about 2 finger widths higher each month. At 3 months, the top of the womb is usually just above the mother's pubic bone (where her pubic hair begins). When the baby is about 5 months old, the top of the womb is usually right at the mother's **navel**. At 8½ to 9 months, the top of the womb is almost up to the mother's ribs. First babies may drop 2 to 3 finger widths lower in the weeks right before birth (see p. 137).

When you measure the womb, you check to see where the top of the womb is. This will tell you 3 things:

1. About how many months the woman is pregnant now.

2. The probable due date. If you were able to figure out the due date from the mother's last monthly bleeding (see p. 78), measuring the womb can help you see if this due date is probably correct. If you were unable to figure out her due date from her monthly bleeding, measuring the womb can help you figure out a probable due date. This should be done during the first checkup.

3. How fast the baby is growing. At each checkup, measure the womb to see if the baby is growing at a normal rate. If it is growing too fast or too slow, there may be a problem.

How to measure the womb

Using the finger method

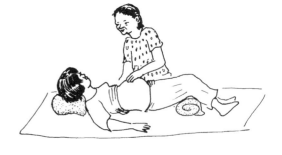

1. Have the mother lie on her back, with some support under her head and knees. Your touch should be firm, but gentle.

2. Find the top of the womb.

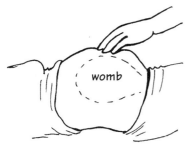

Walk your fingers up the belly.

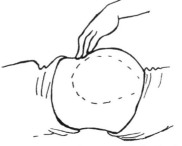

Find the top of the womb (it feels like a hard ball under the skin).

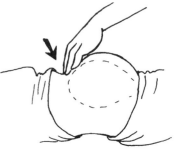

You can feel the top curving into the belly.

3. If the top of the womb is below the navel, measure how many fingers below the navel it is. If the top of the womb is above the navel, measure how many fingers above the navel it is. Then see how many months pregnant the woman is now by comparing the number of fingers with this picture (each line is about the width of two fingers):

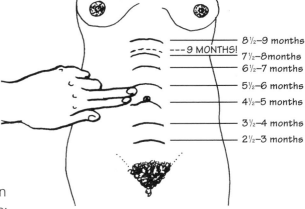

8½–9 months
---9 MONTHS!
7½–8months
6½–7 months
5½–6 months
4½–5 months
3½–4 months
2½–3 months

4. Keep a record of what you find. You can keep a record using one of these methods:

- Draw a picture. Make a circle for the mother's belly, a dot for her navel, and a curved line for the top of the womb. Then draw the number of fingers above or below the navel that you used to find the top of the womb. For example:

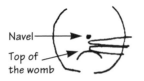

Navel

Top of the womb

This drawing means that the top of the womb is 2 fingers BELOW the navel.

- Use numbers. Write down the number of fingers you used to measure the womb. Put a "+" sign" in front of the number if the top of the womb is above the navel. Put a "–" sign in front of the number if the top of the womb is below the navel. For example: "+3" means that the top of the womb is 3 fingers above the navel.

5. Figure out the due date. For example, if measuring the top of the womb tells you that the woman is 7 months pregnant, you know that the baby will be born in about 2 months. If you have already figured out her due date using her last monthly bleeding, check to see if the 2 dates are about the same. If the 2 dates are not about the same, see p. 120–122.

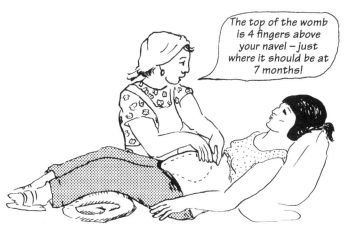

The top of the womb is 4 fingers above your navel – just where it should be at 7 months!

Using a cloth tape measure

1. Follow step #1 above.

2. Find the top of the womb as described in step #2 above. Then lay the measuring tape on the mother's belly, holding the 0 on the tape at her pubic bone. Then follow the curve of her womb up and hold the tape at the top of her womb.

3. Write down the number of centimeters from the top of the pubic bone to the top of the womb. The womb should grow about 1 centimeter per week, or 4 centimeters per month. After 5 to 6 months, the number of centimeters is close to the number of weeks of pregnancy.

4. Follow step #5 above.

Note: Medical people often count pregnancy by weeks instead of months. They start counting at the first day of the last monthly bleeding, even though the woman probably got pregnant 2 weeks later. This makes pregnancy 40 weeks long. During the second half of pregnancy, the womb measures close to the number of weeks that the woman has been pregnant. For example, if it has been 24 weeks since her last monthly bleeding, the womb will usually measure 22 to 26 centimeters.

What to do if you find risk signs

If you are measuring correctly and you do not find the top of the womb where you expect it, it could mean 3 different things:

1. The due date you got by counting from the last monthly bleeding is wrong.

2. The womb is growing too fast.

3. The womb is growing too slowly.

The due date you got by counting from the last monthly period is wrong

There can be several reasons why a due date figured from the last monthly bleeding is wrong. Sometimes women do not remember the date of their last monthly bleeding correctly. Sometimes a woman misses her bleeding without being pregnant, and then gets pregnant later. This woman will really be less pregnant than you figured, so the womb is smaller than you expect. Or, in some cases, a woman has some monthly bleeding after she gets pregnant. This woman is really 1 or 2 months more pregnant than you figured, so the womb is bigger than you expect.

If the due date does not match the size of the womb at the first visit, make a note. Wait and measure the womb again in 2 to 4 weeks. If the womb grows about 2 finger widths a month, the due date that you got from feeling the top of the womb is probably correct. The due date you got by figuring from the last monthly bleeding was probably wrong.

Remember: Due dates are not exact. They can be off by 2 or even 3 weeks.

The womb grows too fast

If the womb grows more than 2 finger widths a month, several different things may be causing the problem:

1. The mother may have twins. See p. 131 to learn how to tell if there are twins.

2. The mother may have too much water in the womb. Any pregnant woman can have too much water. Often too much water is not a problem, but it can cause the womb to stretch too much. Then the womb cannot contract enough to push the baby out or to stop the bleeding after the birth. Or, in rare cases it can mean that the baby will have birth defects.

To see if the mother has too much water, try the *thump test.* Have a helper put one hand on the middle of the mother's womb. Put one of your hands on one side of the mother's belly. Thump the other side of her belly with your other hand. If there is too much water inside, you may feel a wave or ripple cross the belly from one side to the other. (The helper's hand keeps the wave from travelling through the mother's flesh.)

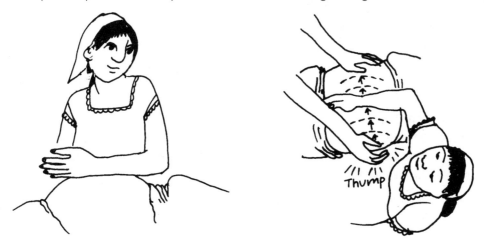

If there is too much water, get medical advice. It may be safer for the mother to deliver in a hospital.

3. The mother may have a tumor in her womb instead of a baby. Sometimes a woman gets pregnant, but a tumor grows instead of a baby. **There is no baby inside.** This is called a molar pregnancy.

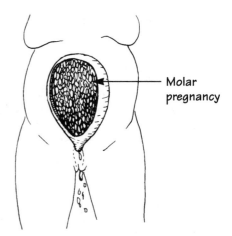

Molar pregnancy

Other signs of a molar pregnancy are: the womb grows faster than expected, the baby's heartbeat cannot be heard, the baby's body cannot be clearly felt, the mother has bad nausea all through pregnancy, and the mother has spotting of blood and tissue (sometimes shaped like grapes).

If you see signs of a molar pregnancy, get medical help as soon as possible. The tumor can become cancer and kill the woman—sometimes very fast. A doctor can remove the tumor to save the woman. If she can see a doctor regularly after the operation, it is usually not necessary to take out the womb. The doctor can just take out the tumor, and then watch to make sure that there is no cancer. However, if the tumor has already turned to cancer, it may be necessary to take out the womb to save her life. Sometimes she will need to take medicine to kill the cancer, too.

The womb grows too slowly

If the mother is very short but wide from front to back, the womb may seem to grow more slowly, even if she and the baby are healthy. (If the woman is short, it is also possible for the womb to seem to grow more quickly.) Or, if the mother is very tall, the womb also can seem to grow slowly. If this is the case, things are probably OK.

But slow growth can also be a sign of one of these problems:

- The mother has high blood pressure (see p. 107). High blood pressure can make the baby starve inside the mother. If you do not have equipment to check her blood pressure, get medical help.

- The mother has a poor diet. Find out what kind of food the mother has been eating. Check p. 50 to see if this is a good diet. If she is too poor to get enough good food, try to find some way to help her and her baby. Healthy mothers and children make the whole community stronger.

- The mother is drinking, smoking, or using drugs. These can cause a baby to be very small and sick. See p. 60.

- The mother has too little water in the womb. Sometimes there is less water than usual, and everything is still OK. At other times, too little water can mean the baby is not normal or will have problems during the labor. It is best for the mother to give birth in the hospital.

- The baby is dead. Dead babies do not grow, so the womb stops getting bigger. If the mother is 5 months pregnant or more, ask if she has felt the baby move recently. Healthy babies 5 months old or more may stop kicking for many hours (or even a whole day), but if the baby has not moved for 2 days, something may be wrong.

If the mother is more than 7 months pregnant, or if you heard the baby's heartbeat at an earlier visit, listen for the heartbeat. If you cannot find it, get medical help. Some health centers may have special equipment to see if the baby is still alive.

If the baby has died, it is important for the mother to give birth soon. If labor does not start in 2 weeks, go to the hospital where she can get medicine to start her labor.

Note: When a mother loses a baby, she needs special love, care, and understanding. If possible, make sure that she does not go through labor alone. Someone should go to the hospital with her and stay with her during childbirth, if this is OK in her culture.

2. Find the position of the baby

Healthy signs

- *There is one baby in the womb.*
- *The baby is head down at the time of birth.*
- *The baby's heartbeat is loudest below the mother's navel.*

Risk signs

- *The baby is breech (buttocks first) at the time of birth.*
- *The baby is sideways at the time of birth.*
- *The mother has twins.*

In the first 7 to 8 months of pregnancy, it is normal for the baby to be in many different positions. Here are some of the positions the baby may be lying in:

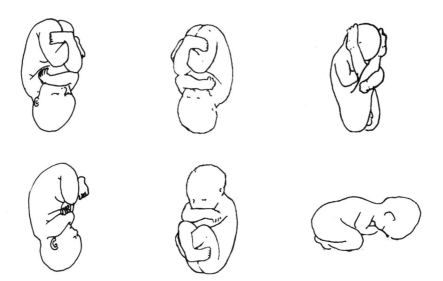

By the last month before birth, most babies are lying with their heads toward the birth opening. This is called a **head down position**. If a baby is head up, with its buttocks toward the birth opening, this is called a **breech position**. If the baby is lying horizontally (side to side), this is called a **sideways position**. The head down position is easiest for childbirth.

It may be difficult to find the position of the baby before the 6th or 7th month. Try anyway, just to get a feeling for the baby and the pregnancy. It will be easier to find the position during the last 2 months of pregnancy.

There are 2 parts to finding the baby's position: *feeling the mother's belly,* and *listening to where the baby's heartbeat is strongest.*

Feeling the mother's belly

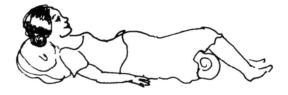

To begin, help the mother lie on her back and give her support under her knees and head. Make sure she is comfortable.

Then feel the mother's belly.
You will be checking for 3 things:

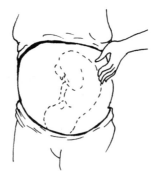

Is the baby vertical? Is the baby lying more on the mother's left or right side?

Most babies are vertical (up and down) by the 7th month. Most babies also lie more on one side of the mother than the other.

To find out if the baby is vertical and which side of the mother the baby is lying on, lay one hand flat on each side of the belly. Press in gently, but firmly, first with one hand, and then with the other.

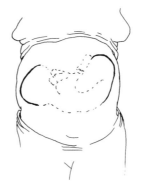

If the baby does not feel vertical, check the shape carefully. Do the ends of the baby seem to be in the mother's sides? If so, the baby is probably lying sideways. Many babies lie sideways in the first months, but most turn head down by 8 months or so. If the baby is sideways after 8 months it must be born in a hospital (see p. 131).

Is the baby lying facing the mother's front or her back?

Next, feel the mother's belly for a large, hard shape (the baby's back). If you cannot feel the baby's back, feel for a lot of small lumps:

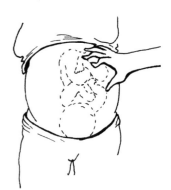

A large, hard shape probably means the baby is facing the mother's back.

If you feel a lot of small lumps, instead of a hard back, the baby may be facing the mother's front.

Is the baby head up or head down?

By the 7th or 8th month, the baby's head has usually moved down in the mother's pubic bones. Here are 4 ways to feel for the baby's head:

1. Find the mother's pubic bone with your fingers. You can feel it just under the skin under the mother's pubic hair.

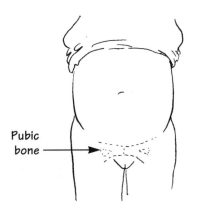

Pubic bone

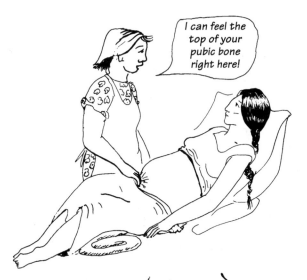

I can feel the top of your pubic bone right here!

Ask the mother to take a deep breath in and then let it out. As she breathes out, press deeply into the flesh just above the pubic bone. Be careful not to hurt her. If you feel a round, hard object that you can move a little from side to side, it is probably the back or side of the baby's head.

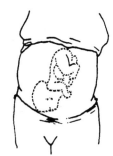

If the shape is not clearly round, it may be the baby's buttocks, or the baby's face. If you do not feel anything in the mother's lower belly, the baby may be lying sideways. Or sometimes the baby's buttocks are up, but the head is not straight down. The head may be bent to the side, or the chin may be up. (These could be signs that the baby is too big to fit through the mother's pelvic bones.)

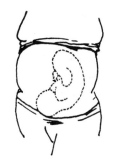
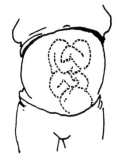

2. Now feel the top of the mother's womb. Does it feel round and hard, like a head? Or is it a different shape— like buttocks, a back, or legs? If the top of the womb feels more like a head than what you felt in the mother's belly, the baby may be breech.

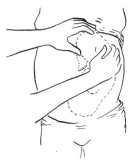

3. Put one hand on the baby's back. At the same time, with your other hand, push the top end of the baby gently sideways. If the whole back moves when you move the top end, the buttocks are probably up.

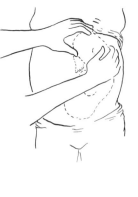

If the back stays where it is while you move the upper part of the baby, you may be moving the head. This is because the neck can bend, while the back stays in place.

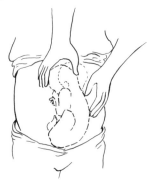

4. If the lower part of the baby is not too deep in the mother's pelvic bones, try moving the baby from side to side. If moving the lower part of the baby makes its whole back move, then the baby may be breech. If the back does not move, then the baby may be head down. If the baby is breech at the time of birth, see p. 262.

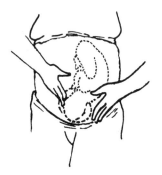

Note: As you feel the mother's belly, try to imagine the different positions the baby might be in. Imagine where the baby's hands and legs might be. Imagine how each position would feel to the mother.

Then ask the mother where she feels the strongest kicks and where she feels smaller movements. Is this where you think the legs and hands probably are? If not, you may not have figured out the baby's position correctly.

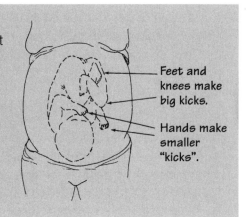

Feet and knees make big kicks.

Hands make smaller "kicks".

During any of these checks of the baby's position, you might feel 3 or more big lumps, or what you think are 2 heads. This might mean the mother has twins. See p. 131.

Listen to where the baby's heartbeat is strongest

The baby's heartbeat also gives you information about the baby's position inside the mother. Listen to the heartbeat at each visit starting at 5 months.

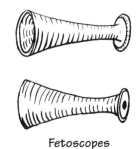

By the last 2 months, you can often hear the baby's heartbeat in a quiet room by putting your ear on the mother's belly. The heartbeat will be easier to hear if you have a **fetoscope** or a stethoscope (like you use for taking blood pressure). You can make a simple fetoscope from wood, clay, or a hollow tube of bamboo. You can also make a stethoscope from homemade materials (see p. 429). Or you can buy a 1-ear or 2-ear fetoscope.

Fetoscopes

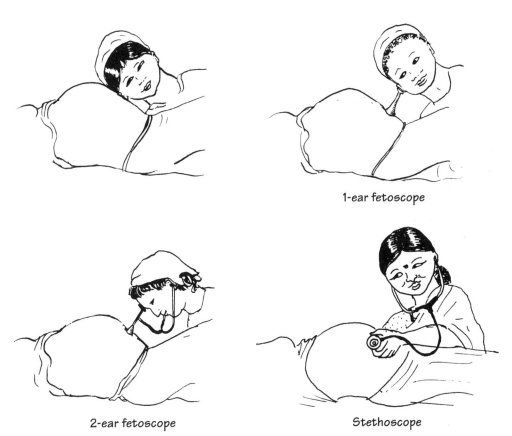

1-ear fetoscope

2-ear fetoscope

Stethoscope

The baby's heartbeat is quiet and quick. It may sound like a watch ticking under a pillow, only faster. The baby's heartbeat is about twice as fast as a healthy adult heartbeat.

Note: If the baby's heartbeat makes a "swishy" sound (shee-oo shee-oo shee-oo), you are probably hearing the baby's pulse in the cord. Cord sounds tell you how fast the baby's heart is beating, but they do not help you find the baby's position.

If the heartbeat sounds slow, you may be hearing the mother's pulse in her belly instead of the baby.

Finding the baby's heartbeat

Think about what you have learned about the baby's position from feeling the mother's belly. Then start listening for the heartbeat near the spot where you think the baby's heart should be. You may need to listen in many places before you find the spot where the heartbeat is the most loud and clear.

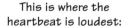
This is where the heartbeat is loudest:

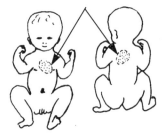

Baby facing front   Baby facing back

Listen to the heartbeat both above and below the mother's navel. If you hear the heartbeat loudest below the mother's navel, the baby is probably head down. If you hear the heartbeat loudest above the mother's navel, the baby may be breech.

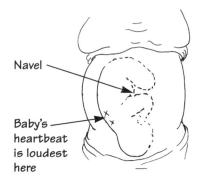
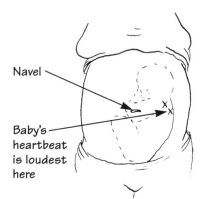

Navel

Baby's heartbeat is loudest here

Navel

Baby's heartbeat is loudest here

Sometimes when the baby is facing the mother's front, the heartbeat is harder to find because the baby's arms and legs get in the way. You may need to listen more towards the mother's sides, or directly in the middle to hear the heart.

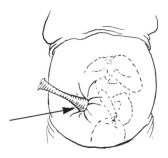

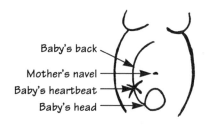

Baby's back

Mother's navel

Baby's heartbeat

Baby's head

If you want to keep a record, you can make a simple drawing. In this picture, the dot in the middle is the mother's navel, the large curved line is the baby's back, the circle is the baby's head, and the "X" shows where the heartbeat was found.

In this example, the baby did not turn head down until 7 months. Even then the baby moved from side to side, so the "X" moves from the left side to the right side of the mother's belly—and then back again. This kind of movement is normal.

5 months	Sept 13	(x)
6 months	Oct 12	(x)
7 months	Nov. 15	(xo) head down
8 months	Dec 10	(x) head down
8 ½ months	Jan. 12	(x) head down
9 months	Jan 28	(xo) head down

Checking how fast the baby's heart beats

When you check the heartbeat to find the baby's position, it is also a good idea to check how fast the baby's heart beats. This can help you know if things are going well for the baby. Things are probably going well if the baby's heartbeat is between 120 and 160 beats per minute. If the baby's heart beat is less than 120 or more than 160 beats per minute, there may be something wrong. If the heartbeat is above 160, wait a few minutes and check it again. Sometimes the heartbeat gets fast when the baby moves. If the heartbeat stays above 160 (especially if it is 170 or more) the mother may have an infection. See if she is hot-to-touch or has a fever. If she is, see p. 105–106.

Follow these steps to check how fast the baby's heart beats:

1. Use a clock or a watch with a second hand, just as you did for taking the mother's pulse (see p. 106). If you do not have a clock or watch, compare the baby's heartbeat to your own pulse when you are resting and calm. (Or make a **timer** out of homemade materials; see p. 427.) The baby's heartbeat should be about 2 times as fast as your pulse.

2. Count the number of heartbeats in one minute. Or you can count for 15 seconds and multiply the number of beats by 4. For example, if the heartbeat is 40 in 15 seconds, then it is 160 beats per minute. If you have trouble watching the clock and counting at the same time, have someone tell you when to start and when to stop counting.

If the baby's heartbeat seems very slow, feel the mother's pulse in her wrist while you listen. If the mother's pulse and the heartbeat you hear are the same, you may be hearing the mother's heartbeat by mistake.

3. Keep a record of where you found the heartbeat and how fast it beats.

Note: A LOUD heartbeat does not mean that the baby is strong. It just means that the baby's back or chest is closer to your ear, or that the mother's belly is easy to hear through. A LIGHT heartbeat does not mean that the baby is weak. It just means that the baby's chest or back is further from your ear, or that the mother's belly is hard to hear through. For example, the wall of the belly might be thick if the mother is fat.

What to do if you find risk signs

Baby is breech

Breech babies are often born without any trouble, especially if the mother has had other children and her births were easy. But there is a real risk for the baby (see p. 262–263).

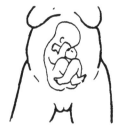

It may be possible to get the baby to turn head down by having the mother try the lifted-hips exercise:

1. The mother lies on her back. Put something soft (like a pillow) under her hips for 15 minutes, 3 times per day. It is best do this when the baby is moving a lot.

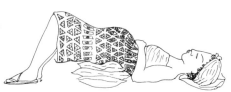

2. After lying this way for 15 minutes, the mother should walk around for about 5 minutes. If she thinks the baby has turned to head down, she should come in to be checked so she can stop the exercise.

> **Caution!** Some midwives have been taught to **massage the womb** to try and turn the baby. This is extremely dangerous! You should try to turn the baby only if you have been taught how to do it properly and can get medical help. Also, do not try and turn the baby if the mother's waters have broken, or if she has ever had vaginal bleeding, high blood pressure, surgery on her womb, or a cesarean section. See p. 407–408 for how to turn the baby.

If the baby does not turn head down by the time of birth, it is safer for the mother to give birth in a maternity center or hospital. Doctors can use pulling instruments *(forceps)* if the baby gets stuck. Or they can do a cesarean section.

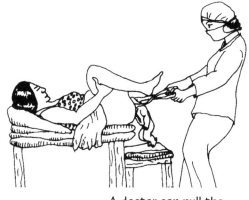

A doctor can pull the baby out with forceps.

If a breech baby is going to be born at home, it is very important for a highly skilled person to be there (see p. 263–265 for how to deliver a breech baby). Also, remember that any of these things will make the birth more dangerous:

- The mother has had long or difficult births in the past.

- This is the mother's first baby (so her flesh will stretch less).

- The baby is big.

- The mother is weak or has been ill, so she cannot push well.

- The midwife is not very skilled or experienced with **breech births**.

Baby is sideways

If the baby is sideways—not head down or head up—by 8 months, you can try the lifted-hips exercise for turning the baby (see p. 130). If the baby does not turn, we suggest you make arrangements for a hospital birth by cesarean section. Sideways babies cannot fit through the mother's bones to be born. If you try to deliver the baby without an operation, the mother's womb will break during labor, and she and the baby could die.

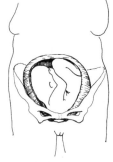

This baby must be born by operation.

If the baby turns head down at any time—even the day the mother goes into labor—it is OK for the mother to give birth at home. But remember that turning a sideways baby by hand (see p. 409) is just as dangerous as trying to turn a breech baby!

Twins

Sometimes it is easy to tell that there are twins, but sometimes it is very difficult, even if you are very skilled. If you think the mother may have twins:

- Watch the growth of the womb. Often the first sign of twins is that the womb grows faster or larger than you expect.

- Feel the mother's belly for 3 or 4 large lumps or 2 heads. Here are some of the positions that twins are likely to lie in:

- Listen for 2 heartbeats. This is not easy, but it is sometimes possible, especially in the last 2 months. You will need 2 good fetoscopes or stethoscopes, a helper, and a quiet room. Here are 2 methods you can try:

1. Find the heartbeat of what you think may be one baby. Then listen for other places where the heartbeat is easy to hear. If you find such a place, have a helper listen to one place while you listen to the other. Each of you can tap the rhythm of the heartbeat with your hand. If the rhythms are the same, you may be listening to the same baby. If the rhythms are not exactly the same, you may be hearing 2 different babies.

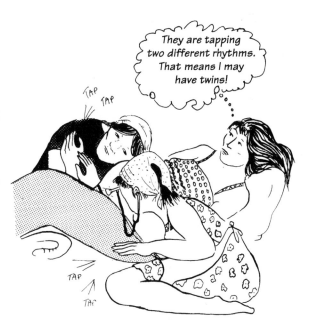

They are tapping two different rhythms. That means I may have twins!

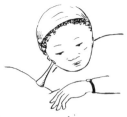

2. If you do not have a helper, but you have a watch with a second hand or a homemade timer (see p. 427), try timing each heartbeat separately. If the heartbeats are not the same, you may be hearing 2 different babies. This method is helpful, but not as reliable as the first method.

If you think there might be twins, get medical help (even if you can find only one heartbeat). A maternity center or hospital can make special tests (like an **ultrasound** or **x-ray**) to see if there are twins.

Since twin births are often more difficult or dangerous than single births (see p. 266–268), we suggest that twin babies be born in a hospital or maternity center whenever possible. Since twins are more likely to be born early, the mother should try to have transportation ready at all times after the 6th month. If the hospital or maternity clinic is far away, the mother may wish to move closer in the last months of pregnancy.

If the babies are to be born at home, it is best to have at least 2 very skilled people at the birth.

Note: There is no truth to the idea that twins have special powers or that one is good and the other bad. They will be children like any others.

After the checkup

Set a time for the next prenatal checkup

After you have finished checking the baby and the mother, find out if she has any more questions, or needs to talk about anything else. If she has any risk signs, carefully explain what the risk sign is, what else to look for, and what she must do to care for herself. If she needs to get medical help be sure she knows who to see, and where and when to go. Before she leaves, set a time for her next prenatal checkup (see schedule on p. 39). Make sure the mother knows when and where the next checkup will be.

Record of prenatal care

Name: _____ Age: ____ Number of children: ____ Ages: ____ Date of last childbirth: _____

Date of last monthly bleeding: _____ Probable due date: _____ Problems with other births: _____

Date of visit	Month of pregnancy	General health and minor problems	Anemia	Risk signs	Swelling Edema (where? how much?)	Pulse	Temp.	Weight (estimate or measure)	Blood Pressure	Protein in urine	Heart beat	Position of baby in womb	Size of womb (how many fingers above (+) or below (-) the navel?

SECTION C

Normal labor, birth and after birth

Introduction

In order for a baby to be born, a woman's body must work hard to move the baby from inside her womb to the world outside. We call this work *labor*.

We divide labor into 5 parts, according to what is happening in the body:

■ Stage 1 begins when labor pains (*contractions*) start to open the cervix; it ends when the cervix is completely open. Stage 1 is usually the longest stage, but the amount of time is different for every birth. Stage 1 could be less than an hour or it could be a day and a night. First babies usually take the longest, but not always.

■ Stage 2 begins when the cervix is completely open and ends when the baby is born. Stage 2 can be as short as a few minutes or as long as 2 hours.

■ Stage 3 begins when the baby is born and ends when the *placenta (afterbirth)* comes out. Stage 3 usually lasts less than one hour.

■ The first 2 to 6 hours after birth. This part begins after the placenta has come out and lasts for 2 to 6 hours. During this time the womb tightens up to slow down bleeding.

■ The first 2 weeks after birth. During this time the mother's womb continues to tighten up and get smaller.

The following chapters will explain what happens inside the mother's body during labor, and how you can help her have a healthy birth:

- What the body is doing during labor (chapter 8)

- Giving good care during labor (chapter 9)

- What to do during stage 1 (chapter 10)

- What to do during stage 2 (chapter 11)

- What to do during stage 3 (chapter 12)

- What to do during the first 2 to 6 hours after birth (chapter 13)

- What to do during the first 2 weeks after birth (chapter 14)

What the body is doing during labor

Chapter 8 contents

What the body is doing during labor

Signs that labor is near

1. The baby drops lower in the belly

First babies often drop lower in the mother's belly about two weeks before birth. When this happens the mother may find it easier to breathe. If a mother has had babies before, this baby may not drop until labor begins.

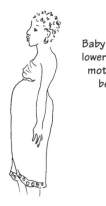 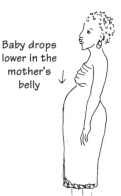

Baby drops lower in the mother's belly ↓

2. Practice contractions get stronger or come more often

During pregnancy and labor the womb will sometimes squeeze up and become hard. This is called a **contraction** because the womb **contracts**, or gets smaller.

There are two kinds of contractions. **Practice contractions** occur throughout pregnancy. They are usually felt high in the belly (or all over the belly) and are mild and irregular. Many women don't even notice when they happen. **Labor contractions** begin closer to the time the baby is born (see p. 139). They are usually felt lower in the belly or back and will get much stronger than practice contractions.

Note: We use the word *contraction* instead of **pains**. In many parts of the world, people use the word *pains* to describe labor contractions. This is because contractions are often very painful. But the contractions of labor and birth do not always hurt. A few women have labors that are strong but painless.

Words are powerful. If we use the word *pains,* the mother expects pain. This can make her more tense and afraid, and labor will hurt even more. If a different word is used, these women may suffer less!

To understand how contractions work, think about what happens when you start to flex your upper arm.

 Before you flex, your arm is relaxed and the muscle is long and soft.

 When you flex, the muscle tightens, and becomes thick and hard.

The womb contracts in the same way. You can see it bunch up, like this:

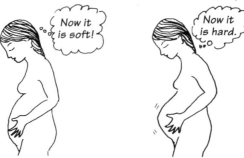

Practice contractions may get stronger and start to come more often a few days before labor contractions begin. Practice contractions may start and stop several times. They will often go away if the mother changes what she is doing. For example, if she stops walking and rests, the practice contractions may stop, too.

3. Show appears

During most of pregnancy, the tiny hole in the cervix is plugged with mucus.

In the last few days of pregnancy, the cervix may begin to open. Sometimes the mucus and a little bit of blood drip out. This is called **show**.

Show may come out all at once, like a plug, or it may leak slowly for several days. It tells you that the cervix is softening, thinning, and beginning to open. Labor will probably start in a day or two.

Be careful not to confuse show with the discharge (wetness from the vagina) that many women have in the 2 weeks before labor begins. This discharge is mostly clear mucus and is not tinged with blood.

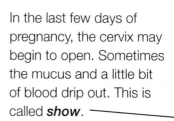

4. The bag of waters breaks

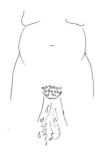

The bag of waters that surrounds the baby usually breaks after labor begins. If the bag breaks before labor begins, it usually means labor will start within a few hours. If labor does not start within 6 hours after the bag breaks, there is a risk of infection. You may wish to do something to get labor started (see p. 377).

5. Stools change

Many mothers get loose stools (diarrhea) before they go into labor. This helps clean out the body so the woman will be more comfortable during labor and birth.

But sometimes mothers get hard stools (constipation) instead. If this happens, the mother may want to have an enema (which cleans the stools out of her body) when labor starts (see p. 174).

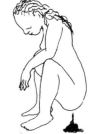

Loose stools are common before labor.

6. The mother feels different

Sometimes a woman can feel that labor is near. She may feel dreamy, very quiet, and aware of her body. Or she may simply feel a strong urge to stay home and wait. All these feelings are normal.

Sometimes women feel a strong desire to clean and rearrange their homes, even late at night. This desire is not dangerous—as long as a woman doesn't work too hard. Since her labor may start at any time, she needs to save her strength. Her family can help her do chores and get rest.

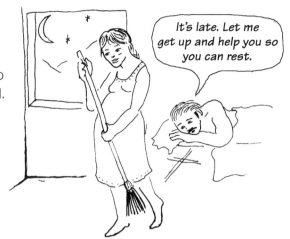

It's late. Let me get up and help you so you can rest.

What the body is doing during labor and birth

1. Stage 1—the cervix opens

During pregnancy the cervix is long, like a big toe. It is also hard, like a flexed muscle. Usually nothing can get in or out of the cervix, because the tiny hole in it is plugged with mucus.

Since the cervix separates the baby from the vagina, it must open for the baby to be born. Towards the end of pregnancy, practice contractions begin to shorten and soften the cervix (so it can open more easily). The cervix may even open a little and the **mucous plug** may fall out.

— Womb

— Cervix

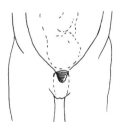

The cervix is long and hard.

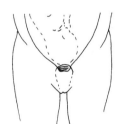

Here it begins to shorten and soften.

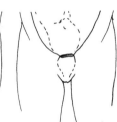

Here it is shorter and softer, so the baby can come out.

When labor contractions start, they do 2 things:

1. Labor contractions push the baby's head down hard against the cervix. This helps open the cervix.

2. Labor contractions slowly pull the cervix open. Each time the womb contracts, it pulls a little bit of the cervix up, out of the vagina and into itself. In between contractions, the cervix relaxes and most of it (but not all of it) comes back into the vagina. This process continues (usually very slowly) until the cervix is completely open.

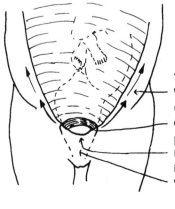

The WOMB pulls up on the CERVIX and pushes baby's HEAD into the VAGINA.

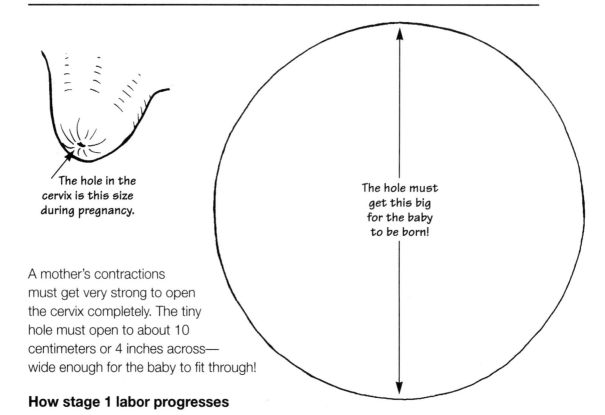

The hole in the cervix is this size during pregnancy.

The hole must get this big for the baby to be born!

A mother's contractions must get very strong to open the cervix completely. The tiny hole must open to about 10 centimeters or 4 inches across—wide enough for the baby to fit through!

How stage 1 labor progresses

Stage 1 labor is divided into 3 parts: light, active, and late labor.

In **light labor**, the contractions are usually short (about 30 seconds long) and come every 15 or 20 minutes. The contractions are often very mild. They are usually felt low in the belly, either in front or in the lower back. The contractions may hurt a little, like the cramps of monthly bleeding or of mild diarrhea. Or the contractions may not be painful at all: they may feel more like pressure or tightening. The mother can usually walk, talk, and even work during these contractions.

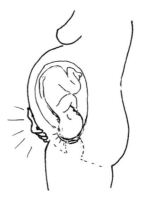

If the baby is facing the mother's side or back, the pain is usually felt in the front.

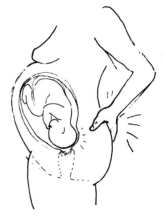

If the baby is facing the mother's front, she will feel pain in her lower back.

As labor continues, contractions get longer, stronger, and closer together. This is called **active labor**. For most women, the labor will usually become very painful. The mother will usually need to stop everything and pay full attention during a contraction. She may feel tired and need to be very still between contractions, or she may want to move about.

In **late labor**, the contractions may last up to $1\frac{1}{2}$ minutes, with only 2 or 3 minutes between them. Sometimes the mother feels that the contractions never stop. But if you put your hand on her belly, you can feel the womb get soft and then hard again.

Labor patterns

Labor can follow many different patterns and still be normal:

- Some labors start with weak contractions and get strong slowly and steadily over several hours.
- Some labors start slowly and suddenly speed up.
- Some labors start strong, then get weaker, and then become strong again.
- Some labors are very light for 2 to 3 days, then suddenly get strong and the baby comes soon after.
- Some labors follow other patterns.

All these labors are normal as long as they get strong enough to open the cervix completely.

2. Stage 2—the baby is pushed out

Once the cervix is open, contractions can push the baby out of the womb and down the vagina. The mother can also begin to help push the baby out.

Each new contraction (and push from the mother) moves the baby's head a little further down in the vagina. Between contractions the mother's womb relaxes and pulls the baby's head back up a little (but not as far as it was before the contraction).

What stage 2 looks like

At first, when the baby is still high in the vagina, all you can see is the mother's *genitals bulging* during a contraction. Her anus (butt hole) may also open a little. Between contractions, you can see her genitals relax.

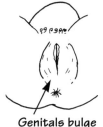

Genitals bulge during a contraction.

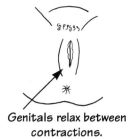

Genitals relax between contractions.

After a while, you will start to see a little of the baby's head when it is pushed down during a contraction. The head will go back inside the mother between contractions. Each push will show a bit more of the head.

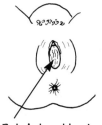

Baby's head begins to show.

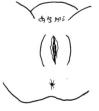

Baby's head goes back inside.

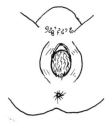

Baby's head shows more with each push.

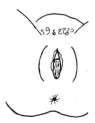

Baby's head between contractions.

When the baby's head stretches the vaginal opening to about the size of the palm of your hand, the head will stay at the opening, even between contractions. This is called *crowning*. The mother should now stop pushing (or push very gently), so that the head can come out slowly. This will help prevent tears in the mother's genitals.

Once the head is born, the rest of the body usually slips out easily with 1 or 2 pushes. In rare cases, there may be a problem with the shoulders (see p. 259).

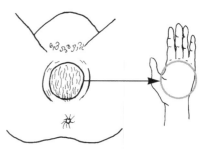

When the head crowns, the vaginal opening is the size of the palm of your hand.

How the baby moves through the vagina

Babies change position as they move through the vagina. Most babies move like this:

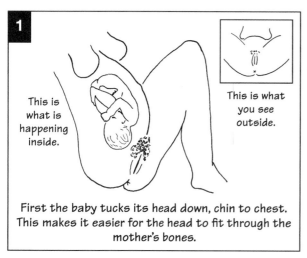

1

This is what is happening inside.

This is what you see outside.

First the baby tucks its head down, chin to chest. This makes it easier for the head to fit through the mother's bones.

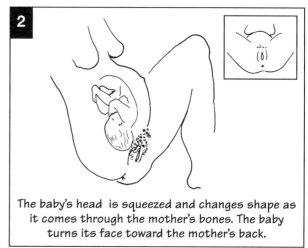

2

The baby's head is squeezed and changes shape as it comes through the mother's bones. The baby turns its face toward the mother's back.

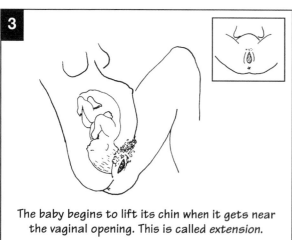

3

The baby begins to lift its chin when it gets near the vaginal opening. This is called *extension*.

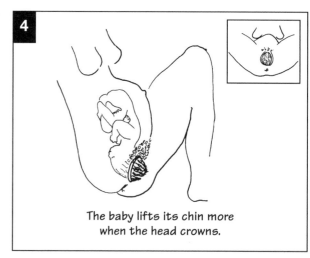

4

The baby lifts its chin more when the head crowns.

5

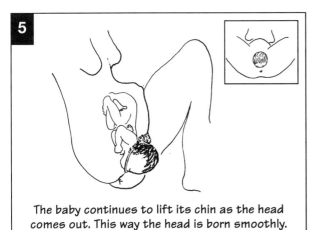

The baby continues to lift its chin as the head comes out. This way the head is born smoothly.

6

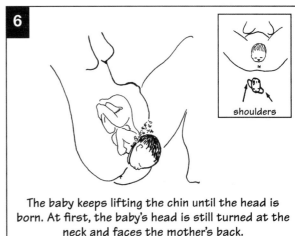

shoulders

The baby keeps lifting the chin until the head is born. At first, the baby's head is still turned at the neck and faces the mother's back.

7

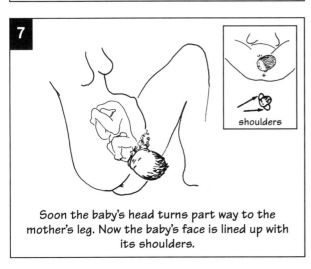

shoulders

Soon the baby's head turns part way to the mother's leg. Now the baby's face is lined up with its shoulders.

8

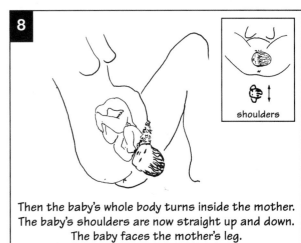

shoulders

Then the baby's whole body turns inside the mother. The baby's shoulders are now straight up and down. The baby faces the mother's leg.

9

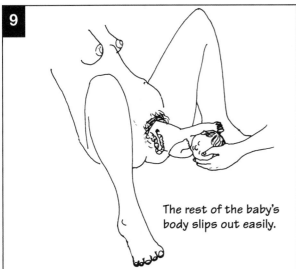

The rest of the baby's body slips out easily.

Note: Most babies move this way, but many do not. For babies facing the mother's front, see p. 240. For forehead-first births, see p. 240. For a breech baby, see p. 262.

3. Stage 3—the placenta is pushed out

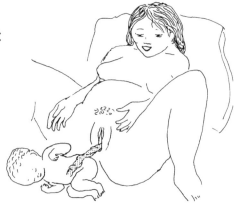

When the baby is first born, its cord is still connected to the placenta inside the mother. The cord will look thick, blue, and pulsing, because the baby is still getting blood from the placenta. This often gives the baby a few extra minutes to learn to breathe.

But the baby can soon breathe on its own and no longer needs the placenta. Now the placenta must do 2 things: **separate** from the wall of the mother's womb and **come out** through the vaginal opening:

1. The placenta usually separates in the first few minutes after birth. There will often be a small gush of blood from the vagina. The cord will become thin, white, and stop pulsing (which means the baby is no longer getting oxygen from its mother). The cord may also get a little longer. Once the cord has become thin and white it can be cut.

2. The placenta may come out right away or it may take a while. The mother's contractions (which continue for a while after birth) may help push the placenta out. Or the mother may need to *squat* and give a little push. Often some blood and *blood clots* will come out, too. The mother usually doesn't feel much pain when the placenta comes out.

Cord is thick, blue, pulsing. The placenta is still attached to the mother's womb.

Cord is thin, white, not pulsing. The placenta has separated.

Placenta comes out.

4. The first 2 to 6 hours after birth—the womb tightens

The place where the placenta was attached to the womb wall is called the *placental site*. After the placenta comes out, the placental site is like an open wound inside the mother's body. This placental site must now be closed off, or the mother will bleed too much.

The contractions which come after birth (sometimes called *after pains*) help close off the wound by squeezing the womb tight and hard. Mothers of first babies often do not feel these pains; other mothers usually do.

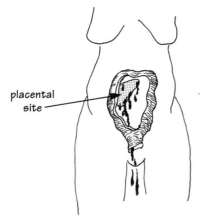

placental
site

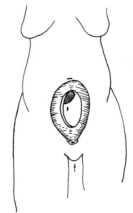

The placental site is like an
open wound that bleeds.

Contractions after birth
help the bleeding slow down.

5. The first 2 weeks after birth—the womb gets smaller

For the first 1 or 2 days after birth, the mother may bleed as much as she would during a heavy monthly bleeding. Over the next 1 or 2 weeks, the mother should slowly bleed less and less—and then stop bleeding completely.

The mother's womb will slowly get smaller during the next 2 weeks. It will get almost as small as it was before she got pregnant.

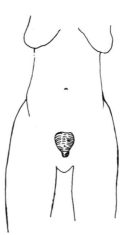

The womb gets
small again.

Giving good care during labor

Chapter 9 contents

Giving good care during labor

When to go to a birth

We recommend that you ask a mother to contact you as soon as she sees signs that labor is near (see p. 137). This way you will know to get ready and to stay in touch.

You should go to the mother when any **one** of these things happen:

- Labor contractions begin.
- The *bag of waters* breaks.
- The mother feels she needs you.

If you go to a birth and find that the mother is in very early labor (and you live nearby), it is usually OK to go home for a while. Ask the mother to call for you when labor gets stronger.

Before leaving, consider these things:

- Is this a first baby? Labor is usually longer for a first baby.
- Were her past births fast or slow? If a past birth was fast, she may have an even faster birth this time.
- How far away is medical help?

Note: When you go to the labor, it is always best to take along a partner or helper. If there is an emergency, one person can take care of the baby while the other takes care of the mother. Or, one person can go for help, while the other helps take care of the problem.

If you do not have a partner or helper, you may want to teach someone (perhaps the mother's sister, husband, mother, or friend) to help you during the birth.

What to bring to a birth

Having the right *equipment* can make the birth safer and easier. The mother will probably have some of this equipment at her home. A midwife will need to bring the rest. It is a good idea for every midwife to assemble a *kit* with this equipment.

The midwife's kit

Caution! Any equipment used during labor and birth must be very clean or *sterile*. See p. 154 for instructions on how to clean or sterilize your equipment.

Equipment that the <u>mother may have</u>.
If she does not have this equipment, the midwife should bring it to the birth.

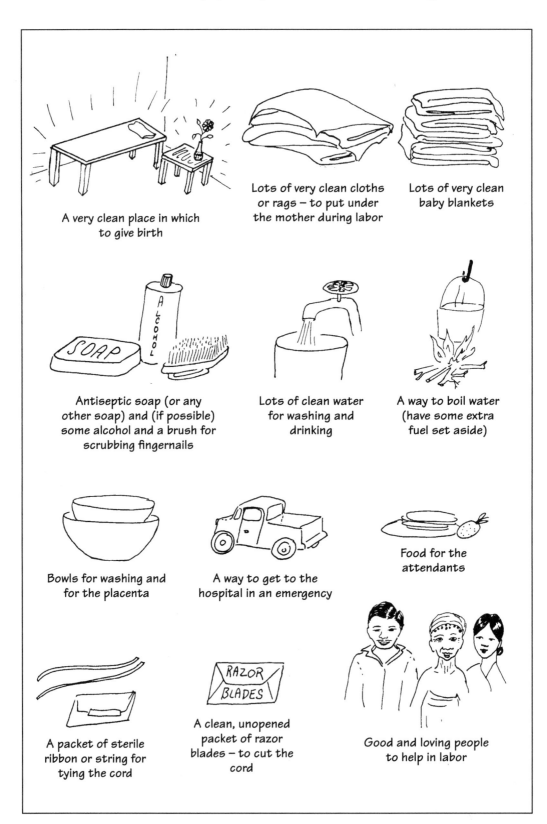

A very clean place in which
to give birth

Lots of very clean cloths
or rags – to put under
the mother during labor

Lots of very clean
baby blankets

Antiseptic soap (or any
other soap) and (if possible)
some alcohol and a brush for
scrubbing fingernails

Lots of clean water
for washing and
drinking

A way to boil water
(have some extra
fuel set aside)

Bowls for washing and
for the placenta

A way to get to the
hospital in an emergency

Food for the
attendants

A packet of sterile
ribbon or string for
tying the cord

A clean, unopened
packet of razor
blades – to cut the
cord

Good and loving people
to help in labor

**Equipment that is <u>very useful for every midwife</u> to carry in her kit.
(Not all midwives will be able to get all of this equipment; some of it is
expensive and difficult to find.)**

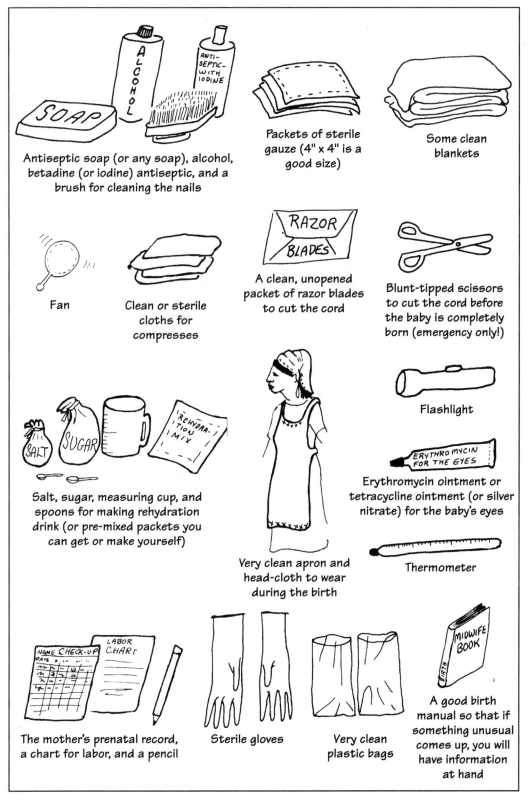

Antiseptic soap (or any soap), alcohol, betadine (or iodine) antiseptic, and a brush for cleaning the nails

Packets of sterile gauze (4" x 4" is a good size)

Some clean blankets

Fan

Clean or sterile cloths for compresses

A clean, unopened packet of razor blades to cut the cord

Blunt-tipped scissors to cut the cord before the baby is completely born (emergency only!)

Flashlight

Salt, sugar, measuring cup, and spoons for making rehydration drink (or pre-mixed packets you can get or make yourself)

Very clean apron and head-cloth to wear during the birth

Erythromycin ointment or tetracycline ointment (or silver nitrate) for the baby's eyes

Thermometer

The mother's prenatal record, a chart for labor, and a pencil

Sterile gloves

Very clean plastic bags

A good birth manual so that if something unusual comes up, you will have information at hand

Equipment that is <u>useful for the midwife</u> to carry in her kit.

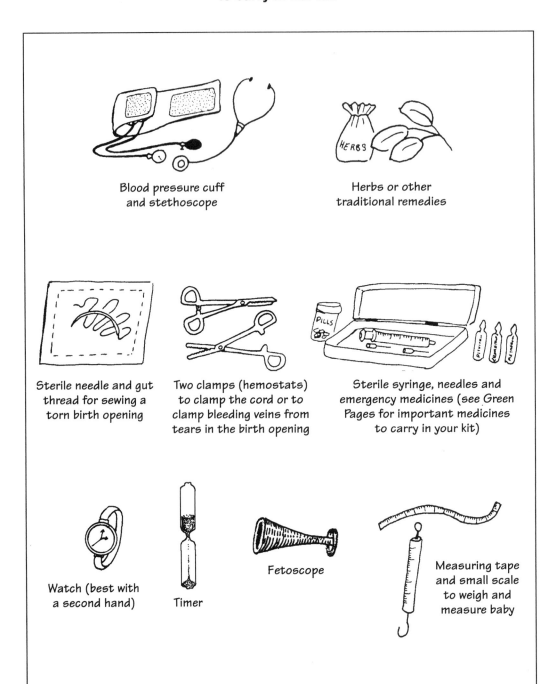

Blood pressure cuff and stethoscope

Herbs or other traditional remedies

Sterile needle and gut thread for sewing a torn birth opening

Two clamps (hemostats) to clamp the cord or to clamp bleeding veins from tears in the birth opening

Sterile syringe, needles and emergency medicines (see Green Pages for important medicines to carry in your kit)

Watch (best with a second hand)

Timer

Fetoscope

Measuring tape and small scale to weigh and measure baby

Preventing infection during labor and birth

A woman in labor or childbirth can easily get germs that cause infection. She can usually get these germs in 2 ways: 1) from contact with other people, and 2) from contact with all kinds of dirt—common house dirt, human or animal stools, or tiny bits of dried blood or body fluids—even dirt so small that you cannot see it.

To prevent harmful contact with people, the midwife should keep anyone with a cold, sore throat, cough, fever, flu, or other illness away from the birth.

Do not let anyone who has an infection or sore on their hands or body touch a new baby. This is especially important if someone has a sore or blister on the lips or nose. Germs that cause simple "*cold sores*" in an adult can harm a new baby.

Also, never put your fingers (or anything else) inside the mother unless there is an important medical reason. Anything that goes inside the mother increases the chance of infection.

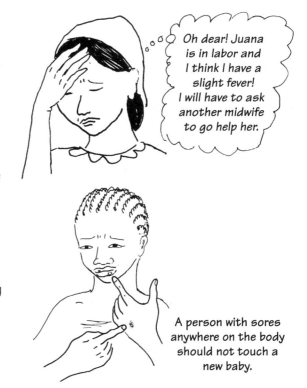

Oh dear! Juana is in labor and I think I have a slight fever! I will have to ask another midwife to go help her.

A person with sores anywhere on the body should not touch a new baby.

Note: Some illnesses, like diabetes and *arthritis*, cannot be passed from one person to another. If you are not sure whether an illness can be spread by contact, ask an experienced health worker about it. If there is no way to find out, the sick person should not attend the birth, if at all possible.

To prevent harmful contact with all kinds of dirt, a midwife must make sure that everything at the birth is clean or sterile. A midwife will need to use 3 different methods: *washing* with soap and water, *sterilizing* (using heat or chemicals to kill ALL of the germs), and *scrubbing* (washing the hands in a special way to kill germs). The sections below will tell you which method to use for the different materials needed at a birth.

1. The birth area

If a woman is giving birth at home, the room where the baby will be born, and the place where the mother will go to urinate (pee), should be cleaned. Sweep these rooms free of dust and dirt, and wash surfaces with soap and water. Put your kit and the mother's birth things on a clean surface.

Note: When cleaning or sterilizing anything, remember to wash your hands first with soap and water.

If the birth is to happen in a maternity center, it is important to be extra careful. Germs can easily be carried from one birth to another. After each birth, try to wash floors and all surfaces with one of these *disinfectants*:

- sodium hypochlorite (household bleach). This solution must be used within 2 hours of making it. Use 1 part bleach to 7 parts water.
- chloramine 2%
- ethanol 70%
- isopropyl alcohol 70%
- polyvidone iodine (betadine) 2.5%
- glutaryl 2%
- hydrogen peroxide 6%

2. Bedding (pads, sheets, and baby blankets)

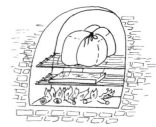

If the woman is giving birth at home, wash bedding in soap and water, and then dry it by hanging it in the sun, or by ironing.

If the birth is to happen in a maternity center, bedding should be sterilized between each use. Wash bedding well first, and then use one of these methods to kill the germs:

- Boil bedding 30 minutes, then dry thoroughly in a clean place.

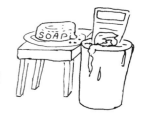

- Iron damp bedding until dry with a hot iron (heat and steam kill germs).

- Fold each piece of bedding, stack them, and wrap all of them together in a large clean cloth. Bake the bedding in the oven for 2 hours at 93°C or 200°F. Put a pan of water in the oven to make steam and prevent scorching.

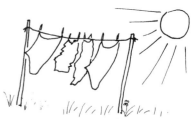

If none of these methods are available, hang bedding in the sun, in a place that is free of dust. The sun should shine on the bedding for one day (turn the bedding so the sun shines on both sides). Never dry bedding on the ground. You should also be careful not to drag bedding across the ground or let it touch the ground.

When the bedding is dry, use one of the larger pieces as a wrapper. Then put a clean plastic bag or clean paper around the outside, if possible. Store in a clean, dry place until needed. **Do not store bedding that is damp or wet. Germs will come back!**

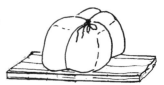

Other kinds of under padding

If you live in an area where there are many newspapers, you can put these under the mother instead of bedding. It is best to bake the newspapers in an oven for 2 hours over a low fire (93°C or 200°F) to kill germs.

If you traditionally use other materials under the mother, try to find a way to get them very clean. For example, banana leaves can be washed with a disinfectant solution, and then smoked for several hours or dried in the sun for 8 hours.

3. Instruments and equipment

All instruments and equipment that you use at a birth should be clean. Be sure that you have washed them carefully between births.

In addition, anything that touches a mother's open wounds, pierces her skin, or goes inside her body must be sterile:

Instruments

- syringes and needles

- scissors or razor blade for cutting the cord

- materials for sewing tears

- clamps or hemostats

Equipment

- gloves

- gauze

- compress cloths

- herbs for wounds

- bulb syringe and mucous trap

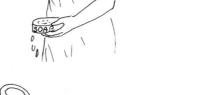

These scissors look clean, but germs are too small to see. I still need to sterilize them.

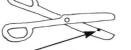

Germs can "hide" in tiny bits of dirt or blood.

At some births there will be plenty of time to sterilize your instruments and equipment at the mother's house. But at other births, you may arrive just as the baby is being born. For this reason we recommend that you sterilize your instruments and equipment at home and always keep them in a sterile container in your kit. A metal box or pot with a tight-fitting lid is probably best. If you cannot get such a container, wrap the instruments and equipment in many layers of sterile cloth.

There are 3 main methods for sterilizing your container, instruments, and equipment:

- **Wet heat** (boiling). This is the best method to use for sterilizing instruments and some gloves.

- **Dry heat** (baking in an oven). This is the best method for sterilizing other equipment. If you cannot use dry heat, wash and boil your equipment, and then dry it in a dust free place.

- **Chemicals** (soaking in a strong disinfectant). If you cannot boil your instruments, use chemicals.

These methods are described below.

How to sterilize your instruments by boiling

Wet heat

1. Wash your container and fill it with water. Boil the water container with the lid on for at least 20 minutes or as long as it takes to cook rice. Start timing **after** the water starts to bubble, not when you turn on the heat. (If you put 1 to 2 grains of rice in the container, you will know the equipment is sterile when the rice is cooked.) Then pour out the water and let the container dry. Do not touch the inside of the container. Once you touch something, it is no longer sterile unless you are wearing **sterile gloves**.

  2. Wash some tools—like forceps, chopsticks, or a couple of spoons or forks. Boil the tools, or let them soak in disinfectant (70% ethanol or 1 part bleach to 7 parts water) for at least 20 minutes. You will need these tools to handle your sterile instruments.

3. Wash your instruments and boil them for at least 20 minutes. Use one end of the sterile tool to pick the instruments out of the water and transfer them to your sterile container. Do not touch the end of the tool that touches the instruments. Anything that you touch is no longer sterile.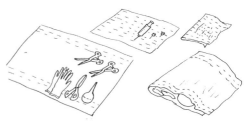

4. Let the instruments dry in the container (with the lid off) in a dust free place with a sterile cloth over the top. (If you are sterilizing your instruments at a birth, you can lay the instruments out on a sterile cloth, then cover the instruments with another sterile cloth to keep the dust off.)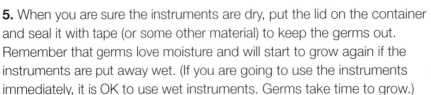

5. When you are sure the instruments are dry, put the lid on the container and seal it with tape (or some other material) to keep the germs out. Remember that germs love moisture and will start to grow again if the instruments are put away wet. (If you are going to use the instruments immediately, it is OK to use wet instruments. Germs take time to grow.)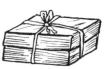

A method from the Philippines

In the Philippines, the Medical Mission Sisters have developed a method for sterilizing instruments by boiling. Follow these steps:

1. Put your clean instruments into a tray. Add a piece of raw cassava wrapped in banana leaf to use as a "timer."

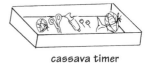

cassava timer

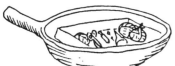

2. Place the tray in a cooking pan.

3. Fill the pan with water until it reaches $\frac{1}{2}$ way up the tray.

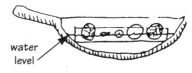

water level

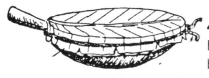

4. Cover the pan with 8 layers of **clean** green banana leaves. Bind the leaves tightly in place with strips of banana leaf or bark. Be careful not to spill water into the tray when you do this.

5. Put the pan on a low fire. After boiling for about 2 hours, carefully remove the banana layers to see if the cassava is soft. Your instruments are sterilized if the cassava is soft.

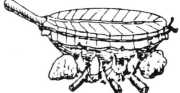

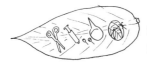

6. Throw away the top layer of the leaves. You can use one of the inner layers as a sterile "cloth" to put your instruments on.

Boiling rubber equipment:

- Most rubber bulb syringes and rubber gloves can be boiled. But some types of gloves fall apart in boiling water. Try to get equipment that can be boiled.

- Be extra careful not to let all the water boil away when cooking. This could cause rubber equipment (and even some metal things) to burn or melt.

How to sterilize by baking

Dry heat

When you use dry heat, you can sterilize with the container already closed (since the equipment does not need to dry), then leave the container closed until you are ready to use it.

To use dry heat, put your clean instruments in a clean container. Tie it shut. Bake at 93°C or 200° F (low fire) for one hour. Put a pan of water into the oven to keep things from burning.

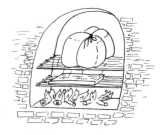

Note: This method does not work for anything made of rubber or plastic. This equipment will melt.

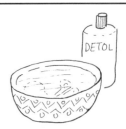

How to sterilize with chemicals

You can soak your container, tools, and instruments in medical alcohol (70% ethanol), or a mixture of 1 part bleach and 7 parts boiled water.

In areas where people cannot get bleach, medical alcohol, or other disinfectants, they sometimes use ordinary drinking alcohol. Strong, clear drinking alcohol is best, but other forms are better than nothing. For example, in parts of India people wash and soak instruments in wine.

To sterilize your container, tools, and instruments with a disinfectant solution or alcohol:

  1. Fill the container with the solution.

  2. Fill 2 bowls with the solution. Put instruments in 1 bowl and tools for handling the instruments in the other bowl.

  3. Soak everything for 20 minutes.

  4. Empty the container. Using the tools, put the sterile instruments into the container.

  5. Let the container and instruments dry completely. Seal the container.

Special equipment needs special care

Thermometer

Wash the thermometer with soap and **cool** water before 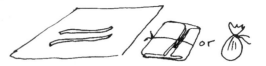 and after you use it. Do not use hot water; the thermometer may break. After washing, it is best to soak the thermometer in alcohol (or a disinfectant solution) for 20 minutes.

Razor blades

Razor blades should stay in their packets until you use them (throw away used blades). Razor blade packets should be wrapped in clean paper or cloth, or kept in a clean, dry box. If the packets get wet or dirty, they are not safe to use anymore—unless you sterilize them first. Sterilize them using one of the methods above.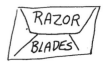

The string for tying the cord

The string for tying the cord should be sterile—or at least *very* clean.

If you want to sterilize string and keep it in your kit, put the string in a piece of paper or cloth. Fold the paper or cloth around the string and tie it closed with another piece of string. Then sterilize the package of string by dry heat (see p. 155).

Sterile packets, gloves and plastic bags

Gauze, *compresses*, gloves, or other equipment sometimes come in *sterile packets*. Since the inside of these packets is already sterile, you can use this equipment directly out of the package. But remember: once you take something out of its sterile package and use it, or if the package gets wet or gets holes in it, the equipment is not sterile anymore.

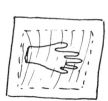
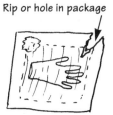

Rip or hole in package

This glove is sterile.

This glove is not sterile.

Things in sterile packets are often meant to be used one time and then thrown away *(disposable)*. But some of these things can be reused if they are carefully cleaned and sterilized before each use. Gauze and compresses can be washed, boiled, and then baked (see p. 155).

Gloves and plastic bags (and other rubber or plastic equipment) that are too delicate to be boiled or steamed can be washed carefully, and then soaked in disinfectant solution (see p. 156).

Needles

If you are going to use *syringes* and *needles*, read p. 384 carefully. Some syringes and needles can be used again and again, but some are disposable and come in sterile packages. Some disposable syringes and needles can be taken apart, boiled, and reused several times before they fall apart.

Throw away after one use.

If you reuse syringes or needles, sterilize by boiling before each use:

1. Draw clean water (or even better, mix 1 part bleach with 7 parts water) up through the needle into the syringe barrel.

2. Squirt out the water several times. Rinse everything with clean water if you use bleach.

3. Then follow the steps on p. 154.

Remember:

If you...

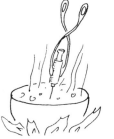
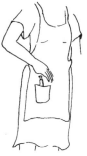
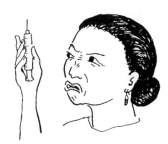

take a sterile needle out of boiling water

and put it in your pocket,

it is not sterile any more. Instead, it is dangerous!

Herbs

Any herbs that will be used at the birth should be sterilized using dry heat.
Never put leaf or plant material *inside* the mother's vagina.

4. People

Anyone who attends the birth—including the mother, midwives, friends, or family—should wash their clothes, hair, and bodies with soap and water. They should wash their hands again whenever they touch the mother or their own hair or clothes. They should also wash again if they get blood, mucus, waters, stool, or dirt on their hands.

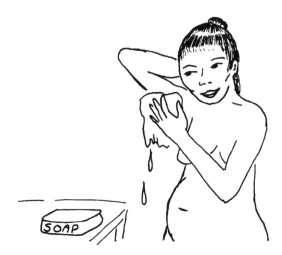

In addition to ordinary hand washing, it is important to use a special hand washing method called the **scrub** during some parts of the birth. You should do a scrub at these times:

Before you

- touch the mother's genitals for any reason

- deliver the baby

- touch sterile instruments

- put your hands inside the mother

- sew up a tear

- touch any wound

During

- any procedure, if you have accidentally touched something unclean

After you

- clean up after the birth

- touch blood or body fluids

How to scrub

You will need:

- Clean or boiled water
- Soap – ordinary soap is good, disinfectant soap is better
- A brush to clean the fingernails

(You can mix disinfectant and regular soap if you want to.)

1

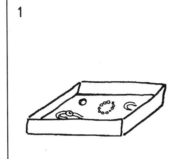

Take off rings and other jewelry and put them away.

2

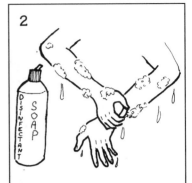

Soap your hands and arms – all the way up to your elbows!

3

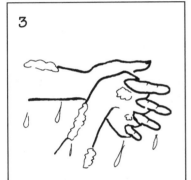

Make sure to scrub in between your fingers.

4

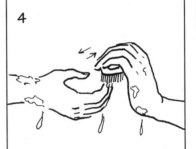

Scrub the nails with a clean brush. (It is even better if the brush has been dipped in disinfectant.)

5

If possible, keep scrubbing, brushing, and washing your hands and arms for 5 whole minutes!

6

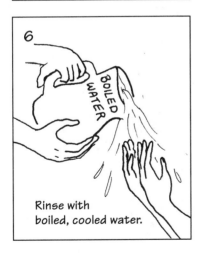

Rinse with boiled, cooled water.

7

It is best to let your hands dry in the air instead of using a towel. Do not touch anything until your hands are dry.

8

In an emergency, when you don't have the time to scrub – or if you don't have clean or boiled water – you can splash and rub your arms and hands with alcohol or disinfectant. This is better than doing nothing to clean the hands and arms.

Gloves

Sterile gloves protect the mother from any germs that may be hiding under your fingernails or on your skin after you scrub. They also protect you. If you have sterile gloves, use them whenever you touch the mother's genitals, or when you handle sterile instruments. It is very important to use sterile gloves if you must put your hands inside the mother.

This is the correct way to put on gloves so that they stay sterile. Practice with the same pair of gloves over and over again until it feels natural:

Note: If you do not have sterile gloves, use plastic bags that have been washed in disinfectant soap instead. In the rest of this book, we will only mention gloves. **Be sure to use plastic bags if you do not have gloves.**

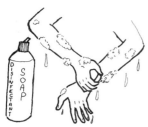

Scrub first (see p. 159).

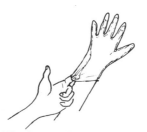

If gloves are in a sterile package, ask a helper to open it for you without touching the gloves.

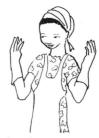

If gloves have been boiled or re-sterilized they can be laid out on a sterile cloth or sit in the water.

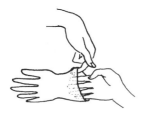

Carefully put a finger into the glove to open it. Do not touch the outside of the glove! Slip your other hand into it.

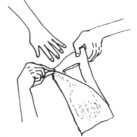

Wiggle your hand in while you pull with your finger.

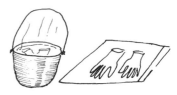

Once the gloves are on, do not touch anything that is not sterile – or the gloves will not be sterile anymore either!

Of course, you will have to touch the mother, but try not to move germs from one part of her body to another. For example, if you must put your fingers inside the vagina, be careful not to touch the mother's anus, where there are many germs. Some of these germs are harmless when they are on the skin or in stools, but they can kill a woman if they get into the vagina or womb.

Remember:

If you...

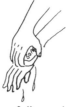

carefully wash your hands

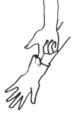

and put on sterile gloves

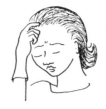

and then scratch your head,

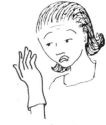

your glove is not sterile anymore.

5. How a midwife can protect herself from infection

It is possible for a midwife to catch an infectious disease from the woman she helps. The danger is greatest in areas where there is a lot of AIDS, hepatitis, or other serious *infectious diseases*. If you know that a woman has a serious illness—whether it is contagious or not—it is probably best for her to deliver in a hospital. The people at the hospital are better equipped to protect themselves against infection, and they will have more ways to help the mother and baby than you will at home.

Unfortunately, it is possible for the mother to have a serious illness and not know it yet, because it takes a while for the disease to show. During this time the woman can pass the disease to others. Since a midwife comes into contact with blood, urine, stool, and other body fluids (where many germs live), you must protect yourself. These precautions will help:

- Wash your hands often. Always wash before and after touching the mother. Washing with ordinary soap is good, but washing with one of these disinfectants is better: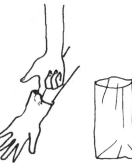

    - polyvidone iodine (betadine) 2.5%
    - hibiclens
    - hydrogen peroxide 6%
    - phisohex
    - dettol
    - local gin

- Always wear gloves or plastic bags when you touch anything bloody (like the placenta), or anything with blood, waters, urine, or stool on it. Gloves are even more important if you have a cut on your hand, since germs could enter your blood through the cut. While we do not recommend that you touch inside the mother's vagina, sometimes it is necessary to save the mother's life. If you need to touch inside the mother, scrub and wear sterile gloves (see p. 159).

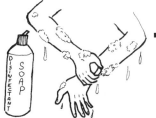

- Try not to get blood, waters, urine, or stool in your mouth, eyes, or in any cuts. Do not touch food or put your fingers in your mouth for any reason until they have been washed with disinfectant, or at least soap.

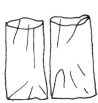

- Be careful not to stick yourself with used needles that have not been sterilized. Carry needles carefully with the point away from your body. Do not leave used needles lying around where someone could poke themselves by accident. Do not put the cap back on a used needle until it has been sterilized again.

What to do during stage 1

Chapter 10 contents

What to do during stage 1

Stage 1 begins when contractions start to open the cervix; it ends when the cervix is completely open. Stage 1 is usually the longest stage, but the amount of time is different for every birth. Stage 1 could be less than an hour or it could be a day and a night.

Overview of healthy signs and risk signs

This list of healthy signs and risk signs gives you an overview of what to look for in stage 1. Healthy signs indicate that stage 1 is going well. Risk signs may mean that something is wrong. If you find a risk sign, turn immediately to the page number following the risk sign to find out what to do next.

Healthy signs

- Contractions get longer, stronger, and closer together.
- Cervix opens in 12 hours or less for a woman who has been pregnant before, 24 hours or less for a first baby.
- Show may come all through labor.
- If the waters break, they are clear (like water).
- Mother's temperature stays below 37.8 °C or 100°F.
- Mother's blood pressure stays below 140/90. Blood pressure does not suddenly drop more than 15 points in the bottom number.
- Mother's pulse is between 60 and 100 beats per minute.

These signs may be uncomfortable, but they are normal:

- Pain or strong pressure in the belly or lower back during a contraction
- Shaking legs or body (in active or late labor)
- Burping
- Sweating
- Tiredness (or a desire to sleep) between contractions in active labor
- Some vomiting (but not constant vomiting)
- Some fears or doubts
- Mild diarrhea

Risk Signs

- Labor begins before the 8th month of pregnancy (see p. 233).

- Mother says she feels hot, she is hot-to-touch, or her temperature is above 37.8 °C or 100°F (see p. 235).

- Waters break but labor does not start within 8–12 hours or $\frac{1}{2}$ day (see p. 236).

- Waters are brown, yellow, or green (see p. 237).

- Strong contractions last more than 12 hours for women with previous pregnancies, or 24 hours for first babies (see p. 237).

- Mother has unusual or heavy bleeding: blood clots, fresh blood, or more than 200 cc of blood during labor (see p. 243).

- Mother feels pain between contractions and the womb does not get soft, or she feels unusual pain during contractions (see p. 244).

- Mother has pre-eclampsia: blood pressure greater than 140/90, swollen face and hands, headaches, vision changes, pain between her ribs, brisk reflexes (see p. 246).

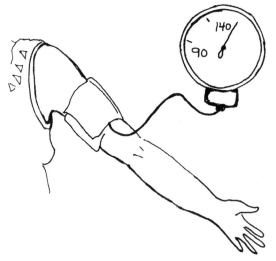

- Mother has convulsions (fits) (see p. 247).

- Mother's pulse is more than 100 beats per minute (see p. 248).

- Baby's heartbeat is more than 160 beats per minute or less than 110 beats per minute (see p. 249).

- Cord comes down in front of the baby (**prolapsed cord**) (see p. 250).

Arriving at the birth place

1. Check the mother's and baby's physical signs

Checking the mother and baby when you first arrive can give you important information about how things are going, and if problems can be expected in this birth. These checks also will be done throughout stage 1. This chart tells how often to do each check:

Checking the mother and baby	
What to check when you arrive	**When to check during stage 1**
Baby's position	
Baby's heartbeat	every $\frac{1}{2}$ hour
Mother's temperature	every 4 hours*
Mother's blood pressure	every hour
Mother's pulse	every 4 hours**
Mother's bag of waters	when the bag breaks

* If the mother's bag of waters has been broken for more than 6 hours, check her temperature every hour.

** If labor is over 12 hours long or if there is a risk of infection (for example, if the woman has had a lot of sexual partners, or if she has a history of sexually transmitted diseases—see p. 361), check her pulse every hour. If the mother is bleeding or **dehydrated** (see p. 171), check her pulse every 15 minutes.

The baby's position

See p. 125 to learn how to tell where the baby's head is. Checking the baby's position can tell you if:

- the baby is lying head down, and which way it faces.
- the baby is moving down through the mother's pelvic bones.

Is the baby lying head down? Which way does it face?

Most babies lie with their head down, facing the mother's back or side. This is the best position for the baby, because the back of the baby's head presses on the cervix and helps labor get stronger. The baby may be born sooner.

If the baby is head down but faces the mother's belly, the labor may be longer. But these babies usually can be born without problems. If the baby is not head down, see p. 262–265.

Is the baby moving down through the mother's pelvic bones?

The baby *floats* above the mother's pelvic bones during most of pregnancy. In late pregnancy or early labor, the baby's head usually starts to settle down through the mother's pelvic bones. When this happens, we say the head is *engaged*. Engagement is a good sign, because it may mean the mother's bones are wide enough to let the baby through.

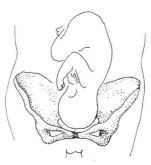 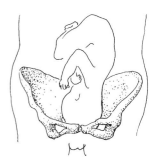

This baby is still high and floating.

This baby is low or engaged.

You can know if the baby is engaged— or if it is still high and floating—by carefully feeling the belly, like this:

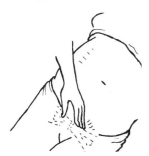 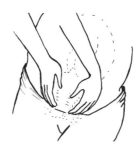 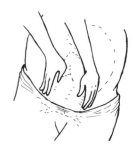

1. Find the mother's pubic bone (just below her hair line).

2. Find the baby's head. If it begins to curve around above the pubic bone, it is not engaged.

3. If the sides of the baby's head go straight down, it is probably engaged.

If a woman is in active labor and the head stays high, there may be a problem (see p. 238). Or if the waters break suddenly while the head is high, the cord may be washed down in front of the baby's head (a prolapsed cord). This is very dangerous for the baby (see p. 250).

The baby's heartbeat

See p. 127 to learn how to check the baby's heartbeat. The best time to listen to the baby's heartbeat is soon after a contraction stops. Listening to the baby's heartbeat can tell you:

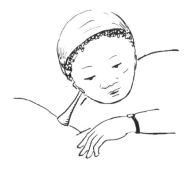

- about the baby's position
- about the baby's health

About the baby's position

Finding the place where the heartbeat is loudest can help you know if the baby is head down, breech (head up), or sideways. See p. 128.

About the baby's health

A healthy baby's heartbeat is between 120 and 160 beats per minute during labor. It may change and speed up or slow down but stay between 120 and 160.

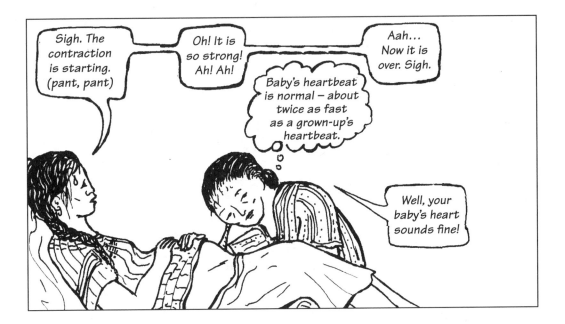

Note: If the heartbeat is less than 110 beats per minute, check the mother's pulse to make sure you are not hearing her heartbeat by mistake.

If you cannot hear the baby's heartbeat during a contraction, it usually does not mean that the heart has stopped! It just means the wall of the womb is so thick that it is hard to hear through, or that the contraction moves the baby away from your ear. If you find the baby's heartbeat after a contraction is over and it is normal, it was probably normal during the contraction, too.

The mother's temperature

See p. 105 to learn how to take the mother's temperature. If you do not have a thermometer, touch her forehead with your lips or hand to feel if she is hot. If she feels **warm**, or if her temperature is above 37°C or 98.6°F but below 37.8°C or 100°F —she may be dehydrated. See p. 171 for other signs of dehydration and check her temperature often to see if it goes up more.

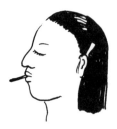

If she feels **hot** or if she has a temperature above 37.8°C or 100°F —turn to p. 235. She may have an infection, or other problems.

The mother's blood pressure

If you have a *blood pressure cuff* and stethoscope, check her blood pressure between contractions (see p. 108). Each time you check her blood pressure, write it down. This way you can watch for changes over time. If it stays below 140/90 and close to her pregnancy blood pressure, check it every hour. If you notice her blood pressure going up (even if it is just a little at a time), check it every 15 or 30 minutes.

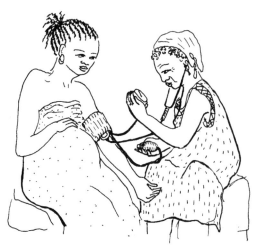

During labor, the top number of the mother's blood pressure should not go up more than 30 points from her pregnancy blood pressure. The bottom number should not go up more than 15 points. For example, if her usual blood pressure during pregnancy was 100/60, it should not go higher than 130/75. (If you do not have a record of her blood pressure during pregnancy, start with the first blood pressure you take in labor.)

Whatever the mother's blood pressure was during pregnancy, if it is more than 140/90 during labor, it is a risk sign (see p. 246). If blood pressure suddenly drops 15 points or more in the bottom number, this is also a risk sign (see p. 243). It may mean she is bleeding inside.

The mother's pulse

In early labor, the mother's pulse should be between 60 and 100 beats per minute between contractions.

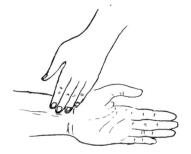

If her pulse is above 100 between contractions, see p. 235 (infection), p. 243 (bleeding shock), and p. 171 (dehydration).

The mother's bag of waters

The bag of waters usually breaks late in stage 1. But it may break at any time—before labor starts or not until the baby is born. Sometimes the waters break with a great gush. Sometimes they just leak a little.

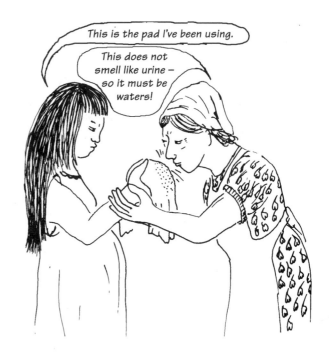

When you arrive at the birth place, ask the mother if her waters have broken. If she is not sure, you can usually find out by checking to see if her genitals and pad are wet. Since this wetness could be waters or urine (pee), smell the pad to see if it smells like urine.

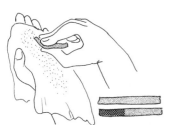

If the paper turns blue or purple, the wetness is waters.

Or, if you have **nitrazine papers**, put the paper into the wetness. If the paper stays orange, the wetness is urine. If it turns blue or purple, the wetness is waters. (Waters and urine can be mixed together. If the paper stays orange or the liquid smells like urine, but you still think the waters have broken, wait and test again later.)

If you decide that the wetness is waters, check their color. Waters should be clear or slightly pink. It is OK if there are white dots in the waters. But if they are brown, yellow, or green, see p. 237.

Once the bag of waters has broken, germs can start slowly moving into the womb. To reduce the risk of infection after the waters break:

- Do not do vaginal exams (except in an emergency).

- Do not put anything into the mother's vagina.

- Do not let the mother sit in water to bathe.

If you are with the mother when her waters break, look at her genitals to be sure the cord is not prolapsed. If it is, see p. 250–251. Listen to the baby's heartbeat right after the waters break. If the baby's heartbeat drops below 110 beats per minute, see p. 249.

2. Plan ahead for the labor and birth

If there are no problems with the mother or baby, now is a good time to plan ahead for the remainder of the labor and birth:

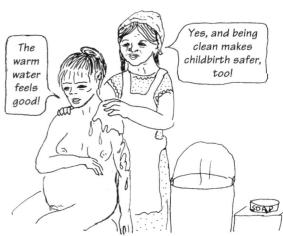

- Make sure the birth place and everyone attending the birth are clean (see p. 152). If the mother has not bathed today, you can help her wash now. If her waters have broken, she should wash by pouring water over her body.

- Make sure your instruments and equipment are sterile and close by (see p. 153–156).

- Check to see if there is enough water, fuel for boiling, and food to last through this labor and birth.

- Check to see if transportation is available for an emergency.

- Ask the mother if anyone should be told that she is in labor.

- Decide if other midwives or medical people need to be told about this labor.

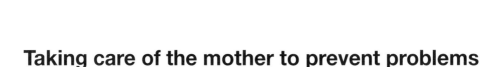

Taking care of the mother to prevent problems

1. Change bedding under the mother when it gets wet or soiled

Most women leak a lot of fluid from the vagina all through labor. This fluid may be show. If the waters have broken, it may be just waters, or waters and show.

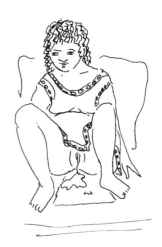

When the mother lies down or sits, you can put clean cloths or pads under her to catch the fluid. When she walks around, she can hold a clean cloth or pad between her legs.

Change cloths and pads when they get very wet or messy. Check them for risk signs—too much fresh blood or blood clots (see p. 243–246), or brown, yellow, or green waters (see p. 237).

2. Make sure the mother drinks at least one cup of liquid each hour

A woman in labor is working hard and can use up the liquids in her body. If she does not drink enough, she may get dehydrated (too little liquid in her body). This can make her labor much longer and harder. *Signs of dehydration* are:

- fast, deep breathing (more than 20 breaths per minute)

- fast, weak pulse (more than 100 beats per minute)

- dry lips

- sunken eyes

- weakness

- *loss of stretchiness* of the skin

- mild fever (less than 37.8°C or 100°F)

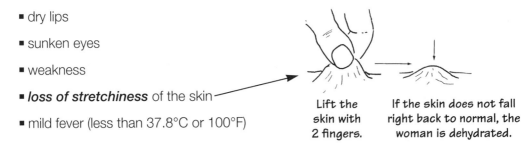

Lift the skin with 2 fingers.

If the skin does not fall right back to normal, the woman is dehydrated.

To prevent dehydration, the mother should drink at least one cup of liquid each hour. Some midwives like to write down when and how much the mother drinks.

If the mother is vomiting and cannot drink one whole cup of liquid at once, have her take small sips after **every** contraction. This way she will get liquid without upsetting her stomach. These liquids may help her feel better: coconut water, fruit juice mixed with water, water with sugar or honey in it, or peppermint or chamomile tea with honey or sugar. There may also be special labor strengthening drinks in your area.

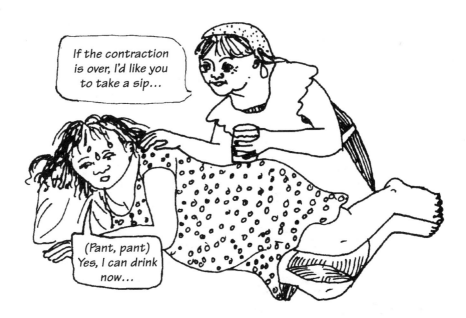

Rehydration drink

If the labor lasts 12 hours or more, or if the mother has trouble drinking liquids, try to give her *rehydration drink*. This drink helps keep the chemicals in the mother's blood balanced.

You may be able to get pre-mixed packets of salts and sugar, such as *Oresal,* for making rehydration drink. If you use these, be careful to mix them correctly and taste the drink. It should be no saltier than tears.

You may also mix the rehydration drink yourself at the labor, or carry the dry ingredients already measured and mixed in little packets in your kit.

---

2 WAYS TO MAKE "HOME MIX" REHYDRATION DRINK

1. With sugar and salt (Raw sugar or molasses can be used instead of sugar.)	**1. With powdered cereal and salt** (Powdered rice is best. Or use finely ground maize, wheat flour, sorghum, or cooked and mashed potatoes.)
In 1 liter of clean **water** put ½ of a level teaspoon of **salt** and 8 level teaspoons of **sugar** 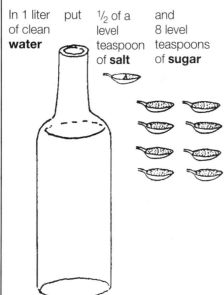	In 1 liter of **water** put ½ of a level teaspoon of **salt** and 8 heaping teaspoons (or 2 handfuls) of powdered **cereal** 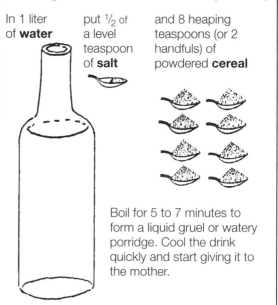 Boil for 5 to 7 minutes to form a liquid gruel or watery porridge. Cool the drink quickly and start giving it to the mother.
Caution! Before adding the sugar, taste the drink and be sure it is less salty than tears.	*Caution!* Taste the drink each time before you give it to be sure it is not spoiled. Cereal drinks can spoil in a few hours in hot weather.

2. To either drink add half a cup of fruit juice, coconut water, or mashed ripe banana, if available. This provides potassium which may help the mother accept more liquid.

Try to adapt the drink to your area. If liter containers or teaspoons are not in most homes, adjust quantities to local forms of measurement. If you don't have a measuring cup or spoons, use a pinch of salt and a small handful of sugar. Where people traditionally give cereal gruels to young children, add enough water to make it liquid, and use that. Look for an easy and simple way.

Note: If the mother feels hungry during labor, it is OK for her to eat. Choose foods that are easy to digest—like bread, rice, or yogurt.

3. Make sure the mother urinates at least once every 2 hours

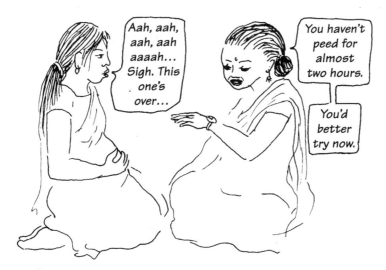

If the mother's bladder is very full, it can make her contractions weaker and her labor longer. A full bladder can also cause pain, problems with pushing out the placenta, and bleeding after childbirth.

When you see or feel a bump like this, the bladder may be too full. Do not wait until the bladder gets this big. Remind the mother to urinate; she may not remember. If you think the bladder is too full and she cannot urinate, see p. 242.

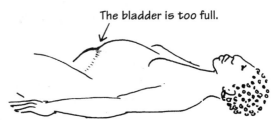

The bladder is *too* full.

4. Make sure the mother rests between contractions

It is important for the mother to rest between contractions, even when labor first begins, so she can save her strength. She does not have to lie down, but she should not waste energy working or fighting against her contractions.

Many women feel very tired when their contractions are strong. They may fear they will not have the strength to push the baby out. But feeling tired is the body's way of making the mother rest and relax. If everything is well, she will have the strength to give birth when the time comes. For ways to help the mother relax, see p. 313–321.

5. Make sure the mother changes position every hour

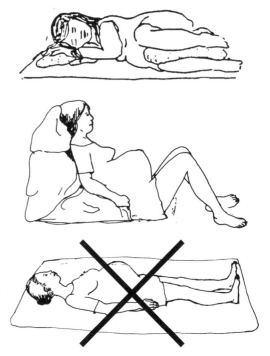

Many women like to walk or move about during labor. A mother can walk, squat, sit, stand, or take other positions. These are all good, because changing positions helps the cervix open more evenly. Sometimes standing or walking makes labor go faster.

The mother should not lie flat on her back. This squeezes the blood vessels that bring blood to the baby and mother. But it is OK for her to lie on her side with a pad between her legs, or on her back with her upper body propped up—as long as she changes position every hour (see p. 317).

6. Give the mother an enema if she wants one

An *enema* washes the stool out of the body with clean water. In some areas it is the custom to give an enema to a woman in labor, but we do not recommend this. If water from the enema gets into the vagina, or onto other things that must stay clean, the mother may get an infection. Also, some women have a little diarrhea before going into labor, so there is no need to give an enema.

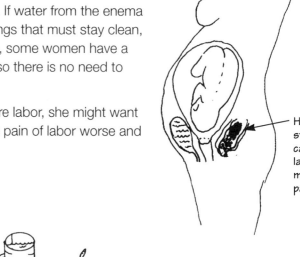

Hard stools can make labor more painful.

But if a woman was constipated before labor, she might want an enema—hard stools can make the pain of labor worse and keep the baby's head high.

To give an enema, you will need:

- a *rectal tube*

- a hose (60 cm or 2 feet long) that attaches to the rectal tube

- a can or container that can attach to the tube, or a funnel to pour the water into the hose

- about 500 ml or 2 cups of clean, warm water

When the equipment is ready:

1. Ask the mother to lie on her side.

2. Put some oil on the rectal tube.

3. Insert the tip of the tube gently into the mother's **rectum**.

4. Hold the container just high enough so that the water runs into the rectum.

5. Ask the mother to hold the water until she feels she must move her bowels.

6. Stay with her in case the bag of waters breaks or the baby comes while she is moving her bowels.

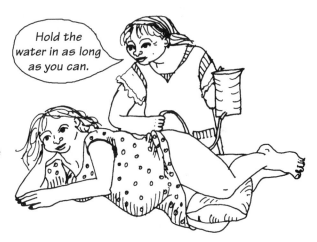

Hold the water in as long as you can.

Caution! Never give an enema to a woman:

- if her bag of waters has broken.

- if she is in active or late labor.

- if the baby's head is floating (see p. 166).

- if she does not want one.

---

7. Support, guide, and guard the labor

Support the labor

When you support the labor, you help the mother relax and welcome her labor, instead of fighting against it. Although labor support will not make labor painless, it can make labor easier, shorter, and safer. Labor support can be given by the mother's husband, family, or friends. It can also be given by the midwife or her helper.

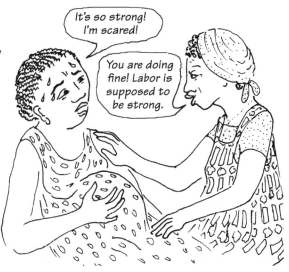

It's so strong! I'm scared!

You are doing fine! Labor is supposed to be strong.

What you do depends on the needs of the woman, and on the birth beliefs and practices of your area. But every woman needs kindness, respect, and attention. Be aware of her emotions and feelings. Encourage her, so she can feel strong and confident in labor. Help her relax and welcome her labor. (See p. 313–321 for other ideas.)

Guide the labor

When you *guide the labor*, you help the labor stay on a healthy path. For example, if the labor is slow because the mother is tired or afraid, you may be able to help her rest, or lessen her *fear* by talking with her. You may also guide the labor by making sure the mother does not *push* too soon (see p. 253).

Guard the labor

When you *guard the labor*, you protect it from wrong *interference*. Here are some examples:

- Sometimes you must protect the mother from other people who would interfere with the labor. Keep rude or unkind people away—the mother should not have to worry about family problems. Do not let anyone make the mother feel she has to hurry the birth. Do not let anyone bring fear to the birth.

- Do not use unnecessary drugs, instruments, or procedures. If you do not find any risk signs, it is best to assume that this birth will be normal.

Do not let anyone give the mother plant medicines or drugs to hurry the labor; these can add useless risks. *Injections* that are supposed to hurry the birth can cause bleeding inside the womb. These injections can make labor more painful, and can kill both the mother and the baby.

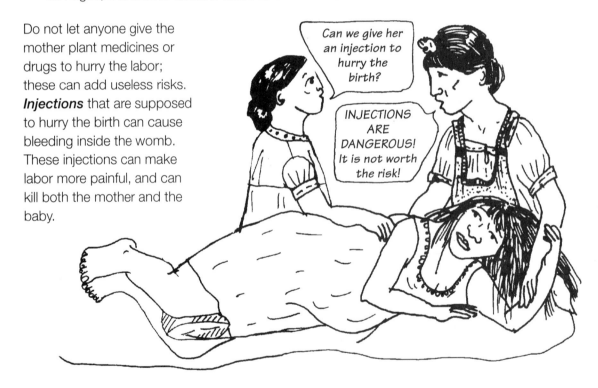

> Can we give her an injection to hurry the birth?

> INJECTIONS ARE DANGEROUS! It is not worth the risk!

Caution! There is a correct way to give a medicine called *pitocin* or *syntocinon (oxytocins)* when a labor is too long. But since it must be given slowly in the *vein*, it should be done in the hospital to be safe (see p. 420). Doctors or others who give oxytocins by injection in the muscle or by mouth are not practicing medicine correctly. They are doing something dangerous!

8. Check for signs of progress

In stage 1, progress means the cervix is opening so that the baby can come out.

The only way to know for sure that the cervix is opening is to do a vaginal (internal) exam. But since vaginal exams increase the risk of infection (and you need special training and gloves to do them), do not do these exams unless there is a good reason and you have had proper training (see p. 389–391). Good reasons to do a vaginal exam are:

- A long, hard labor with no signs of progress. A vaginal exam can tell you if the cervix is opening.
- The baby's heartbeat cannot be heard. A vaginal exam can tell you if there is time to go to the hospital before the birth.
- A prolapsed cord. In a vaginal exam, you can push the baby's head away from the cord.
- Any medical emergency. A vaginal exam can tell you if there is time to go to the hospital before the birth.

Never do a vaginal exam if there is heavy bleeding from the vagina (see p. 101).

Fortunately, vaginal exams are not usually necessary. Most women have other signs of progress. As labor gets stronger, you will see more and more of these signs:

- Contractions get longer, stronger, and closer together.
- Mother says contractions feel stronger.
- Womb feels harder when you touch it during a contraction. In light labor, contractions may make the womb feel as hard as a flexed arm muscle. Later, stronger contractions make the womb feel almost as hard as bone.
- Amount of show increases.
- Bag of waters breaks.
- Mother burps, sweats, vomits; her legs shake.
- Baby's head seems to be moving down through the mother's pelvic bones.
- Mother feels tired and dreamy between contractions, and her eyes get glassy. This is a sign of late labor (but make sure there are no signs of shock—see p. 243).
- Mother wants to push. This may indicate that stage 2 is near or starting. Do not let the mother start pushing until you are certain stage 2 is beginning (see p. 180). Pushing too soon can tear the cervix, cause it to swell or bleed, cause problems at future births, and waste the mother's energy. (Usually, if she cannot help but push, she is already in stage 2.)

Note: Experienced midwives often use intuition or feeling to tell if labor is progressing normally. If you are being taught by an experienced midwife, ask her to help you learn this. The intuition comes from being present at a lot of births.

If the labor lasts longer than 12 hours for women with previous pregnancies, or 24 hours for first babies, something may be wrong (see p. 237).

What to do during stage 2

Chapter 11 contents

What to do during stage 2

Stage 2 begins when the cervix is completely open and ends when the baby is born. Stage 2 can be a short as a few minutes or as long as 2 hours.

Overview of healthy signs and risk signs

This list of healthy signs and risk signs gives you an overview of what to look for in stage 2. Healthy signs indicate that stage 2 is going well. Risk signs may mean that something is wrong. If you find a risk sign, turn immediately to the page number following the risk sign to find out what to do next.

Healthy signs

- Mother pushes well.

- Bag of waters breaks (if it has not already).

- Baby's head begins to show more and more during contractions, then crowns.

- Skin on baby's head is wrinkled.

- Baby's head is born (usually face down), and then turns to face mother's thigh.

- Baby's shoulders and body are born in the next 1 or 2 contractions after the head is born.

These signs may be unpleasant, but are normal:

- Mother may feel pain in her ***tail bone*** as the baby's head comes down the vagina.

- Mother may have a burning feeling as her skin stretches to let the baby's head out.

Risk signs

- Baby is not born after 1 or 2 hours of strong contractions and good pushing (see p. 253).

- Blood gushes out **before** the baby is born (see p. 257).

- Waters are brown, yellow, or green (see p. 258).

- Cord wraps tightly around the baby's neck (see p. 258).

- Baby's heartbeat is more than 160 or less than 90 beats per minute (see p. 259).

- Baby gets stuck at the shoulders (see p. 259).

- Baby is breech (see p. 262).

- Unexpected twins appear (see p. 266).

- Baby is very small or more than 5 weeks early (see p. 269).

Watch for signs that stage 2 is near or starting

When you see 2 or more of the following signs, stage 2 is probably near or starting. The mother can now begin to push the baby out.

- Contractions that have been very strong and close together get farther apart. But the contractions stay strong or get stronger.

- Mother feels a **strong** urge to push. Sometimes she even starts pushing without knowing it. When this happens you may notice her holding her breath or grunting during contractions. (Even if the mother feels no need to push, pushing will feel good if she is really in stage 2.)

- Mother suddenly feels more alert.

- Mother's outer genitals begin to bulge during contractions.

- Mother feels the baby's head begin to move into the vagina.

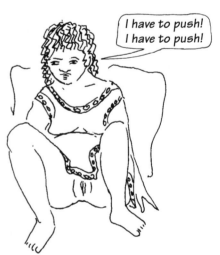

I have to push!
I have to push!

The only way you can be certain that the cervix is open all the way is to do a vaginal exam. But remember that vaginal exams can be dangerous (see p. 389). With experience, you can usually tell when the mother is ready to push without doing an exam.

Help to make the birth safer and easier

1. Make sure everything is clean and ready for the birth

If you have not already cleaned the mother's genitals and sterilized your equipment, do it now (see p. 154–156).

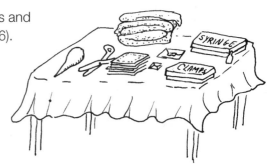

When the birth is near, lay out your equipment in a clean place where it will be easy to reach. If you do not have a partner or helper, explain the equipment to someone who will be at the birth. Then they can hand you something when you need it.

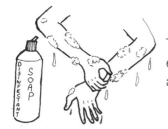

The midwife and anyone who may touch equipment, the mother's genitals, or the new baby and cord, should scrub (see p. 159).

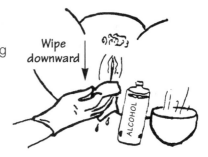

Wipe downward

Clean the mother's genitals gently and carefully, using clean or boiled water. Use disinfectant if you have it (see p. 161). When cleaning, wipe away from the vagina toward the anus (butt hole) so the soiled material does not enter the vagina.

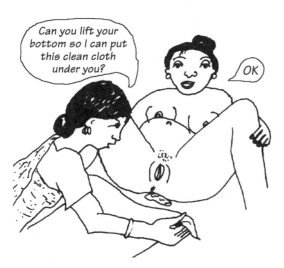

Can you lift your bottom so I can put this clean cloth under you?

OK

Keep a clean cloth under the mother and extra clean cloths close by, in case they are needed during the birth. If any stool comes out during pushing, remove the stool with a clean cloth, change gloves (if possible), and gently wash the mother's bottom again. If there is no time to remove the stool, cover it with a clean cloth and make sure the vaginal opening is clean.

Note: Clean hands do not stay clean for long. If you or a helper touch anything other than the mother's genitals or sterile equipment, you will need to scrub again. For example, if you touch your own hair or clothes, or pick something up that has not been freshly washed, you will need to scrub again.

2. Check the mother's and baby's physical signs

The mother's physical signs

It is wise to check the mother's blood pressure and pulse every $\frac{1}{2}$ hour or so during stage 2. If stage 2 lasts more than 1 hour for a woman who has given birth before, or 2 hours for a first baby, check her blood pressure and pulse every 15 minutes.

If the mother's blood pressure is 140/90 or higher, or suddenly drops more than 15 points in the bottom number, see p. 243 and 246. If her pulse is more than 100 beats per minute between contractions, see p. 248.

The baby's physical signs

The baby's heartbeat is harder to hear in stage 2 because it is usually lower in the mother's belly, near her pubic bone. Do not worry if you cannot find the baby's heartbeat.

A very skilled midwife with good equipment may be able to hear the baby's heart—especially between contractions. It is normal for the heartbeat to go as low as 70 beats per minute **during** a pushing contraction. But it should come right back up to **at least** 90 beats per minute as soon as the contraction is over.

If the baby's heartbeat does not come back up within one minute, the baby may be in trouble. Ask the mother to change position (see the next page) and take the baby's heartbeat again. If it is still low, see p. 259.

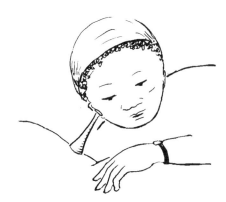

3. Help the mother push effectively

Help the mother get in a good *pushing position*

These positions are good for pushing:

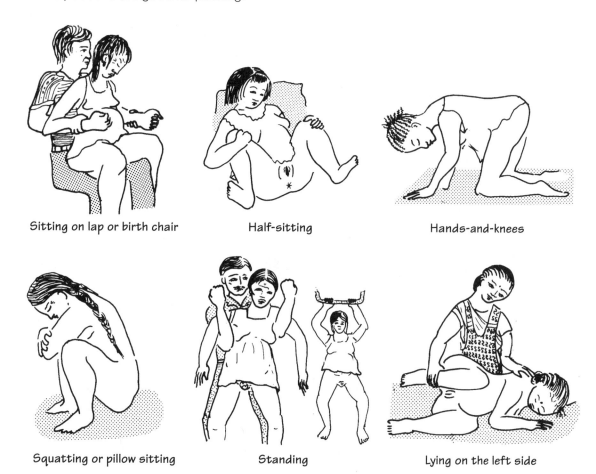

Sitting on lap or birth chair   Half-sitting   Hands-and-knees

Squatting or pillow sitting   Standing   Lying on the left side

These positions have special benefits:

Sitting or half-sitting. This position is often the most comfortable, and makes it easier for the midwife guide the birth of the baby's head.

Hands-and-knees. This position is good when the woman feels her labor in her back. It can also help when the baby's shoulders get stuck (see p. 259).

Squatting or standing. This position can help bring the baby down when the birth is slow.

Lying on the left side. This position is relaxing and helps prevent torn skin.

Note: If things are going well, let the mother choose her own position.

It is usually not good for the mother to lie flat on her back during a normal birth. Lying flat can squeeze the blood vessels that bring blood to the baby and the mother, and make it harder for the mother to push. But if the baby is coming very fast, it is OK for the mother to lie on her back.

Note: There are some medical emergencies in which a woman must lie on her back so the doctor can do a procedure. But many doctors make all women lie flat to deliver—even in a normal birth. This may make things easier for the doctor, but it usually makes birth harder for the mother and baby. **We believe that lying flat during a normal birth is a harmful modern practice.**

Help the mother push correctly

Page 321 explains 3 ways to push correctly. The mother can:

- pant and give several short, strong pushes during each contraction (*pant pushing*).

- take a deep breath and give a long, hard "*push-moan*" *(moan or growl pushing)*.

- take two deep breaths, hold the second breath, and push as hard and long as she can (*hold-the-breath pushing*). This may be the best method if the baby is coming slowly.

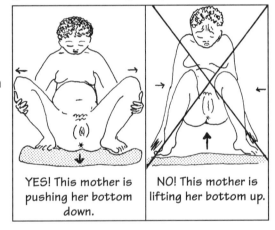

YES! This mother is pushing her bottom down.

NO! This mother is lifting her bottom up.

In all of these methods, the mother should keep her mouth and legs relaxed and open, her chin down on her chest, and her bottom down during pushes.

If the mother is tightening her bottom or having trouble pushing correctly, these things may help:

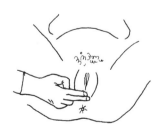

aaargh!

- Asking the mother to change position.

- Asking the mother to push with her mouth open, and jaw loose and forward.

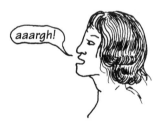

- Applying clean, warm, wet cloths to her genitals (see p. 187). **Do not burn her!**

- Applying light pressure to her genitals with your gloved fingers, while asking her to push toward your fingers.

Support the mother's pushing

If a mother has difficulty pushing hard or correctly, do not scold or threaten her. Upsetting or frightening her can slow the birth. Instead, explain how to push correctly. If necessary, urge her again and again to push hard. Praise her for trying.

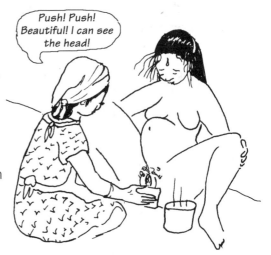

You can encourage the mother by telling her when you see her outer genitals bulge. Explain that this means the baby is coming down. When you see the head, let the mother touch it. This may help her push better.

4. Judge the speed of the birth

When you judge the speed of a birth, you are judging how fast the baby's head is moving down through the birth canal. The baby can move down at a *fast, average,* or *very slow* speed.

Fast birth. If you can see the baby's head after just 1 or 2 pushes, the baby is coming very fast. Tell the mother to stop pushing right away. Ask her to blow out or pant when she feels like pushing (see p. 188, 322).

Average birth. If the mother's genitals start to bulge after a few good pushes, and then slowly bulge more and more, the baby is coming at an average speed. After about $1/2$ hour, you should start to see a little of the head during a push. Tell the mother to stop pushing right before the head crowns.

Very slow birth. If you do not see more and more bulging of the genitals after $1/2$ hour of strong pushing, the baby is coming very slowly. The mother may need to stand or squat to push, and use the hold-the-breath method for pushing (see p. 321).

As long as the baby continues to move down (even very slowly), and the mother has strength, things are probably OK. She should continue to push until the head crowns. Make sure she continues to drink liquids and urinates. A full bladder can slow down the birth.

If there is **no** bulging after $1/2$ hour of strong pushing, or if the mild bulging does not increase, the head may not be coming down. If the baby is not coming down at all after one hour of pushing, this may be a risk sign (see p. 253–256).

> **Caution!** It is dangerous to push on the mother's belly to make the baby come out. You can break the womb or cause other damage (see p. 245).

5. When the baby's head is about to crown, help the mother get in a good birthing position

These 4 positions are
good *birthing positions*:

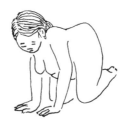

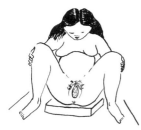

- hands-and-knees

- half-sitting, sitting (Be sure the mother's bottom is up on something, so that the midwife can get to the baby as soon as the head is born.)

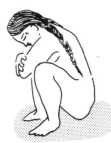

- squatting

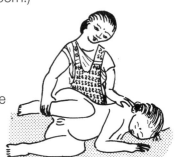

- lying on the left side (as long as there is someone to help hold up the mother's right leg)

6. Help prevent tears around the vaginal opening

Sometimes the birth of the head can tear the mother's vaginal opening. This is more common with first babies, tense women, or women who have been circumcised. To help prevent tears, you can massage the vaginal opening, use very warm cloths, slow the birth of the head, or cut a *circumcision scar* if necessary (see p. 406).

Massage the vaginal opening

To massage the vaginal opening:

1. Scrub your hands before touching the mother (see p. 159).

2. Wear sterile gloves if you have them. **If you must massage and do not have sterile gloves, wear plastic bags and keep your fingers on the outside skin only!**

3. Pour a little clean (unused) vegetable oil onto your fingers.

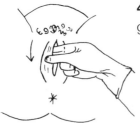

4. Put the tips of two fingers into the vagina (only if you have gloves on). Keep your thumb on the outside.

5. Start at the top, and move your fingers gently, but firmly, to pull the skin down and outward. Try to help the mother's muscles relax and stretch.

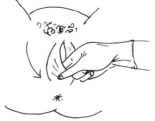

6. If the head starts to crown, you can stroke downward, away from the vaginal opening, with oiled fingers. If you see a white line appear at the bottom of the vaginal opening, this means the skin is stretched very thin. Gently try to move the skin downwards.

Note: If the mother says the massage hurts, you are massaging too hard. A hard massage will make the mother tense and increase the chance of tearing.

If she does not want the massage, do not do it.

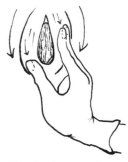

Stroke downwards with oiled fingers.

Use very warm cloths

Warm cloths around the vaginal opening help bring blood to the skin, making it more soft and stretchy:

1. Use only boiled or very clean water. If possible, add a little disinfectant (like iodine or betadine).

2. Dip a clean or sterile cloth in the water and wring it out. Touch the cloth to the inside of your wrist to see if it is too hot.

3. Press the cloth lightly on the mother's genitals. **Be careful not to burn her.**

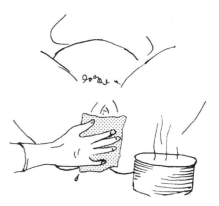

You can also help prevent tears by supporting the mother's skin with a warm cloth while the baby's head comes through.

Slow the birth of the head

If the head is born slowly, the mother's skin has more time to stretch and is less likely to tear. To slow the birth of the head, help the mother stop pushing.

When the mother should stop pushing

- If the baby is coming very fast, the mother should stop pushing right away, or the baby's head may tear her skin in one push.

- If the baby is coming at an average speed, the mother should stop pushing right before the baby's head crowns.

- If the baby is coming very slowly, the mother should keep pushing until the baby's head crowns.

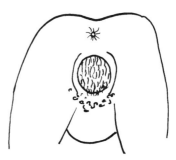

This mother should STOP PUSHING. The baby's head is about to crown.

How to help the mother stop pushing

The need to push can be very strong, so it is not always easy for the mother to stop pushing. It is best to teach the mother about how to stop pushing before she goes into labor (see p. 322).

To keep the mother from pushing, tell her to blow hard and fast. (It will be hard for her to blow and push at the same time.) Or, if the baby's head is not coming out and the mother can control her pushing, ask her to give a very small push—and then stop and blow. This gives her skin time to stretch. Each small push should move the head no more than one centimeter farther out of the mother. A centimeter is this long: |←→|

After the widest part of the head comes out, the rest of the head may come out without any pushing at all.

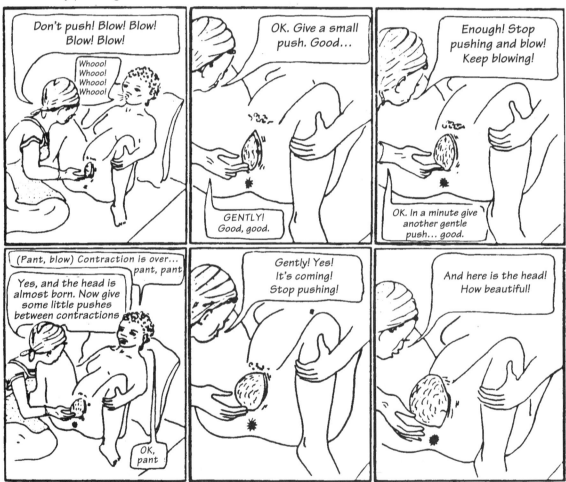

Caution! Do not slow the birth of the head if:
- there is a gush of blood before the birth (see p. 257).
- you have any reason to believe that the baby is in trouble.
- there is a prolapsed cord (see p. 250).

Cut a circumcision scar

In many parts of the world—especially Northern Africa, South Asia, and some parts of Egypt and Western Africa—many women have been circumcised. Circumcision causes scars that may not stretch enough for the baby's head to come out.

To avoid tearing and pain to circumcised women, most doctors recommend cutting the circumcision scar during stage 2, before the baby's head starts to crown. See p. 406.

If circumcision is done where you live, try to learn about delivering babies from someone who is experienced with circumcisions.

7. Check for a cord around the baby's neck

Often there is a short rest between the birth of the head and the birth of the shoulders. Check to see if the cord is wrapped around the baby's neck. If it is, slip it over the baby's head or shoulders after they come out.

If the cord is very tight, or seems to be wrapped around the neck more than once, see p. 258.

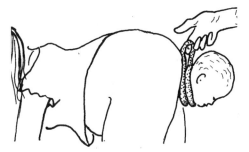

Usually, you can gently loosen the cord and slip it over the baby's shoulder as it is born.

8. Clear the baby's nose and mouth if necessary

If the baby's nose or mouth is clogged with fluid or mucus, you can clear them with a **bulb syringe** (sometimes called an ear syringe) or a **suction trap**. Both the syringe and suction trap should be sterile before you use them.

This is how to use a bulb syringe:

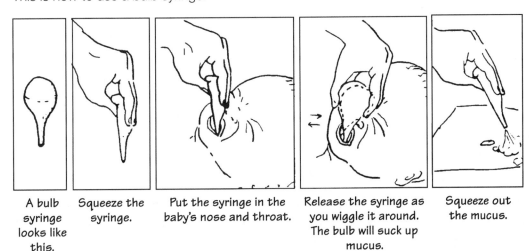

| A bulb syringe looks like this. | Squeeze the syringe. | Put the syringe in the baby's nose and throat. | Release the syringe as you wiggle it around. The bulb will suck up mucus. | Squeeze out the mucus. |

You should keep suctioning the baby's nose and throat until its breathing is clear.

A suction trap works even better than a syringe. To make one, you need a small jar, a cork, and some thin, soft tubing that can be cleaned easily. Make 2 holes in the cork, and push one tube through the cork till it almost touches the bottom of the jar. Push the second tube through until it is just below the cork.

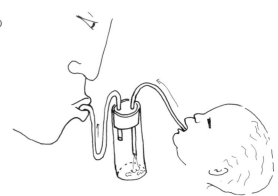

To use the trap, put the tube that goes to the bottom of the jar in the baby's mouth or nose (no more than 7 centimeters or 3 inches). Put the other tube in your own mouth. Wiggle the first tube around in the baby's mouth or nose while you suck on the other tube. The fluid in the baby's mouth or nose will go into the jar, but not into your mouth.

If you do not have a bulb syringe or suction trap, you can gently clear the baby's mouth and nose with a clean cloth wrapped around your finger.

9. Deliver the baby's shoulders

After the baby's head turns to face the mother's leg, wait for the next contraction. Ask the mother to give a gentle push as soon as she feels the contraction.

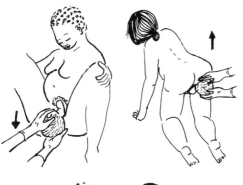

To prevent tearing, it is usually best to deliver one shoulder at a time. To deliver the top shoulder, gently move the baby's head toward the mother's tailbone.

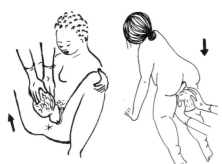

To deliver the bottom shoulder, gently move the baby's head toward her belly. If the shoulders are stuck, see p. 259.

Caution! Do not bend the baby's neck too much or too hard. Do not pull on the head. If the baby must come out quickly because there is a problem, have the mother push hard.

10. Deliver the baby's body and hand it to the mother

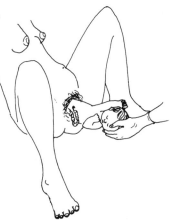

After the shoulders are born, the rest of the body usually slides out without any trouble. Remember that new babies are wet and slippery. Be careful not to drop the baby!

If everything seems OK, give the baby to the mother right away. You can put the baby on her stomach or in her arms (if the cord is long enough). You do not have to wait until the placenta comes out or the cord is cut. If the room is cold, put a clean blanket over the baby to keep it warm.

11. Cut the cord when it turns white and stops pulsing

When the baby is born, the cord is fat and blue. If you put your finger on it, you will feel it pulsing. This means the baby is still getting oxygen from its mother.

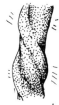
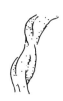

WAIT! OK to cut

When the placenta separates from the wall of the womb, the cord will get thin and white and stop pulsing. Now the cord can be cut. (In some places it is the custom to wait until the placenta is born before cutting the cord. When there is no medical emergency, this custom is not harmful.)

How to cut the cord

1. Use a sterile string or sterile clamp to tightly tie or clamp the cord about 2 finger widths from the baby's navel. The chance of the baby getting tetanus is greater when the cord is cut far from its body. Tie a square knot.

2. Put another sterile string or clamp a little further up the cord.

3. Cut the cord between the strings or clamps with a sterile knife, razor blade, or scissors. (Anything that is sharp enough to cut the cord will work, as long as it has been boiled for 20 minutes. If you have a new, unused razor blade in its original wrapper, it does not need to be boiled.)

4. Leave the string or clamp on until the cord falls off.

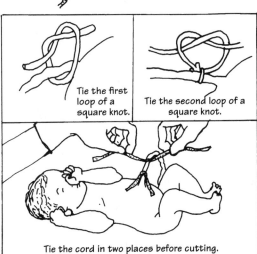

Tie the first loop of a square knot.

Tie the second loop of a square knot.

Tie the cord in two places before cutting.

Caution! To avoid tetanus, AIDS, and other infections, the cord and anything that touches it must be very clean. Never put dirt or animal dung on the cord stump.

What to do during stage 3

Chapter 12 contents

What to do during stage 3

Stage 3 begins when the baby is born and ends when the placenta comes out. Stage 3 usually lasts less than one hour.

Overview of healthy signs and risk signs

This list of healthy signs and risk signs gives you an overview of what to look for in stage 3. Healthy signs indicate that stage 3 is going well. Risk signs may mean that something is wrong. If you find a risk sign, turn immediately to the page number following the risk sign to find out what to do next.

Healthy signs

The mother

- Small gush of blood comes from vagina.
- Cord gets longer.
- Cord may be fat and blue at first, then turns thin and white.
- Mother remains awake and alert.
- Placenta is born whole, in one piece, and attached to cord.
- Womb stays up in the mother's belly and remains hard.

The baby

- Baby may be blue at first, but "colors up" soon.
- Baby starts breathing within a few minutes.
- Baby's arms and legs are active—not limp.
- Baby has good reflexes.
- Baby's heartbeat is strong.
- Baby sucks at the breast.

Risk signs

The mother

- Heavy or constant bleeding **before** the placenta comes out (see p. 271).

- Mother has signs of shock (see p. 275).

- There is no sign that the placenta has separated after $1/2$ hour, or the placenta has not come out after one hour (see p. 275).

- Heavy or constant bleeding **after** the placenta comes out (see p. 276).

- Womb comes out with the placenta (see p. 279).

Risk signs for the baby

- Baby does not breathe at all (see p. 280).

- Baby has no heartbeat, or heartbeat is less than 80 beats per minute (see p. 281).

- Baby has trouble breathing (see p. 282).

- Baby is very pale or stays blue after the first few minutes (see p. 283).

What to do for the mother

If you are working alone, you will need to decide whether to care for the mother or the baby first:

- If the mother shows risk signs, you probably need to care for her first, and the baby later.

- If the mother is OK, it is usually best to care for the baby first. If you put the baby on the mother's belly, it will be easier to watch the mother and baby at the same time. It is also good for the mother and baby to be together as much as possible.

- In an emergency where both mother and baby are in trouble, we believe the mother's life is more important and that she should be helped first.

If you have a partner, one of you can give her full attention to the mother, and the other can take care of the baby.

1. Watch for heavy bleeding

Some bleeding is normal during stage 3. There will usually be a small gush of blood when the placenta separates and perhaps some blood from a tear in the mother's skin. But if there is more bleeding than a monthly bleeding **before** the placenta comes out, this is very dangerous.

If the mother is bleeding, you may see blood coming out the vagina. But sometimes the blood will stay inside the womb where you cannot see it. If the womb gets larger and softer than usual, it may be filling with blood. (Remember that when the placenta separates from the womb, the womb changes shape and rises in the belly. Do not confuse this with the womb getting larger.) If you see blood coming out of the vagina, or if you think that the mother may be *bleeding inside*, see p. 276.

If the mother is feeling faint or dizzy, help her lie down and put her legs and feet up. Check her pulse and blood pressure every 15 minutes for a while. It is normal for a new mother to feel this way if she gets up quickly after the birth, but it may also be a sign of shock and bleeding inside (see p. 275). If there are no other signs of shock, she may be fine and able to get up slowly after more rest. If you see other signs of shock, follow the treatment for shock on p. 243.

2. Watch for convulsions

If a woman had pre-eclampsia during pregnancy or labor, she may still have convulsions in the first 24–48 hours after giving birth. Watch her carefully (see p. 247).

3. Watch for signs that the placenta has separated

The placenta usually separates in the first few minutes after birth, but it may not come out for a while after that. It is OK for the woman to lie on her back while waiting for *signs of separation*. This is usually more comfortable for her.

These are signs that the placenta has separated from the womb:

Small gush of blood comes from vagina. A gush is a handful of blood that comes out all at one time, then stops. It is not a trickle or a flow. If blood keeps flowing after (or before) this gush, there may be a problem (see p. 271).

Cord gets longer. When the placenta comes off the wall of the womb, the placenta drops down closer to the vaginal opening. This may make the cord seem a little longer, since more of it is outside the mother's body.

After the cord stops pulsing and gets white, there is a way to tell if more of the cord comes out of the mother's body. Mark the cord with a piece of sterile string (or a sterile clamp) about a hand's width from the vaginal opening. When the placenta separates, the string will be farther away from the mother's body.

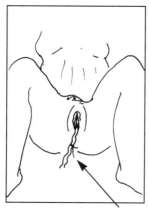

String marks the length of the cord.

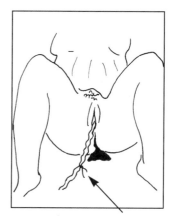

String moves farther from the mother's body, and there is a small gush of blood. The placenta has probably separated.

Womb changes shape and feel. Before the placenta separates, the womb is usually round but a little flat on top. The top of the womb is a little below the navel.

After the placenta separates, the womb usually rises to the navel or a little above. It may feel rounder or lean toward the front of her belly. It may also feel harder. If you use 2 fingers to push the womb gently to the side, the womb moves a little.

If it has been at least $\frac{1}{2}$ hour since the birth and there are no signs that the placenta has separated, see p. 275.

4. Deliver the placenta

Normal delivery

Once the placenta has separated, it can and should come out. To deliver the placenta:

1. Ask the mother to let someone else hold the baby for a while. Assure her that delivering the placenta will not hurt, because it is much smaller and softer than the baby. She should also feel more comfortable once the placenta is out.

2. Put on clean gloves or plastic bags.

3. Have the mother sit up or squat over a bowl. Ask her to push when she gets a contraction. It sometimes even helps for her to push between contractions. Usually the placenta slips out easily.

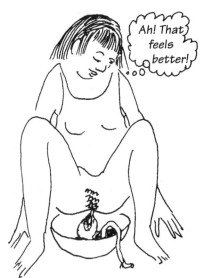

If the mother is having trouble pushing the placenta out, put the baby to breast to get a contraction. This contraction will help push the placenta out. If the baby will not nurse, try *nipple stimulation* (see p. 378).

If the placenta does not come out in 10 to 15 minutes, it may help to have the mother urinate (pee). A full bladder can slow the birth of the placenta.

4. The *membranes* from the bag of waters surrounding the baby should also come out with the placenta. If some of the membranes are still inside the mother after the placenta comes out, hold the placenta in 2 hands. Turn it slowly and gently until the membranes are twisted. (When they are twisted, they are less likely to tear inside.) Then **slowly** and **gently** pull the membranes out.

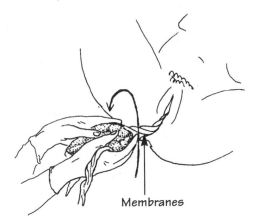

Membranes

5. Feel the mother's womb to make sure it is small and hard. If it is not small and hard, see p. 209–210.

The *cord-guiding* method

Sometimes a midwife will need to **gently** guide the placenta out by the cord. This should be done if the mother has trouble delivering the placenta herself, if she is too weak to sit or squat, or if she is bleeding a lot while the placenta is still inside. Guiding the placenta out is only done when you are sure the placenta is no longer on the womb wall, but is sitting in the vagina and the mother is unable to push it out herself. It is usually better, if the mother is not bleeding, to just let her push it out herself.

> **Caution!** Many midwives and traditional birth attendants are told to never pull on the cord. That is because pulling on the cord can cause bleeding, cause the cord to break off the placenta, or even pull the womb inside out. If midwives in your area have been taught to never pull on the cord, do not use this method.

This is the correct way to help the placenta out:

1. Make sure the cord is marked with a piece of sterile string (see p. 196). Then check for signs of separation by pushing the womb up from below. If the cord and string move up with the womb, the placenta is probably still attached. **Wait and try again later.** If the cord does not move up, the placenta is probably separated.

Find the bottom of the womb.   Push the womb up.

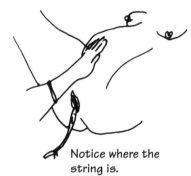

Notice where the
string is.

If the string stays in the
same place, the placenta may
be sitting in the vagina.

If the string moves up with
the womb, the placenta
may still be attached.

2. If you see signs of separation, press one hand beneath the womb to help hold the womb in place and feel if it moves. Wait for a good contraction—the womb will get tight and the mother can also tell you when a contraction comes.

3. Gently guide the placenta downward and outward by the cord. Be steady and smooth—a sudden or hard pull can tear the cord. Ask the mother to push while you are guiding out the placenta.

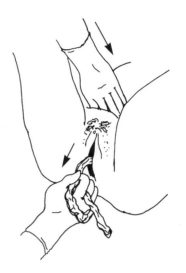

4. If the womb seems to move down as you pull the cord, **stop!** If the mother says it hurts, or if the placenta will not come, **stop!** The placenta may still be attached. Wait a few minutes and try again. If the womb still seems to move down, the placenta will not come, and there is no bleeding, **wait**. If the woman is bleeding, see p. 275.

5. If the womb stays up, and the cord is getting longer as you guide, continue to guide **gently** until the placenta comes out.

Caution! Pulling on the cord can be dangerous! If you pull too strongly on the cord and the placenta is still attached to the mother, the cord may break and cause bleeding. Or you can pull the womb out and **kill the mother**.

Never pull on the cord if the baby was born at least one month early, or seems small. The cord is likely to break.

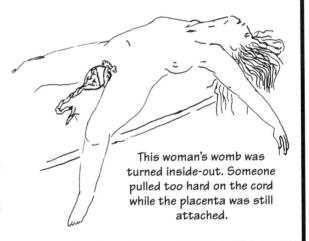

This woman's womb was turned inside-out. Someone pulled too hard on the cord while the placenta was still attached.

5. Check the placenta and cord

Usually the placenta comes out whole, but sometimes a piece gets left inside. This could cause bleeding or infection later. To see if everything has come out, check the top and bottom of the placenta, and the membranes from the bag of waters. This is also a good time to check the cord to see if it is normal.

Be sure to wear gloves or plastic bags when checking the placenta and membranes. If you do not have either gloves or plastic bags, use spoons or chopsticks to handle the placenta and membranes.

Top of the placenta. The *top of the placenta* (the side that was toward the baby) is smooth and shiny. The cord goes in on this side, and then spreads out into many deep blue blood vessels, like tree roots.

In rare cases there is an extra piece attached to the placenta. Check for blood vessels trailing off the edge of the placenta and going nowhere. This may mean that an extra piece is still inside the mother.

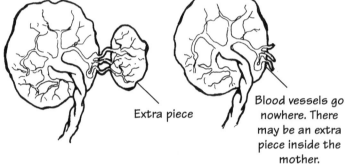

Extra piece

Blood vessels go nowhere. There may be an extra piece inside the mother.

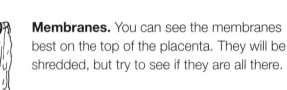

Membranes. You can see the membranes best on the top of the placenta. They will be shredded, but try to see if they are all there.

Bottom of the placenta. The *bottom of the placenta* (the side that was attached to the womb wall) has many lumps. To check this side, cup your hands and hold the placenta, so that all the lumps fit together. See if there is a hole where a piece seems to be missing. This piece may still be inside the mother.

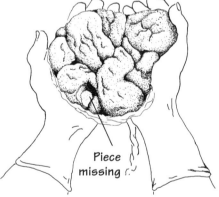

Piece missing

If you think pieces or membranes are missing, ask the woman to sit or squat—and then push or cough. If this does not bring the pieces out, see p. 278.

Note: The placenta of a baby who is born early is often very smooth. The placenta of a baby who is born late may have a lot of small white spots (like tiny rocks) on the lumpy side. These are *calcium deposits*. They are normal.

Cord. If you look carefully at the end of the cord, you should see 3 holes—1 large hole and 2 small holes. These are the arteries and vein that carried the baby's blood to and from the placenta.

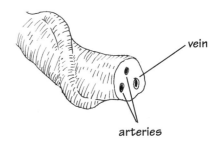

vein

arteries

If there are only 2 vessels in the cord, there is a small chance that the baby may have some problems. If possible, the baby should be checked by a doctor soon.

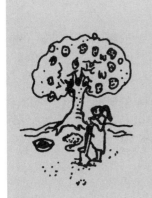

What to do with the placenta

There are different customs in different places. Some people burn it. Some cook and eat it. Some bury it in a corner of the house, or in the garden as fertilizer. Some dry the placenta and make medicine. Some use it for healing or protective magic. Some just throw it away.

In many areas of the world, the placenta should be buried deeply or burned (because of the risk of the AIDS virus in body waste, like blood). If the placenta is just thrown away, it should be wrapped tightly in a plastic bag.

What to do for the baby

In most cases, you can put the baby on the mother's belly as soon as it is born—even before you cut the cord. You can also check the baby while it is on the mother's belly.

Most babies are fine, but some need a little help getting started. Treat the new baby gently. Birth is difficult for a baby, too.

1. Check the baby's health

Some babies are alert when they are born. Other babies start slow, but as the first few minutes pass you can see that they are breathing and moving better, getting stronger, and becoming less blue.

Medical people often check for the following signs when the baby is one minute old, and again when the baby is about 5 minutes old. But be aware of them at all times. Notice whether the signs are getting better, worse, or staying the same.

Breathing

A new baby should be trying to breathe within 1 or 2 minutes after birth. Some healthy babies even cry at birth. A strong cry means that the baby is breathing well. But many healthy babies do not cry—especially if they are not upset. Never hit or hurt a baby to make it cry.

Watch the baby's nostrils and chest as it tries to breathe. If you see any of the following signs, the baby is having trouble breathing:

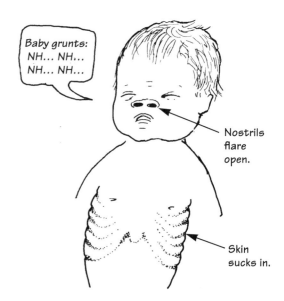

- Baby's nostrils *flare* (get larger) as it tries to take in air.

- Baby's skin between or below the ribs sucks in as it tries to breathe.

- Baby takes more than 60 breaths per minute in the first 2 hours after birth when it is resting. Count breaths by watching its tummy rise and fall.

- Baby grunts or makes a noise when it breathes out.

If you see any of these signs, turn to p. 282.

Heartbeat

A new baby's heart should beat between 120 and 160 beats per minute. You can check the baby's heartbeat by listening with a stethoscope.

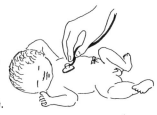

Or you can place 2 fingers over its heart. Count the heartbeat for one minute.

If the baby's heartbeat is between 80 and 100 beats per minute, get medical help to see if the baby is OK. If the baby's heartbeat is less than 80, it needs help **now!** Even if there is **no** heartbeat, it may still be possible to save the baby (see p. 281).

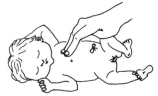

Muscle tone

If a healthy baby holds its arms and legs tight and close to its body, and its elbows and knees are bent, we say this baby has good *muscle tone*. A limp baby seems very relaxed. Its arms and legs are loose and open. But even if a baby is born limp, it should gain strength in its arms and legs within a few minutes.

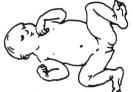

This baby has
good muscle tone.

The longer the arms and legs stay limp, the more likely it is that the baby is in trouble. If the baby is just a little limp, try rubbing its back and talking to it. This may help the baby wake up and try harder to breathe. If the baby is very limp, especially after the first minute, suction or try to wipe out its mouth and nose.

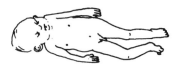

This baby is limp.

Reflexes

Reflexes are the body's natural and unthinking reactions to things. For example, when you fall down, you put your hands out to catch yourself— without even thinking about it. Or, when an insect flies at your eye, you blink. Good reflexes are a sign that the brain and nerves are working well.

At birth, a baby should have these reflexes:

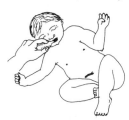

Grimace

Grimace. The baby should make a face when you put a finger in its mouth, or when you suction its mouth and nose (see p. 189).

Moro reflex. If the baby is dropped gently backward, or if it is moved suddenly or hears a loud noise, the baby stiffly flings its arms wide and opens its hands.

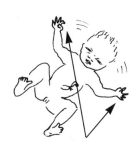

Moro reflex:
arms open wide

Sneeze. A sneeze means that the baby is reacting to the waters and mucus in its nose. (Of course, if there is no mucus or fluid in the nose, even a healthy baby will not sneeze.)

If the baby does not have any of these reflexes, but is breathing and its heartbeat is greater than 100 beats per minute, get medical advice.

Color

Most babies are blue or even purple when they are born, but they quickly become a more normal color in 1 to 2 minutes. Sometimes their hands and feet stay blue a little longer than the rest of the body. If the baby stays blue, see p. 283. If the baby is born very red, see p. 291. If the baby is born very pale, see p. 291.

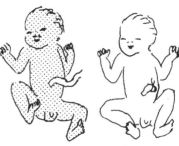

The baby may be born blue.

In a few minutes, most babies become a normal color.

2. Keep the baby warm and dry

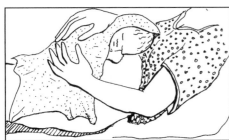

Dry the baby with a clean cloth or towel and keep it covered. If the baby is on the mother's body, this will be just the right temperature for the baby.

If the weather is hot, do not wrap the baby in heavy blankets or cloths. Do not make the room too hot. Too much heat can cause the baby to get dehydrated.

3. Help the baby begin breast feeding

The mother's milk will not come in for at least several days after the birth. But before the milk comes, her breasts make a liquid that nourishes the baby (*colostrum*). It is good to let the baby breast feed soon after birth, even before the placenta comes out.

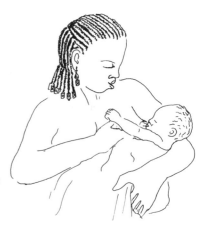

Early breast feeding has these advantages:

- Breast feeding makes the womb contract. This helps the placenta come out, and it helps prevent heavy bleeding.

- Breast feeding is a good way for the mother and baby to begin to know each other.

- Breast feeding comforts the baby.

- Breast feeding can help the mother relax and feel good about her new baby.

If the baby does not want to suck right away, try again later. If the mother has trouble getting the baby into a good position, prop the baby (or the mother's arms) up with something soft. If the baby still has a lot of mucus, lay the baby across the mother's chest with its head down before and while it nurses. This will help the mucus drain.

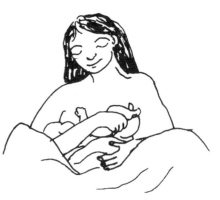

4. Put medicine in the baby's eyes to prevent blindness

A mother can have an infection in her vagina that she does not know about. When the baby is born, the infection can get in the baby's eyes and make it blind.

To prevent blindness, put a small amount of erythromycin 0.5% *eye ointment* (also called Ilotycin) or a little tetracycline 1% eye ointment (also called Latycin) in each of the baby's eyes. **Do this for every baby within 4 hours of its birth, even if the mother seems very healthy!**

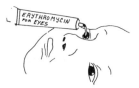

In some areas, people use *silver nitrate* (or other "silver" eye medicines) in the baby's eyes. These medicines stop *gonorrhea blindness*, but they do not stop other forms (for example, the blindness that comes from Chlamydia). Silver nitrate also irritates the baby's eyes for a few days. If you can get erythromycin or tetracycline eye medicines, use one of them. If you can only get silver nitrate medicine, use that or whatever your health ministry recommends.

Caution! If you see *pus*, swelling, or redness in the baby's eyes in the first few days, seek medical help immediately!

---

5. Give the baby a vitamin K injection

When babies are born they are not able to make their blood clot to stop bleeding. In many areas all new babies are given an injection of vitamin K to help them make blood clots. This is very important for all babies, but especially for those who had long labors or a lot of swelling in the head, for small babies, or for babies who will be *circumcised*. Check with your local health authorities to see if you should be giving new babies vitamin K. (See p. 386 for how to give a baby an injection.)

o

What to do during the first 2 to 6 hours after birth

Chapter 13 contents

What to do during the first 2 to 6 hours after birth

This part of labor and birth begins after the placenta has come out. It lasts for the first 2 to 6 hours after birth.

Ideally the midwife or another trained person should stay with the mother for 6 hours, but this is not always possible. Before the midwife leaves, she should make sure that the mother's womb is firm and hard, with only a little bleeding; that the mother has urinated (peed); and that the baby has begun to breast feed.

Overview of healthy signs and risk signs

This list of healthy signs and risk signs gives you an overview of what to look for during the first 6 hours after birth. Healthy signs indicate that things are going well. Risk signs may mean that something is wrong. If you find a risk sign, turn immediately to the page number following the risk sign to find out what to do next.

Healthy signs

The mother

- Mother is alert and interested in the baby.
- Genitals are not torn.
- Bleeding is no heavier than monthly bleeding.
- Womb stays tight and hard, and does not get bigger.
- Mother is able to urinate.
- Mother takes food and drink.

The baby

- Baby begins to breast feed.
- Baby continues to have good color, breathing, reflexes, muscle tone, and heartbeat.
- Baby urinates and has bowel movements (shits).

Risk signs

The mother

- Mother bleeds more than heavy monthly bleeding (see p. 285).

- Bleeding has stopped, but the mother has lost a lot of blood during the birth (see p. 286).

- Cervix can be seen at the vaginal opening (see p. 286).

- Mother has pain in the birth area or a growing blood blister (hematoma) in the vagina (see p. 287).

- Mother feels ill, is hot-to-touch (or her temperature is above 38°C or 100.4°F); her pulse is fast and her womb is tender (see p. 287).

- Mother cannot urinate after 4 hours (see p. 287).

- Mother cannot (or will not) eat or drink after 2 or 3 hours (see p. 288).

- Mother is not interested in the baby (see p. 288).

- Mother cannot (or will not) breast feed (see p. 289).

- Mother has convulsions (fits) or had signs of pre-eclampsia before the birth (see p. 289).

The baby

- Baby has trouble breathing, or takes more than 60 breaths per minute (see p. 290).

- Baby is limp, weak, or cannot seem to wake up (see p. 290).

- Baby is still blue, yellow, pale or red one hour after birth (see p. 291).

- Baby is limp, cold-to-touch (or its armpit temperature is less than 36°C or 97°F $1/2$ hour after birth) (see p. 291).

- Baby makes a strange, high-pitched cry (see p. 292).

- Baby shows signs of infection: baby takes more than 60 breaths per minute $1/2$ hour after birth; baby is cold-to-touch (or armpit temperature stays below 36°C or 97°F); baby seems ill, sucks poorly, and has a weak, fast heartbeat (see p. 292).

What to do for the mother

1. Prevent heavy bleeding

After the birth, it is normal for a woman to bleed like heavy monthly bleeding. The blood comes out in little spurts when the womb contracts, or when the mother coughs, moves, or stands up. The blood should also look just like monthly blood—old and dark, or pinkish.

If the mother bleeds more than heavy monthly bleeding, it can be dangerous. To check for heavy bleeding in the first 2 to 3 hours after birth, do the following:

- Check the womb right after the placenta is born, and then every 15 minutes for one hour and every $1/_2$ hour for the next 1 to 2 hours. If the womb is hard, this probably means it is contracting as it should. Leave it alone between checks. If it is soft, see the section below for what to do.

- Check the mother's pads often.

- Take the mother's pulse and blood pressure every 15 minutes for one hour, and then every hour for the next 4 hours. Watch for signs of shock (see p. 243).

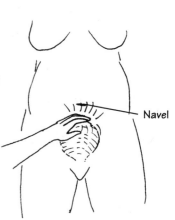

Navel

How to help a *soft womb* contract

If the womb is soft, there are natural ways to help it tighten up:

- Check the mother's bladder. An over-full bladder can keep the womb from contracting properly. If the bladder is over full, help the mother urinate. If she cannot urinate after 4 hours, she may need to have a tube (**catheter**) put into her bladder to help her urinate (see p. 391).

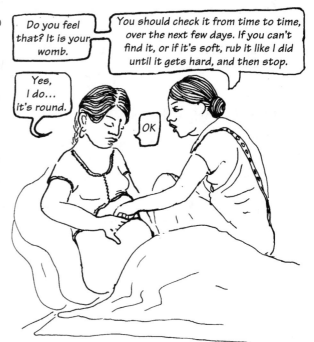

Do you feel that? It is your womb.

Yes, I do... it's round.

You should check it from time to time, over the next few days. If you can't find it, or if it's soft, rub it like I did until it gets hard, and then stop.

OK

- Massage the womb: Gently put your hand on top of the womb and make a circular motion while squeezing the womb. Check the womb every 1 or 2 minutes for a while. If it gets soft again, rub it until it tightens up again. Teach the mother and her family how to check the womb and how to rub it to make it hard (see p. 326).

■ Push on the womb to squeeze out clots. If there are clots in the womb, they can keep it from contracting properly. Squeeze them out by pushing on the womb like this:

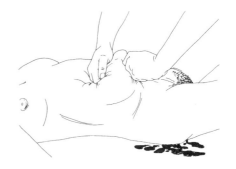

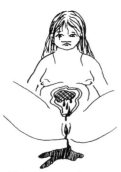 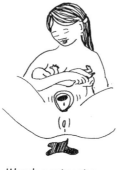

Womb stays large.   Womb contracts.

■ Encourage the mother to breast feed. When the baby sucks, it helps the mother's body make oxytocin. Oxytocin makes the womb contract or squeeze tight (just as it did during labor); this will help slow the bleeding. Explain the importance of breast feeding to the mother and her family.

If the womb continues to stay soft, if bleeding is heavier than a heavy monthly period, or if there is fresh, red blood that does not look like monthly bleeding, see p. 285.

> **Caution!** If the womb feels firm but is growing larger, it may be filling with blood. This is dangerous! The more blood that fills the womb, the more difficult it is for the womb to contract and stop bleeding. If the womb stays soft and does not tighten up, squeeze the womb to make the blood come out.

Judge whether the mother has lost too much blood

Even if a mother's bleeding has stopped, she may have lost enough blood to cause problems. It may take her longer to get her strength back after childbirth, and she is more likely to get infections of the womb.

The amount of blood loss that is dangerous for the mother depends on her general health. A healthy woman can lose more blood than an ill or malnourished woman and still be OK. Check how the woman feels, not just the amount of blood lost.

If a woman feels very weak, faint, or dizzy, even while lying down, she may have lost too much blood (especially if she still feels this way after 1 to 2 hours). See p. 243.

2. Clean the mother's genitals, belly, and thighs

The mother may want to wash after the baby is born. If she is not ready to get up, you can make her more comfortable by changing her bedding and washing her body.

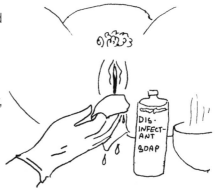

You should scrub and put on gloves before you touch the mother's genitals, just as you did before the birth (see p. 159). Clean her genitals very gently, using very clean or boiled water, and a sterile cloth. If you have some disinfectant, like betadine, add a little to the water. (Do not use alcohol or any other disinfectant that might sting the mother.) Use soap if you do not have disinfectant.

Wash downwards, away from the vagina. Be careful not to bring anything up from the anus (butt hole) towards the vagina. Even a piece of stool that is too small to see can cause infection.

3. Check for tears and other problems

Gently examine the mother's genitals for tears, a blood clot or a blood blister under her skin (**hematoma**), or a cervix that has dropped down to the vaginal opening (**prolapsed cervix**). If you find a hematoma, see p. 287; a prolapsed cervix, see p. 286; a tear, see p. 395.

4. Make sure the mother urinates

A mother's bladder will probably be full after birth, but she may not realize it. Try to get her to urinate within the first 2 to 3 hours.

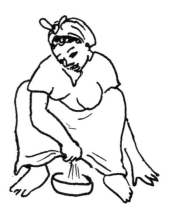

If the mother can get up and walk to urinate, make sure someone goes with her in case she faints. If she is too tired to get up and walk, she can squat over a bowl in the bed or on the floor. She can also urinate into a clean towel or other material while lying down.

It may be hard for her to relax her bottom enough to urinate. Sometimes it helps to pour clean, warm water over her genitals while she tries to urinate.

If she cannot urinate for 4 hours after the birth, or if her bladder seems over full and she cannot urinate, see p. 391.

5. Give liquid and offer food to the mother

After the birth, the mother can eat every kind of nutritious food. Customs that restrict the mother's diet after birth (like those that allow her to eat only the main food) are very harmful. Avoiding certain foods can lead to anemia, infection, and even death for the mother. Also, it will be harder for her to make milk.

If she is hungry right away, it is OK for her to eat whatever she wants. If she is not hungry, she should at least have something to drink. Fruit juice is good because it gives energy. Some juices also have vitamin C, which reduces the chance of heavy bleeding. Encourage her to eat soon, within the first few hours, and to drink often.

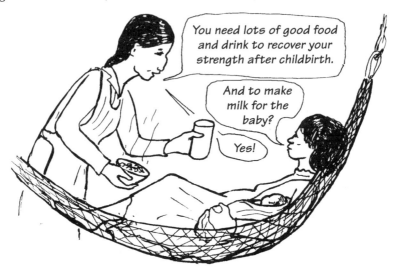

> You need lots of good food and drink to recover your strength after childbirth.
>
> And to make milk for the baby?
>
> Yes!

Note: If a mother gets constipated easily, she should eat whole grains, and lots of fruits and vegetables. She should avoid constipating foods, for 1 to 2 days.

7. Give the new family some time alone

While you are taking care of physical things, also try to be aware of the emotional needs of the new family. The mother may feel many different things after the birth. She may feel weak and tired, or very excited. She may wish to spend time with her baby. Many women cannot sleep for several hours after a birth.

The new parents often need a few minutes alone with each other and their new baby. A good time for them to be alone is when you examine the placenta. The parents also may need to talk, laugh, cry, or celebrate in some way. Traditional rituals are sometimes very comforting and helpful to the new family.

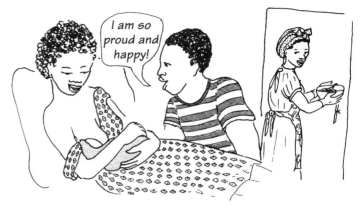

> I am so proud and happy!

What to do for the baby

If the baby does not have any risk signs, and the mother seems OK, it is time to give the baby a more complete exam. Many health problems can be prevented or cured if you find them quickly and take care of them.

Make a clean place to put the baby as you examine it. Then scrub your hands, just as you did for the birth, and put on gloves (if possible). It is easy for a new baby to get an infection, so everything that touches the new baby must be as clean as possible. Wearing gloves until the baby is bathed will also help prevent you from getting an infection.

Write down what you find at each step on a chart. A chart will help you remember to do each step and to notice changes that happen over time. Here is an example of a chart you can use:

16 steps to a newborn baby exam

1. General appearance						
2. Physical signs	Hour 1	Hour 2	Hour 3	Hour 4	Hour 5	Hour 6
breathing						
heartbeat						
temperature						
3. Weight and length	kilos/pounds			cm/inches		
4. Skull	cm/inches					
5. Ears						
6. Eyes						
7. Nose and mouth						
8. Neck						
9. Chest						
10. Shoulders, arms, and hands						
11. Belly						
12. Genitals						
13. Hips						
14. Legs and feet						
15. Back						
16. Skin						

Remember! If you find any risk signs while examining the baby, turn immediately to the page number listed after the risk sign.

1. General appearance

The way a baby looks and sounds can tell you a lot about its health. Notice everything! Is the baby small or large? Fat or thin? Do its arms, legs, feet, hands, body, and head seem to be the right size? Is the baby tense or relaxed? Active or still?

Listen to the baby's cry. Every baby's cry is a little different, but a strange, high, piercing cry can be a sign of illness (see p. 292).

2. Physical signs: breathing, heartbeat, temperature

It is very important to watch the baby's physical signs, since it cannot tell you how it feels. Take these signs every hour for 2 to 6 hours after the birth.

Breathing rate

A new baby should take between 30 and 50 breaths per minute while it is resting. **Count the baby's breaths for one full minute by watching its belly rise and fall.** It is normal for breathing to slow down and speed up from moment to moment.

A baby who is breathing too fast or too slow, or is having difficulty breathing, may be having trouble getting enough air, or may be having other problems. See p. 290.

Heartbeat

A new baby's heart should beat between 120 and 160 beats per minute. If you have the equipment or have homemade supplies (see p. 429), you can take the baby's heartbeat by listening with a stethoscope, or you can place 2 fingers over its heart. Count the heartbeat for one minute.

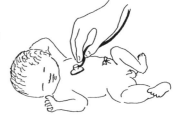

If the baby's heartbeat is above 160 beats per minute, it may have an infection (see p. 292). If the heartbeat is between 80 and 100 beats per minute, get medical help. If the heartbeat is below 80 beats per minute, the baby may not be getting enough air and **needs help *now!*** See p. 281.

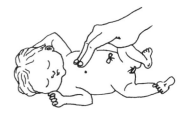

Temperature

A new baby's temperature taken under its arm is usually between 36° and 37.2°C, or 97° and 99°F. An ill baby is more likely to have a low temperature than a fever.

To take the baby's temperature, gently put the silver end of the thermometer into its armpit. Then press the baby's arm against its body. Hold it there for 5 minutes. If you do not have a thermometer, feel the back of the baby's neck while you touch a healthy person. If the baby does not feel as warm as the healthy person, its temperature is too low.

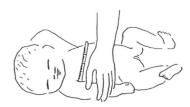

A baby may have a little trouble making its own heat at first, since the mother's body kept it warm before birth. A baby whose temperature is **between 35.5° and 36°C or 96° and 97°F should be warmed *quickly*.** Do not wait. See p. 291.

If the baby's temperature is below 35.5°C or 96°F, or stays between 35.5° and 36°C or 96° and 97°F for more than one hour, the baby may have an infection or other problems. See p. 292.

3. Weight and length

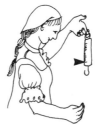

Weight

It is best if a new baby weighs between 2.5 and 4 kilograms (between 5.5 and 9 pounds). (See p. 430 for how to make a homemade scale.)

If you have a hanging scale, follow these steps:

1. Adjust the scale so that it is at 0 when nothing is on it. If there is no knob to adjust the scale, write down the number that the scale is at when nothing is on it.

2. Weigh the baby's blanket.

3. Weigh the baby and the blanket (or baby wrapper) together.

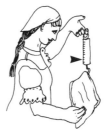
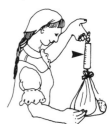

Nothing is on this scale, so it reads 0.

The blanket weighs .25 kilograms.

The baby and blanket together weigh 3.25 kilograms.

4. Then figure out the baby's weight like this:

Baby and blanket together weigh	3.25 kilograms
Blanket alone weighs	−.25 kilograms (take away this)
Baby alone weighs	3.00 kilograms

If you have a scale that you stand on, follow these steps:

1. Weigh yourself, and write down the weight.

2. Get off the scale.

3. Get back on the scale holding the baby without its clothes or blankets. Write down the weight.

4. Subtract your weight from the combined weight of you and the baby. For example: If you weigh 59 kilograms (130 pounds) and the combined weight is 62 kilograms (137 pounds), then the baby weighs 3 kilograms (7 pounds).

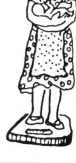

If the baby weighs less than 2.5 kilograms (5.5 pounds), see p. 292. If the baby weighs more than 4 kilograms (9 pounds), see p. 294.

Note: Before you weigh the baby, look at it, feel it, and guess its weight. Then weigh the baby and see whether you are correct. This will help you learn how to guess the size of a baby that is still inside the mother.

Length

Gently stretch the baby. With a tape measure, measure from the top of its head to the bottom of its heel. Most babies are between 45 and 53 centimeters, or 18 and 21 inches.

4. Skull

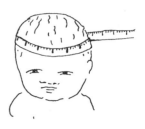

While you have the tape measure out, measure the baby's head. The normal size for a baby's head is 35 centimeters or 13 to 14 inches. Write down the head size. When you measure the head a few days later, you can look at this number and know how much the head has grown.

Head shape, suture lines, soft spots

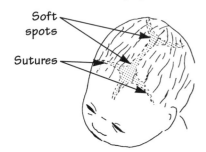

Soft spots

Sutures

The skulls of children and adults are solid, but the new baby's skull is made of 5 separate pieces. The soft areas between these 5 pieces are called **sutures** or **suture lines**. The baby's skull also has 2 larger soft areas called soft spots or **fontanels**.

The suture lines and soft spots help the baby's head change shape so it can move through the mother's vagina. Sometimes the skull bones even have to overlap for the head to be born. This is called **molding**. When the baby is first born, its head often stays the same shape that it was during birth (but will usually become its regular shape in 1 to 3 days). Here are some of the different shapes you might see at birth:

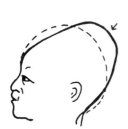
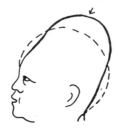
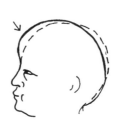
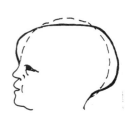

Molding is normal, but the suture lines and soft spots can alert you to other problems. Feel the suture lines with your fingers. The front suture should stop at or near the top of the forehead. Notice if the lines are a normal width or unusually wide. Also feel the soft spots: are they soft, or tense and bulging?

If the sutures are unusually wide, if the front suture goes down to the middle of the forehead, or if the soft spots are tense or bulging, the baby may have *water on the brain* (**hydrocephalus**). Hydrocephalus can make a child mentally slow, or cause other serious problems. Get medical advice. An operation can help the baby.

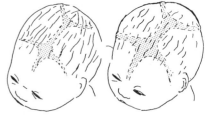

OK   Not OK

Caputs and hematomas

Some babies have swelling (a **caput**) in the area that was pressed against the cervix during labor and birth. A caput usually crosses a suture line. It will go away in 1 or 2 days.

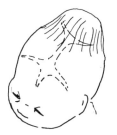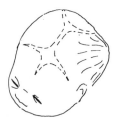

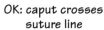

If you find a swelling on the head that does not cross a suture line, it may be a hematoma. This means that the birth was difficult for the baby. It also can cause the baby to get yellow eyes and skin (**jaundice**) as it heals. Jaundice can be dangerous to the baby.

OK: caput crosses suture line　　　Not OK: hematoma

If you find a hematoma, check the baby every day for signs of jaundice (see p. 303) until the hematoma is gone.

5. Ears

To check the baby's ears, look straight into its face. Imagine a line across its eyes. Some part of each ear should be above this line.

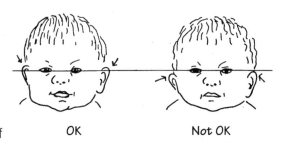

OK　　　Not OK

If the ears are uneven or low, there may be a problem with the baby's insides. The baby should be watched carefully. If both ears are below the line, the baby may have kidney problems and should see a doctor.

6. Eyes

Look at the baby's eyes. Notice if they seem normal, and if they move together. A little bit of blood under the surface of the eye is OK, if it is not in the **pupil** (the dark spot in the center of the eye). The blood should go away in a few days.

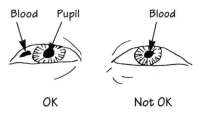

Blood　Pupil　　　Blood

OK　　　Not OK

7. Nose and mouth

First see if the baby can breathe easily through its nose. If not, try suctioning the baby again (see p. 189).

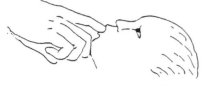

Baby sucks well

Then gently stroke the baby's cheek. It should turn its head toward your finger. This is called the **rooting reflex**. Put your clean finger inside the baby's mouth. The baby should suck on your finger. If there is no rooting reflex, and if the baby does not suck, it may be very sick (see p. 306).

8. Neck

Check the neck for swelling and lumps. Make sure to notice if the **thyroid** (the lump in the front of the throat) is swollen. If you find any problems, get medical advice.

9. Chest

Shape

First look to see if the shape and size of the chest seems normal. Watch the baby breathe. If the skin between and under the baby's ribs sucks in when it takes a breath, the baby is having trouble breathing (see p. 189, 282).

Breath sounds

Listen to the baby's breathing. Use a stethoscope or fetoscope if you have one. If not, just use your ear. You should hear breathing sounds on both sides of the chest, and on both sides of the back. If you do not hear breathing sounds on both sides, one lung may not be working. **Get medical help immediately.**

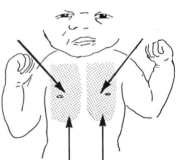

Breath sounds should be the same on both sides.

Heart sounds

If you have a stethoscope or fetoscope, use it to listen to the baby's heart sounds, too.

It is hard to describe heart sounds in a book. We recommend that someone teach you, if possible. But listen to the baby's heart sounds even if you are not skilled. Over time you will learn what sounds normal, and will be able to notice unusual sounds. If the heart sounds unusual, get medical advice.

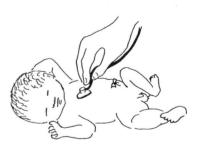

10. Shoulders, arms, and hands

Take a look at the baby's arms and hands. Do they look normal? Does the baby move them normally?

Sometimes a baby's shoulders, collar bones, or arms break during the birth. Feel them to see if there are any odd lumps or breaks. A baby with a broken bone may be crying in pain, but it may not. Or it may be crying for other reasons.

Next, check the Moro reflex again (see p. 203) to see if the baby's arms open wide and move in the same way.

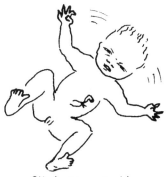

OK: Arms open wide

If you find any problems, get medical advice.

11. Belly

Look at the belly. Does it look normal? Has the cord stopped bleeding? If it is still bleeding, try clamping or tying it tighter. If this does not work, get medical help.

What happens to the area around the cord when the baby cries? If some of the baby's insides push the skin out, this means the belly wall is not fully formed. This is called an **umbilical hernia**. The baby should be seen by a doctor.

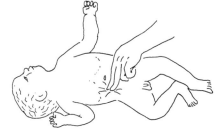

Next, feel the belly. When the baby is not crying, the belly should be soft. Check for lumps, round sacks of fluid (**cysts**), or other odd shapes. If you find anything odd, the baby should be seen by a doctor.

12. Genitals

Spread the baby's legs to look at its genitals. All babies' genitals will look swollen. If the baby was breech, the genitals may be very swollen.

For a boy

First look at the baby's balls (**scrotum**). The scrotum will probably look large for the baby's body. This is normal.

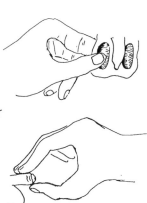

The scrotum contains 2 sacks. Inside each sack, there is a smooth, round **testicle** (where the boy's seed is stored). Sometimes, especially if it is cold, the testicles will be up high and not actually in the sacks. You should be able to feel the testicles and move them down with your fingers. If you cannot find one or both testicles, try warming the baby.

Next, check to see if the hole at the end of the **penis** seems in the right place.

If the penis does not look normal, or if there are any problems with finding the testicles, get medical advice.

Male circumcision

Circumcision is an operation to remove the skin around the tip of the penis *(foreskin)*. Circumcision is not medically necessary, but it is important in many cultures or religions. Sometimes the baby boy is circumcised right after birth, or a few months after birth. Sometimes he is not circumcised until he is 13 years old.

Only a very skilled person should circumcise a baby. Anything used to cut the foreskin must be sterile.

The risks of circumcision are infection, bleeding, injury to the penis, and pain and trauma to the baby. Serious bleeding is less likely if you wait until the baby is 8 days old. However, some people believe that younger babies (about one week old) suffer less than older ones (over one month old). Cultures which wait until the boy is 13 years old may believe the pain is an important part of becoming a man.

If a boy is not circumcised, he may get more infections of his penis if it isn't kept clean. Teach the parents to gently clean the skin around the tip of the penis from time to time and clean away the white cream underneath. At first, the skin may not move back very far. Over the next weeks and months the skin will move farther back, but it can take as long as 3 to 5 years for it to go all the way back. Also encourage the parents to teach young boys to clean under the skin at least 2 times each week.

For a girl

Make sure that the girl has both outer and inner "lips" of her genitals. She should also have a small opening to her vagina. If she does not have an opening, she may need an operation. She should see a doctor immediately. It is normal for girls to have a small amount of blood from the vagina for 1 to 2 days after birth.

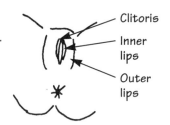

Girls are often circumcised, too, when they are older. In this procedure, the clitoris (pleasure spot) at the front end of the vagina is cut out. Sometimes part of the vaginal lips is also cut away. This is a dangerous procedure and should be avoided. Girls who have been circumcised may have frequent urinary and vaginal infections, and difficulty during childbirth.

For both boys and girls

Make sure that the anus is really an opening, and not covered over with skin. If the baby has had a bowel movement, you know that this part of the body works. **If the baby has no anus, or if it is closed, the baby needs to see a doctor immediately or it will die.**

If the baby has no opening for urinating, it should see a doctor immediately.

13. Hips

To check the hips, hold the baby's legs like this:

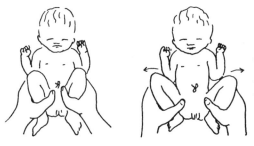

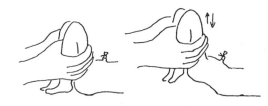

Gently move the hips straight out to the sides. Listen or feel for a click as you move the legs.

Next, gently move each leg up and down. Again, listen or feel for a click as you move them.

If you find a click with either of these tests, the baby should see a doctor or skilled health worker for an x-ray during the first month after birth. The baby may need to wear a special cast or extra thick diapers for a while so its joints can grow properly.

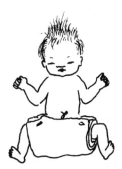

Also, see if you can find the baby's pulse in the place where the leg and genitals come together. A skilled person may have to teach you. If a skilled person cannot find this pulse, the baby may not have good blood flow to the legs. Get medical advice.

14. Legs and feet

Check to see if both legs look normal. Are they the same length? If one of the baby's feet turns inward and cannot be straightened, it may have a *club foot*. This can be helped if the baby sees a doctor.

15. Back

Turn the baby over and look at its spine. Look for holes, sores, cysts, growths, or tufts of hair.

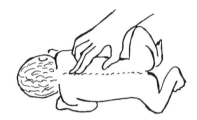

Move your fingers down the baby's spine to feel the bumps of its spinal bones. Can you feel a flat spot in the spine? Are there any holes in the skin at the bottom of the spine where the baby's buttocks begin?

If you find any of these signs, get medical advice.

16. Skin

Look carefully at the baby's skin. Some babies have spots on the skin that are darker than the rest of the skin. Some of these spots are OK, and some may be a sign that something is wrong. If you are not sure, get medical advice.

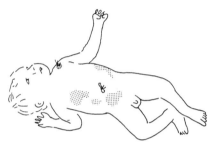

Also, check the baby's skin color. If the baby's body is still blue, yellow, pale, or red after one hour, see p. 291.

Note: Before you leave, make sure the mother and family know what is normal to expect in the next few days, what risk signs to look for, and what to do if risk signs appear.

Giving BCG *immunizations*

In some places, where there is a lot of tuberculosis (TB), a vaccination is given to all babies at birth. In other places this vaccination is given at birth only to babies of mothers who have TB. The dose of BCG for infants is 0.05 cc intradermally (between the layers of skin). If you do not give the BCG yourself, remind the mother to have the baby immunized in the first month at the nearest health center.

What to do during the first 2 weeks after birth

Chapter 14 contents

What to do during the first 2 weeks after birth

The last part of labor begins 6 hours after the birth. It lasts for 2 weeks after birth.

Overview of healthy signs and risk signs

This list of healthy signs and risk signs gives you an overview of what to look for during the first 2 weeks after birth. Healthy signs indicate that things are going well. Risk signs may mean that something is wrong. If you find a risk sign, turn immediately to the page number following the risk sign to find out what to do next.

Healthy signs

The mother

- Womb stays small and hard.

- Bleeding gradually grows less (although it may increase when the mother gets up or is more active).

- Mother may have mild contractions (after pains) from time to time for the first few days, especially when she breast feeds.

- Mother's milk comes in within 2 to 4 days, if she breast feeds often.

The baby

- Baby loses weight in the first 2 days after birth, but is back to its birth weight by 10 days after birth.

- Baby sleeps a lot.

- Baby urinates (pees) 7 to 10 times per day.

- Baby has a bowel movement (shits) at least one time per day.

- Baby cannot lift its own head.

Risk signs

The mother

- Womb does not stay round and hard, and it does not get slowly smaller (see p. 297).

- Mother bleeds a lot (see p. 298).

- Mother has signs of shock (see p. 297, 243).

- Mother has signs of womb infection: bleeding starts again or gets worse, blood or discharge smells bad or has an unusual color, mother feels ill, is hot-to-touch (or has a temperature above 38°C or 100.4°F), or has chills or pain in the belly (see p. 298).

- Mother has signs of vaginal infection: pain "down below"; pus; a swollen, hard, red lump in the vagina (see p. 299).

- Mother's breasts are painful, red, or swollen (see p. 300, 333–334).

- Mother feels extreme depression (sadness), anger, fear, or craziness (see p. 301).

- Mother's legs are red, hard, and swollen (see p. 301).

- Mother's urine or stool seems to leak out of the vagina (see p. 302).

The baby

- Baby does not have a bowel movement within 24 hours after birth (see p. 302).

- Baby does not urinate within 24 hours after birth (see p. 303).

- Baby gets yellow (jaundice) (see p. 303).

- *Vomit "shoots" out* when the baby spits up (see p. 303).

- Baby does not gain weight normally, or appears thin and stays small (see p. 304).

- Baby has signs of dehydration (see p. 305).

- Baby has signs of infection (see p. 306).

- Baby has signs of tetanus (lockjaw) (see p. 308).

What to do for the mother

We suggest that you visit the mother and baby the day after the birth, and then again at least once in the next week. During these visits you can check for healthy signs and risk signs.

A midwife can also help by:

- Encouraging the mother to eat every kind of nutritious food she can get (see p. 46–56).

- Encouraging the mother to get plenty of rest. It is OK for her to do light work when she feels well enough. Do not make her stay in bed all day unless she is very ill.

- Encouraging the mother to stay clean. It is good for her to bathe, and to keep her genitals and breasts very clean. If plant medicines are used to help her genitals heal, they should be clean (boiled is best). **Do not put plant medicines inside the vagina.**

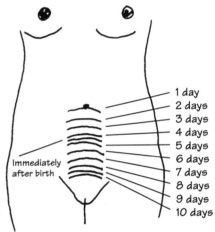

- Allowing the mother's womb to return to its normal size. Do not give her any herbs or medicines that will stop her contractions for 2 to 3 days after birth. These contractions help the womb close down. It is OK to give acetaminophen or paracetamol for pain at any time if everything else is going well. This picture tells you about where the top of the womb should be for the first ten days after birth:

- Giving the mother emotional support. Traditional customs and rituals that honor the mother, celebrate the birth or thank the midwife are often very good for everyone.

In addition, the family can help prevent problems by:

- Massaging the mother's womb if it gets soft. A midwife should teach the mother and her family how to check the womb by feeling it, and to rub it to make it contract.

- Checking the mother's temperature 2 times a day for the first week. If her temperature is above 38°C or 100.4°F, have the mother or family notify you immediately.

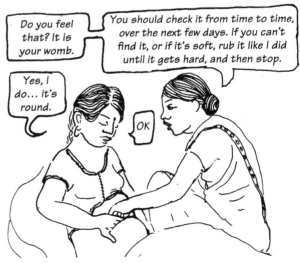

What to do for the baby

It is not complicated to take care of a healthy baby. Here are some basic rules the mother and family should know:

- Keep the baby clean. Anything that goes in the baby's mouth should be very clean.

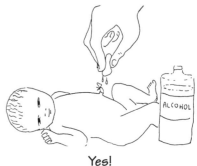

Yes!

- Keep the cord stump clean and dry. Always clean your hands before touching the cord stump. Wash the cord gently 3 to 4 times a day with alcohol, gin, or gentian violet. This will kill germs and help the cord dry and fall off. Do not put anything else, especially animal dung, on the cord. This can cause tetanus and kill the baby. If the baby is wearing diapers, ask the mother to keep the diaper folded below the cord.

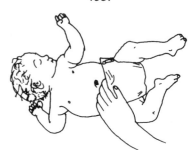

Yes! Diapers are below cord stump.

If the cord or the area around the cord gets red, drains pus, or smells bad, see p. 306. The drying cord may smell a little odd—like dried meat—but it should not smell foul.

The cord should fall off in about 5 to 7 days after birth. When the cord falls off, there is often a smooth, silvery mucus underneath that should go away in 1 to 2 days. If the mucus is white, yellow, grainy, or foul smelling, see p. 306.

There also may be a few drops of blood when the cord falls off. If the baby continues to bleed, put pressure on the cord area—just enough to stop the bleeding. Do not press too hard. If the bleeding does not stop, keep pressure on the cord area and get medical help.

- Let the baby breast feed often, starting from the very first day (see chapter 21).

- Take the baby's temperature (see p. 214) if it is not feeling well or is not breast feeding well.

- Check to see that the baby is back to its birth weight 10 days after birth.

- Keep the baby warm but not hot. Too much heat can lead to dehydration (see p. 305).

- Take the baby out in the sunlight (sunlight is good for the baby), but avoid sunburn.

- Encourage the mother to take the baby to the health clinic for **immunizations** and well baby checkups. The first visit should be in the first month. The baby should receive BCG (if it hasn't been immunized at birth) and TT (tetanus toxoid), or DPT (a combination of immunizations given together).

Check with your local health authorities, if possible, because the schedule of immunizations can change. This chart gives one immunization schedule:

Vaccine	Minimum age at 1st dose	Number of doses	Minimum interval between doses
BCG*	Birth or any time after birth	1	
DPT	6 weeks	3	4 weeks
Hep. B	6 weeks	3	4 weeks
Polio	6 weeks	3	4 weeks
Measles	9 months	1	

* Given in places where there is a lot of tuberculosis.

SECTION D

Complications of labor and birth

Introduction

Although most babies are born without problems, sometimes things can go wrong. When things go wrong, we call these problems **complications**. There will usually be risk signs to warn you of complications.

Some risk signs are more serious than others. A risk sign may mean there is nothing wrong now, but that there is a danger that **something might be wrong soon** (for example: waters break but labor does not start within 8–12 hours). Or it may mean that **something *might* be wrong** (for example: a long labor). Or it may mean that **something is *already wrong***, that there is a great danger, and the woman or baby needs medical care immediately (for example: too much bleeding).

When you find a risk sign:

- Stay calm.

- Find out what is causing the risk sign (different problems can cause the same risk sign).

- Decide if a remedy is needed. Sometimes it is more dangerous to use a remedy than to do nothing.

- Get help when you need it. If the instructions in this book say *go to the hospital,* get help as soon as you see the risk sign. Do not wait to see if things get worse. If you cannot get to the hospital, or if the hospital is far away, there may be instructions on how to lessen the danger or deal with the emergency.

The next five chapters are arranged by risk sign and explain the signs that may appear during each stage of labor and childbirth:

- Complications in stage 1 (chapter 15)

- Complications in stage 2 (chapter 16)

- Complications in stage 3 (chapter 17)

- Complications in the first 2–6 hours after birth (chapter 18)

- Complications in the first 2 weeks after birth (chapter 19)

Complications in stage 1

Chapter 15 contents

Complications in stage 1

1. Labor begins before the 8th month of pregnancy

A baby in its mother's womb grows until the day it is born. During the last weeks of pregnancy, the baby's body gets ready for life outside the womb. Its lungs develop so it can breathe. The baby gets bigger and stronger so it can breast feed, digest food, and resist illness.

A baby that is born at 8 months—or even as early as 7 months—can live and become healthy if it has good care. But the earlier the baby is born, the harder it will be for it to survive. Also, the baby will face a greater danger of brain damage and illness. A baby that is born before 7 months usually cannot live without very advanced medical care in a good hospital.

Judging the baby's age

If you think that labor is beginning early:

- Check the mother's due date again by counting from the last monthly bleeding (see p. 78).

- Feel the mother's belly. Sometimes the due date you get by counting from the last monthly bleeding is wrong, so it is important to also check the size of the baby. A baby who can be delivered safely should reach $1/2$ way between the lower ribs and the **breast bone** (the bone between the mother's breasts). If you are not very skilled at judging the size of the baby, get help from someone who is.

If the due date says the woman is less than 7 months pregnant, but the baby feels as big as a 7 month baby (or bigger), it might be worth trying to save its life. The mother may really be 7 or 8 months pregnant.

Note: To learn how to guess the size of the baby before it is born, remember to practice these things:

- Guess the size of every baby when its mother starts labor.

- After every baby is born, weigh it and see if you guessed right. If you don't have a scale, look at the baby and remember how it felt inside its mother.

When to get medical help

If you decide that a baby is less than 8 months and a hospital is nearby, go immediately. The hospital may be able to give the mother medicine that will slow or stop the labor. If the baby is born anyway, the hospital will be better able to care for it.

You should also go to the hospital if you see any of these signs:

- Baby seems smaller than 2.0 kilograms or 4.5 pounds.
- Mother has signs of infection (see p. 235).
- Mother has unusual bleeding or pain (see p. 243–244).
- Mother's waters have broken.

When to stay at home

If the hospital is far away, or very expensive—or if there are other circumstances that make the chances of saving the baby small—the mother may prefer to stay at home. For example, if the baby is less than 7 months old it is likely to die, even in many hospitals. The mother also may decide not to go to the hospital if there is no heartbeat or movement from the baby for more than one day. The baby may be dead.

There are still some things that can be done at home. You may be able to help slow or stop the mother's labor by having her lie in bed with her hips up. She should stay in bed and remain quiet.

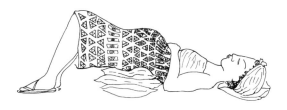

In addition, you can give her at least one liter (about one quart) of water, tea, or juice immediately—and then as much as she can drink every hour. Or if you know of an herbal tea in your area that is known to stop labor or to relax the body, give this to her now. You may consider giving her 200 cc or one cup of an alcoholic drink (beer or whatever is used in your area) every hour until the contractions stop. Be aware that the mother may become **intoxicated** (drunk). If she becomes too agitated or starts vomiting, stop giving her the alcoholic drink. Don't give her more than 3 glasses (don't try this for more than 3 hours).

If the labor does stop, the mother should not do much physical work for the rest of the pregnancy. She should rest, and avoid worry and strain, if possible.

2. Mother says she feels hot, she is hot-to-touch, or her temperature is above 37.8°C or 100°F

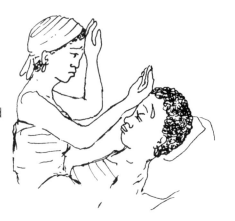

These are symptoms of fever. Fever is usually a sign of infection, which means that harmful germs have entered the womb, bladder, or kidneys and are poisoning the mother. Fever can also be caused by malaria.

Other signs of infection are:

- Mother's vagina smells bad.

- Mother has pain in the waist area—either in the front, on the sides, or in the back.

- Mother's belly is sore or tender to the touch.

- Mother's pulse is more than 100 beats per minute.

- Baby's heartbeat may be more than 160.

What to do

If the mother has a fever and one of these signs, she will need help immediately. Begin by giving her lots of fluids—water, rehydration drink (see p. 172), or herbal teas known in your area to reduce fever. You may give the mother 500 mg of paracetamol (acetaminophen) every 3 to 4 hours by mouth to reduce the fever. This medicine does not stop the infection, but it will help bring down fever.

If possible try to go to the hospital for intravenous (IV) fluids (see p. 414) and *antibiotics*. If medical help is more than an hour away, give one of the following antibiotics on the way:

- ampicillin 2 grams, every 6 hours

- penicillin VK 1 gram, every 6 hours (give only by mouth)

- penicillin G 2 million units, every 6 hours

- procaine penicillin 1.2 million units, every 6 hours

It is best to give these medicines (except penicillin VK) by *intramuscular injection* (IM), but it is still useful to give them by mouth (see p. 383–387). **Do not combine these medicines!** Be sure to ask the mother if she has ever had an allergic reaction to antibiotics (see p. 388). If she has, do not give her any but get to the hospital as quickly as you can.

If you cannot go to the hospital, give one of the antibiotics for at least 5 days, even if the mother's temperature goes down. After 5 days have passed, stop giving the antibiotic when the mother's temperature has been normal for 2 days.

Note: Some infections can only be cured by special antibiotics. You may want to talk to local health authorities to see if there are any special medicines you should carry in your kit.

3. Waters break but labor does not start within 8–12 hours or $\frac{1}{2}$ day

Once the bag of waters has broken, germs can start slowly moving into the womb. To avoid infection, the baby should be born within one day and one night (24 hours) after the waters break. Therefore, to have time for the labor and birth, the labor should start within 8–12 hours after the waters break.

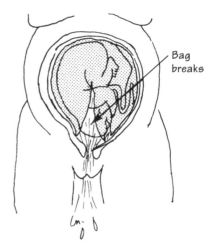

Bag breaks

When the bag breaks, the barrier to the womb is gone. Infection can start slowly creeping into the womb.

> Note: It is a good idea to check with the local doctor or health center to see how long they recommend waiting for labor to start after the water breaks. The amount of time may vary from area to area.

What to do

If labor has not started in 8–12 hours, or if it has started but stays weak, do the following:

- While waiting for labor, advise the mother not to have sex, not to put anything in her vagina, and not to sit in water. The mother should wipe her genitals from front to back after having a bowel movement (shitting).**The midwife should never give a vaginal exam. It might cause an infection.**

- If there are no signs of infection, you may wish to use a *"home method"* to help labor start or get stronger (see p. 377–382). Do not give the mother modern medicines like oxytocins at home to start labor. These medicines should only be used in a hospital.

- Watch the mother closely for signs of infection. If you have a thermometer take her temperature every 2 hours. If any signs of infection develop, see p. 235.

- Go to the hospital immediately if the baby is less than 8 months, if there are **any** other risk signs, if the woman has had many sexual partners, if her sexual partners have had many sexual partners, if she has recently had urine infections or infections of the vagina, or if she has put anything in her vagina since her waters broke.

  Remember to consider the time it takes to get to the hospital. For example: If the hospital is 4 hours away, you should start for the hospital after 4–8 hours have passed.

- You might want to go to the nearest hospital even if there are no risk signs or signs of infection. The hospital has medicine that can start the labor.

- If you cannot go to the hospital, give the mother antibiotics to prevent infection (see p. 298–299).

4. Waters are brown, yellow, or green

Stools begin to form in the baby's intestines (tubes the stool moves through) during pregnancy, but the baby usually does not have a bowel movement until after birth. Baby's stool is black, tarry and sticky. It is called **meconium**.

If the waters are green or brown, it probably means that the baby has already had a bowel movement. This is common when the baby is breech, but for other babies it may be a sign that the baby is having problems.

There is also a danger that the stool can get in the baby's mouth and nose. If the baby breathes the sticky stool into its lungs, it can be hard for the baby to get enough air. This sometimes causes a lung infection, brain damage, or death.

What to do

Find out if the baby is breech by feeling the mother's belly (see p. 123–128). (If the baby is breech, the stool will be dark green or black, and somewhat formed.) Follow the advice on p. 262–265.

If you know that the baby is head down, check the color of the waters. If they are a very light green and there are no other risk signs, there may not be a problem. Continue to listen to the baby's heartbeat throughout the labor and watch for risk signs.

If the waters are darker than light green and you can get to a hospital before the baby is born, it may be safest for the mother to give birth there. Also, the baby may have trouble during the labor and may need to be born by forceps or by operation. The hospital may have special equipment to clear the baby's mouth and lungs when it is born, and can treat it if there is a problem with its lungs.

If you cannot get to a hospital, you will need to take special precautions for this birth (see p. 258).

5. Strong contractions last more than 12 hours for women with previous pregnancies, or 24 hours for first babies

Sometimes a long labor is normal, and there is no danger as long as the mother rests between contractions, drinks liquids frequently, and urinates (pees). But a long labor can also be an important risk sign! Observe the mother closely. Are the pains getting further apart? Is she getting signs of infection? Is she getting exhausted? Is the baby's heartbeat still normal?

Check the mother to see if any of the following problems may be causing a long labor. If you are trained and permitted to do vaginal exams, do one now to help you decide what the problem is.

Baby is too big to fit through the mother's bones

If the baby is too big to move between the mother's pelvic bones, the baby cannot come out. The mother will labor until the womb tears and she dies of bleeding inside, or until she and the baby die of exhaustion.

Sometimes you can tell if the baby is too big by feeling the mother's belly, but often you must rely on other information. A woman is more likely to have a baby that is too big if the:

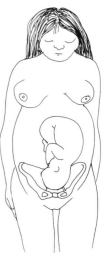

- Baby's father is very big (especially if the woman is very small, or if the father is from a different, larger race of people).

- Mother is very short compared to other women in her area.

- Mother is very young and her hips are not fully grown.

- Mother has a deformity of the hip bones.

- Mother has diabetes.

- Baby feels very big, or grew unusually fast during pregnancy.

- Baby has an unusually big head.

- Baby's head was still high and "floating"—can be felt above the pubic bone—when labor started (see p. 166).

- Mother had a hard time pushing out her last baby, and this one is bigger.

- Mother has been in labor a long time without progress.

Since you cannot tell for sure if the baby is too big to fit, let the mother labor a few hours first and see what happens. Sometimes a baby seems too big but comes out fine. If the woman has been in strong labor for more than 12 hours without signs that the birth is near, take her to the hospital. She may need to have an operation for the baby to be born.

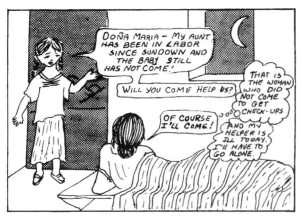

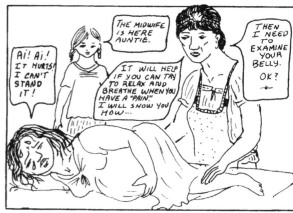

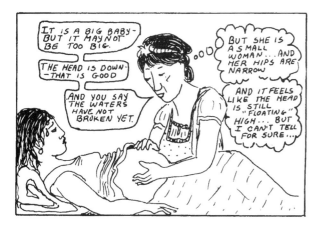

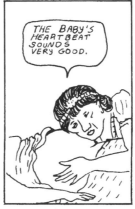

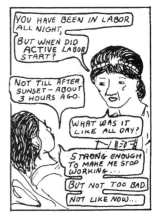

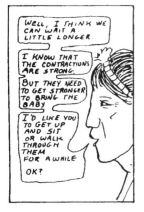

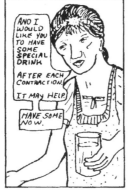

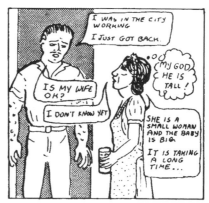

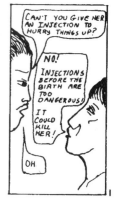

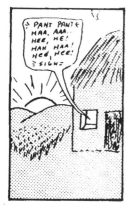

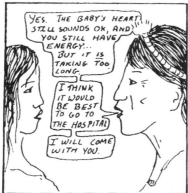

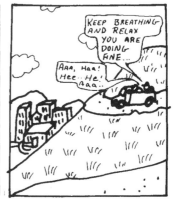

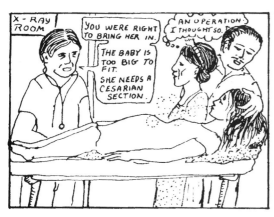

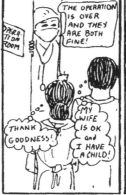

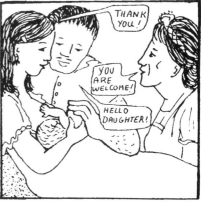

Baby is in a difficult or impossible birth position

Labor is usually shortest when the baby is lying head down, facing the mother's back. If the baby is in another position—like *facing the mother's front, face first, forehead first* or *sideways*—it may be difficult or impossible to deliver.

A baby that lies facing the mother's stomach

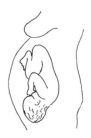

If a baby faces forward, it can often be born without problems but the labor is usually longer. You may want to try and make the labor stronger. Try using **nipple stimulation** or other gentle, natural methods, like walking (see p. 377). It may also be helpful to:

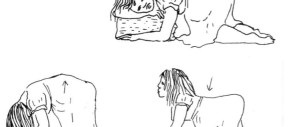

■ Put the mother in a hands-and-knees position for an hour or more. (It is OK if she needs to walk and stretch her legs between contractions.)

Arch back.   Straighten back.

■ Have the mother do the angry cat exercise between contractions (see p. 69).

If you see no signs of progress after 12 hours of active labor, or if progress stops for several hours, take the mother to a hospital—especially if the hospital is more than one hour away.

A baby whose head is face first or forehead first

Sometimes the way the baby holds its head can slow or prevent the birth.

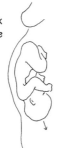 Most babies tuck their heads in like this. This makes it easier for the head to fit through the mother's bones.

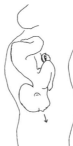 But sometimes the baby is face first. This makes it much harder to fit through the mother's bones.

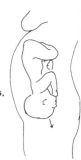 This baby is forehead first. This baby usually cannot fit through the mother's bones.

If you think the head is either **face first** or **forehead first**, go the hospital now. Do not attempt to change this baby's position.

A baby that lies sideways

A baby that lies sideways in its mother's womb cannot be born in this position.

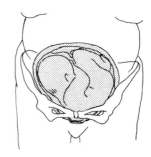

If the mother has had babies before, if her contractions are more than 20 minutes apart, **and** if you are skilled at turning the baby or can find someone who is, the baby may turn easily (see p. 409). If it does not, go to the hospital immediately!

A baby that lies sideways will not fit through the mother's pelvic bones.

> **Caution!** Do not try to turn the baby if you have not been taught by a very skilled person, if this is a first baby, or if the mother has regular contractions every 10 minutes.

Mother is dehydrated or exhausted

It is normal for a mother to get very tired and sweat a lot in strong labor. But if a mother gets exhausted or dehydrated (not enough water in the body), it can cause a longer, more dangerous labor. Dehydration can also make a woman feel exhausted.

If you arrive at a labor and find the mother is very tired and has signs of dehydration (see p. 171), immediately give her weak tea with lots of sugar or honey, fruit juice, or a rehydration drink (see p. 172).

If the mother is exhausted, find out whether she is in light, active, or late labor (see p. 140).

- If light labor goes on for many hours or days, the mother can get too tired to give birth, even before active labor begins. If birth is still far away, it may help if the mother rests or sleeps between contractions. Help her get comfortable and relax.

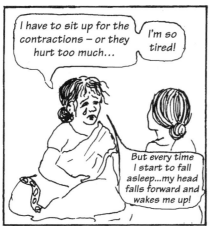
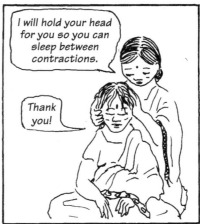

There may be traditional medicines or plants (for example, valerian) in your area that midwives use to help women rest in early labor. If you know that these will not harm the baby, you can try them now.

Sometimes emotions—like fear, not wanting another baby, or loneliness—can slow a labor. Companionship and support can sometimes help a mother find comfort.

- If the mother is in active labor but is not making progress—and the birth seems many hours away—give her liquids, encouragement, and perhaps a massage and a bath (if the bag of waters is still intact). If she has been in active labor for more than 12 hours and birth is not near, take her to the hospital.

Mother's bladder is full and cannot be emptied

To check if the bladder is full, feel the mother's lower belly. A full bladder feels like a plastic bag full of water. Usually you can see the shape of the bladder clearly under the mother's skin.

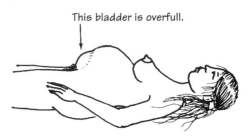

This bladder is overfull.

If the mother's bladder is full, she **must** urinate. If the mother cannot get out of bed, perhaps she can squat over a bowl in bed. If it is hard for her to get up, try putting a towel or extra padding between her legs and have her urinate where she is. Some women say it helps to dip a hand in warm water while urinating (see p. 391).

If the mother cannot urinate at all, she needs help. A trained health worker can put a sterile tube *(catheter)* into the mother's bladder to help the urine come out (see p. 391). If this person can come to the house, the mother can stay home. If not, the mother should go to the hospital.

Mother is tense or afraid

Sometimes the more a woman fears her labor, the more she fights against it. This can make labor longer and more painful. Good labor support and companionship can often solve the problem (see p. 313–321). Unfriendly family members or neighbors should not attend the birth.

It is very common for the mother of a first baby to get tense or afraid when labor starts to get very active. This can cause good labor to slow down or get stuck in the middle. Help her understand that active labor is normal and helps bring the birth closer. Explain that the more she resists, the longer the labor will be.

6. Mother has unusual or heavy bleeding: blood clots, fresh blood, or more than 200 cc of blood during labor

Any unusual bleeding

If a mother bleeds heavily, she may go into *shock*.

Shock

Signs of shock

- Mother feels faint, dizzy, and weak.

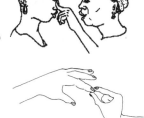

- Mother gets pale and has a cold sweat. Women with dark skin who are bleeding also get pale, but it helps to check their eyes and nails. Pull down the eye and look for pale pink instead of red around the rim of the eye. You can also push on the nail. If it does not turn white, the mother may already have lost a lot of blood.

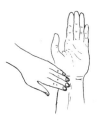

- Mother's pulse is more than 100 beats per minute and feels fast, thin, and faint.

- Mother's blood pressure drops below 80/40, or either number in her normal pregnant blood pressure drops more than 15 points.

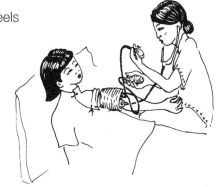

How to treat shock

1. Put the mother's head down, and her legs and hips up. This sends more blood to her brain and internal organs.

2. If you know how, start an IV using *normal saline* or *Ringer's lactate*, or give rectal fluids (see p. 409).

3. Go to the hospital. The mother may need a *transfusion* (blood given by IV). Try to send a relative to the hospital who can donate blood for the mother.

IV fluids

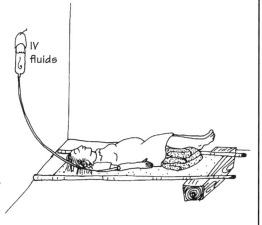

Unusual bleeding without pain

If a mother is bleeding but has no unusual pain, it may be a sign of placenta previa (see p. 101). Although there are usually signs of placenta previa in late pregnancy, sometimes

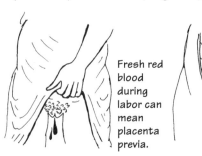

the first sign is bright red bleeding (enough to soak a pad) while the mother is in light labor. Go to the hospital immediately. The mother could bleed to death very fast once the cervix is open, so it is not safe to wait and see if the bleeding gets worse. Treat for shock along the way (see p. 243).

Fresh red blood during labor can mean placenta previa.

If the placenta covers the cervix like this, the placenta will bleed when the cervix opens.

> **Caution!** Never do a vaginal exam if there is unusual bleeding! You could poke a hole in the placenta with your finger and make the bleeding much worse.

7. Mother feels pain between contractions and the womb does not get soft, or she feels unusual pain during contractions

Pain **between** contractions or unusual pain **during** contractions can be a very serious risk sign. It can mean that the placenta is coming off the wall of the womb (detached placenta), that the womb is torn, or that the womb is infected.

Detached placenta (abruption)

If the placenta starts to separate from the wall of the womb, both the mother and baby are in danger. The mother may die from loss of blood because the place where the placenta was attached (placental site) starts to bleed. The womb cannot squeeze this place closed while the baby is inside. The baby may die or have severe problems because it can no longer get enough air from the mother.

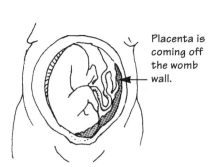

Placenta is coming off the womb wall.

Signs of bleeding in the womb:

- Mother has pain between contractions (it may be very mild at first, so pay close attention to any unusual pain). The danger is greatest if the pain is getting worse.

- Mother may be bleeding (but sometimes no blood comes out).

- Womb is hard between contractions, or hard all the time.

- Belly is sore and tender to the touch.

- Mother has signs of shock (see p. 243).

- Baby's heartbeat can be very fast (more than 180 beats per minute) or very slow (less than 100 beats per minute), or the baby could be dead (no heartbeat).

Unless the birth is happening very fast, get the mother to a hospital now! Do not wait! On the way to the hospital, treat the mother for shock (see p. 243).

Torn womb

A **torn womb** is one that has torn open, like this:

Any one of these things can
cause a torn womb:

- Mother has had a cesarean section in a past birth.

- Mother has had 5 or more babies.

- Mother's labor is very long and strong.

- Mother has been given strong medicine (either by
  mouth or by injection) to start labor or make it stronger.

- Someone has been pushing on the mother's belly,
  or her belly has been hit or injured.

- Baby is too big, or is lying in a difficult position.

*You cannot see a torn
womb because it is inside.
But it can kill a mother
and baby!*

Since a torn womb is inside the mother, you cannot see it. But these signs tell you that
the womb may be torn:

- Mother has very bad pain between contractions, then a "tearing feeling," then less
  pain.

- Mother's contractions stop.

- Mother may be bleeding (although sometimes no blood comes out).

- Mother has signs of shock (see p. 243).

- Baby feels loose (and sometimes higher) in the belly and has no heartbeat.

**If you see the signs of a torn womb, get the mother to the hospital now—even
if it is far away!** She can bleed to death very quickly, and the baby will also die. On the
way, treat the mother for shock (see p. 243). The mother will need an operation to stop
the bleeding, blood to replace what she has lost, and antibiotics to prevent infection. Be
sure to send a friend or relative with her to donate blood for her.

Infected womb

Sometimes an infection of the womb will also cause pain between contractions. An
infected womb means that harmful germs have gotten inside the womb and are
poisoning the mother. The signs of an infected womb are similar to the signs of other
infections. See p. 235 for what to do next. An infected womb can also cause shock
(see p. 243).

8. Mother has pre-eclampsia: blood pressure greater than 140/90, swollen face and hands, headaches, vision changes, pain between her ribs, brisk reflexes

If the mother has **any** signs of pre-eclampsia (see p. 112) during labor, she may have convulsions, detached placenta, bleeding in the brain, or a severe hemorrhage. The baby might die.

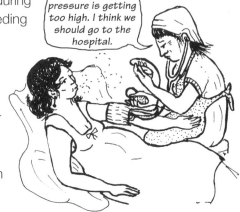

Your blood pressure is getting too high. I think we should go to the hospital.

Going to the hospital

It is best for a mother with pre-eclampsia to go to the hospital immediately. On the way to the hospital, have her lie on her left side and help her stay quiet and calm. If possible, keep the vehicle dark inside. Usually these labors are very fast. Stay with her in case the baby is born or she has a convulsion (see p. 247).

Staying at home

If it is impossible to get to the hospital, have the mother stay in bed on her left side. Help her stay as calm and quiet as possible. Keep the room dark. Give her plenty of fluid to drink. Be prepared for convulsions (see p. 247).

There are several medications that can be used to treat pre-eclampsia and prevent convulsions. But there are many different beliefs about what kind to give, how much to give, and when to give these medicines. Each country or health district may have different rules, so you should discuss what medicines you can carry in your kit with your local health officer.

We believe that all of these medicines are best used in a hospital because they have many dangerous side effects. However, since these medicines are permitted in several areas, we have included some recommendations about when to use them. You should use these medicines only if you have training and permission to use them. A drug called magnesium sulfate is the best medicine for preventing hard convulsions, but it is difficult to use and can make the mother stop breathing. Find out from your local health authorities if you can use magnesium sulfate and how to give it.

If you do not have a blood pressure cuff

You may give the mother **one** of these medicines by intravenous injection (IM) to prevent convulsions (see p. 383–388):

diazepam (valium) 10 mg IM, every 6 hours (this can also be given rectally if you do not have needles or syringes)   OR

amobarbital 250 mg IM   OR

phenobarbital 130 mg IM (first dose), then 30–60 mg. IM every 6 hours

> **CAUTION!** Do not give more than this amount of diazepam. Too much diazepam can make the mother stop breathing. Diazepam also sometimes makes the baby too sleepy to breathe at birth. Be ready to do *rescue breathing* (see p. 280) if necessary.

If you have a blood pressure cuff and know how to use it

- If the mother's blood pressure is between 140/90 and 160/110, give her either diazepam, amobarbital or phenobarbital as mentioned above.

- If the mother's blood pressure is 160/110 or higher, give either diazepam or phenobarbital as above AND one of the following to prevent bleeding in the brain. Give one time only!

> aldomet 250 mg by mouth
>
> > OR
>
> hydralazine 25 mg by mouth
>
> > OR
>
> hydralazine 10–25 mg IM

You may give both one of the medicines to prevent convulsions and one of the medicines to prevent bleeding in the brain, but do not give them in the same syringe.

9. Mother has convulsions (fits)

When a woman has a convulsion, she may fall *unconscious*. Her eyes may roll, and her hands and face may twitch. She may become stiff. Her body may shake, sometimes violently. She may turn blue or breathe with a loud, bubbly sound. She may bite her tongue, urinate, or have a bowel movement. Then she may sleep for a while. When she wakes up, she may be confused and not know what happened.

A convulsion may last from a few seconds to many minutes. Some convulsions are stronger than others, but they are all dangerous. Over half of the women who have convulsions in labor will die, or lose the baby, or both. Get the mother to the hospital as soon as possible when the convulsion is over.

What to do during a convulsion

1. Remain calm.

2. Do not let the mother put anything in her mouth. Keep her throat clear so she can breathe.

3. Put a padded stick between the mother's teeth to keep her from biting her tongue (but don't block her breathing).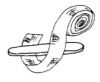

4. Put the mother on her side, so that she won't breathe fluids or vomit.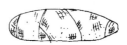

5. Give the mother oxygen, if you have it.

6. Give the mother medicine (see the next page).

7. Remove hairpins or other sharp objects which could harm the mother.

Medicines for convulsions

During a convulsion, you can give daizepam in one of these forms:

- Injectable diazepam. Since a woman having convulsions cannot swallow pills, and diazepam may not work well when injected into a muscle during a convulsion, it may be best to put injectable diazepam in the mother's rectum. Give 20 mg after the first convulsion. If there are other convulsions, give 10 mg after each one.

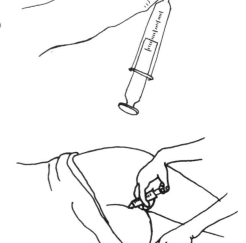

To give injectable diazepam, first fill your syringe and **take off the needle**. Put the whole barrel of the syringe up into the rectum and empty it inside the mother. Keep the barrel of the syringe in the rectum for at least 5 minutes. It will act as a plug to keep the medicine from coming out. (If some fluid leaks out of the rectum, it is OK to give 5 mg more diazepam—15 mg in all.)

- Diazepam pills. If you cannot get injectable diazepam, you can crush diazepam pills and mix them with water. (The pills won't dissolve but mix them with water anyway.) Give the same dosage as injectable diazepam.

Draw the water up into a syringe and put it in the rectum—the same as above. If you do not have a syringe, you can stick the pills up into the mother's rectum with your finger. But they will take a long time to dissolve. Please wear gloves.

10. Mother's pulse is more than 100 beats per minute

When a woman in labor is resting between contractions, her pulse should be about the same as it was during pregnancy.

A fast pulse can be caused by different problems:

- fever (see p. 235)

- blood loss (see p. 243)

- dehydration (see p. 171)

- fear (see p. 242)

To find out what is causing the mother's fast pulse, turn to the pages following each of these problems. If the mother has any other signs described there, follow the instructions given.

11. Baby's heartbeat is more than 160 beats per minute or less than 110 beats per minute

The best time to listen to the baby's heartbeat is right after a contraction is over. Make sure it is really the baby's heartbeat you are hearing and not the mother's (see p. 127–128).

Slow baby heartbeat

These things can cause the baby's heartbeat to drop below 110 beats per minute:

- Placenta does not work well. This is more likely when the mother has high blood pressure or when the baby is late.
- Placenta is starting to separate from the womb.

If you notice that the baby's heartbeat is slow for a few seconds **immediately after** a contraction but then goes back to normal, the baby may be having trouble. Listen to several contractions in a row. If the heartbeat is normal after most other contractions, things may be OK. Try putting the mother in different positions, to help take pressure off the cord (see p. 317). Listen again to see if this helps. Keep checking the baby's heartbeat often during the rest of labor to see if it slows down again.

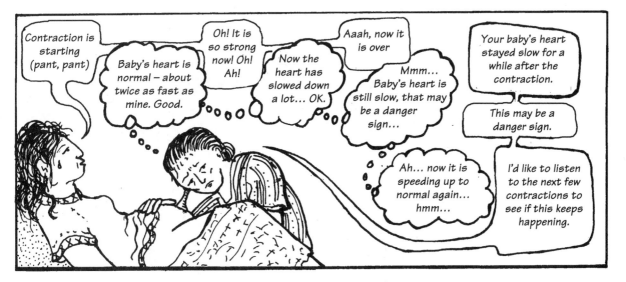

If the baby's heartbeat seems to stay slow after a contraction the baby may be in danger. If the baby's heartbeat goes below 90 beats per minute and stays slow until the next contraction—or almost to the next contraction—the baby is in danger. This is especially true if there are other risk signs, like green waters or a long labor. The baby could be very weak at birth or suffer brain damage.

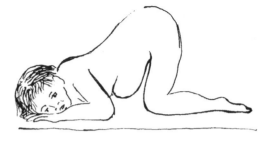

You must decide how far you are from a hospital and how soon you think the mother will deliver. If the birth is near and the mother has the urge to push, it may be better to stay home and deliver the baby quickly. If you decide to take the mother to the hospital, put her in the **knee-chest position**, or in some other position with her hips up. This may help increase the amount of blood and oxygen to the baby.

Fast baby heartbeat

These things can make the baby's heartbeat speed up to more than 160 beats per minute:

- Mother is dehydrated (see p. 171).

- Mother's womb is about to tear (torn womb; see p. 245).

- Mother has a fever (see p. 235).

- Mother is bleeding (see p. 243).

If the baby's heartbeat stays fast for 20 minutes (or 5 contractions) and at least one of these signs listed above is also present, go to the hospital.

12. Cord comes down in front of the baby *(prolapsed cord)*

When the bag of waters breaks, the cord will sometimes come down the vagina in front of the baby's head. This is more likely if there is lots of water, the baby is small or less than 8 months, or the baby is in a difficult position. If the cord gets caught in front of the baby's head, or on the side of the head, it can be squeezed between the head and the mother's bones. This makes it hard for blood to get through the cord and bring air to the baby. The baby suffocates.

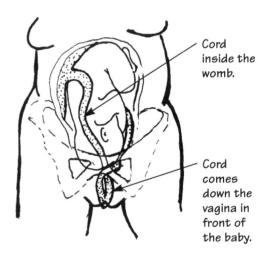

Cord inside the womb.

Cord comes down the vagina in front of the baby.

Signs of a prolapsed cord:

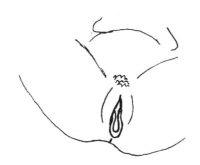

- You may see the cord come out of the vagina (but not always).

- The baby's heartbeat drops suddenly—especially right after the waters break—and does not return to normal.

- The baby's heartbeat gets very slow (less than 90 beats per minute) during each contraction.

What to do

1. If you can see the cord, touch it gently to check for a pulse. If the cord has a pulse, get the mother to a hospital right away. She will need an operation to save the baby. When you travel, wrap the cord in a clean cloth and put the mother in a knee-chest position with her hips high in the air. This will take some of the pressure off the cord. Do not touch the cord again. If you have sterile gloves, do a vaginal exam and try to push the baby's head up, away from the cord.

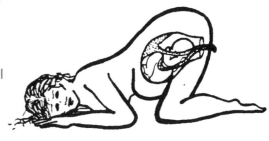

2. If you cannot see the cord and are trained (and allowed) to do a vaginal exam, scrub and put on sterile gloves. Then check inside the mother to see if you can feel a cord in front of the baby's head. Put your gloved hand on the baby's head and gently push it up, away from the cord. Try not to touch the cord very much. While you travel, put the mother in the knee-chest position and push up on the baby's head with your fingers.

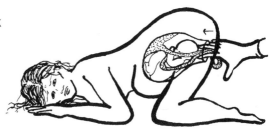

If it is impossible to get the mother to the hospital, deliver the baby as quickly as possible. If the baby is born alive, it may need oxygen, *rescue breathing*, and medical help (see p. 280–282). But there is a good chance that the baby will die.

3. If the cord has no pulse, stay at home to deliver the baby. The baby is probably dead, so prepare the mother to deliver a stillborn baby.

Complications in stage 2

Chapter 16 contents

Complications in stage 2

1. Baby is not born after 1 or 2 hours of strong contractions and good pushing

Even when the baby is moving down, it may take several hours of strong contractions and good pushing for the baby to be born. First babies often take a full 2 hours of pushing (and sometimes more than 2 hours). Second and later babies do not usually take more than one hour of pushing.

If you do not see signs that the baby's head is coming down—or if the baby seems to get stuck, or progress stops—you need to find out what is causing the slow birth. Ask yourself the following questions to try and find out:

Is it time for the mother to push?

If the mother starts pushing before her cervix is fully open, the baby cannot get out because the cervix is in the way.

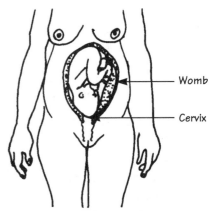

If the mother has been pushing without progress for more than $1/2$ hour and you have had training in vaginal exams, you may wish to do an exam now (see p. 389–391). If you find the cervix in the way, put the mother in the knee-chest position. This position takes the baby's weight off the cervix so that the swelling can go down, and the cervix can start opening again.

Womb

Cervix

If there is too much cervix in the way, the baby cannot get out — no matter how hard the mother pushes. Pushing will only make the cervix swell and get bigger.

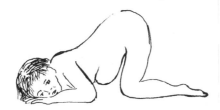

Help the mother to labor in this position without pushing for an hour or so. When you see signs that the cervix is thin and fully open (see p. 390, 140), she can try regular pushing again.

Is the mother pushing correctly?

Sometimes women push down and pull up at the same time. If this happens, a woman is holding the baby in while she pushes. This slows progress and often makes labor more painful. Encourage the mother to push correctly by holding her bottom down and keeping her thighs relaxed and open (see p. 184). She can also try the hold-the-breath method for pushing (see p. 321).

Is the mother afraid, upset, or tense?

A woman who has fears or emotional pain may hold the baby back—even without meaning to. Here are some of the common causes of fear and tension:

- This is a first baby.
- The mother's last baby was born dead or damaged, or died later.
- The mother has many children and is too poor to feed another one.
- The mother has no husband, partner, or family to help her.
- There are family problems.
- There is a history of sexual abuse.

Since most women will not say they are scared, you usually must use your intuition to decide whether fear or tension is a problem. If you think either of these is causing a longer labor, you can:

- Try talking with the mother to ease her fears or help solve the problem. Treat her with care and respect.
- Give her a massage.
- Give her a warm bath, or apply warm cloths to her body.

Does the mother need to change position?

A *squat* is often the best position for bringing the baby down to the birth opening. Squatting opens the hip bones wider, and it uses gravity to help the baby move down. Sometimes it helps to give the mother something to hold on to. (For example, she can hold onto the back of a chair or a friend's hands. Remember that the person or object that supports the mother must be strong and balanced.)

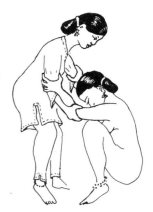

If the mother cannot squat, have her try one of these positions: *sitting squat*, *sitting straight* up, or *standing* (see p. 183).

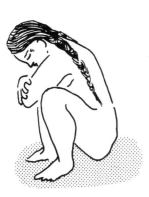
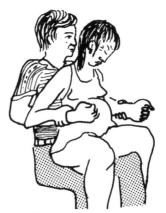
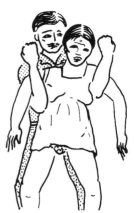

Sitting squat   Sitting straight up   Standing

Is the mother exhausted or dehydrated?

See p. 171 and 241 to learn about exhaustion and dehydration. If the mother has signs of dehydration, give her rehydration drink (see p. 172) or one of the liquids described there.

If the mother is truly exhausted and her contractions remain strong but without progress, take her to a hospital.

If the mother's contractions get fewer and farther apart, let her rest for a while. If strong contractions start again in one hour and she makes progress, stay at home. If contractions do not start in one hour, or if they start but she does not make progress, take her to the hospital.

Is the baby unable to fit through the mother's pelvic bones?

Three different problems can make it difficult for a baby to fit through the mother's pelvic bones:

- Sometimes the baby's head is a normal size, but the mother's pelvic bones are too narrow. The head cannot fit through.

- Sometimes the pelvic bones are big enough at the top but too narrow at the bottom. The baby may start to come down and get stuck.

- Sometimes the baby's head is very big. It may not fit through the mother's bones, even if they are normal size.

If the mother has one of these problems, the first stage of labor probably has been longer than normal, too. The mother's womb may tear open, or the mother and baby may die of exhaustion.

If you have tried the different methods for bringing the baby down—better pushing, different positions, emptying the bladder, rehydration drink, massage, and so on—and still see no progress after one hour of good pushing, take the mother to the hospital. It is not safe to wait until more risk signs appear.

While you are traveling, help the mother to stop pushing (see p. 188, 322). Put her in the knee-chest position (or some other position with her hips up) to take some of the pressure off the baby's head.

Is the baby in a difficult or impossible birth position?

See p. 240–241 for a description of difficult or impossible birth positions.

If the baby is lying facing the mother's stomach, it may be easier for the mother to push in either the hands-and-knees position, or in the squat position. This may also help the baby turn to face the mother's back as it comes down.

If the baby is face first or forehead first, the birth may be very difficult or impossible. If you suspect this problem, take the mother to the hospital right away. While you are traveling, help the mother stop pushing (see p. 188).

If you have asked all of the questions above and are still unsure about what is causing the slow birth, you may want to take the mother to the hospital. Consider these things in making your decision:

- *Does the mother or baby have any other risk signs (see p. 164, 180)?*

- *Does the mother still have energy to push?*

- *Is the baby continuing to move down, or is it stuck?*

- *How far is the hospital?*

- *Is the baby's heartbeat normal?*

- *Was the first stage longer than normal?*

If the baby is moving down slowly and all other signs are good, you may want to stay home for a while longer. If there are any signs of risk, if the mother is exhausted, or if the hospital is nearby, take the mother to the hospital. The baby may need to be born with forceps or by operation.

Caution! Never push on the mother's belly to hurry the birth. Pushing on the belly can make the placenta separate from the womb, or make the womb tear. These problems can kill the mother and baby.

2. Blood gushes out *before* the baby is born

During pushing, there is often a little bleeding from small tears in the mother's skin or cervix, or from show. But a gush of blood could be a sign of a detached placenta, a torn womb, or a torn cervix.

Detached placenta (abruption)

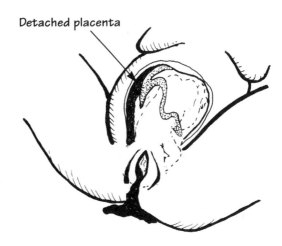

Detached placenta

If there is a sudden gush of blood from the birth opening and the baby's heart-beat is either very fast or very slow, the placenta may be detaching from the womb (see p. 244).

If you think you can get to a hospital before the birth, take the mother now. Watch for signs of shock and treat her if they appear (see p. 243).

If the birth is near and you cannot get to the hospital, have the mother push as long and as hard as she can. Get the baby out fast so that it can start to breathe, and so that the womb can start to contract and slow down the bleeding. Don't waste time slowing the birth of the baby's head. If necessary, cut the mother's birth opening to make it larger so that the baby can come out faster (see p. 393–397).

Be ready! This baby may need extra help to start breathing (see p. 280), and the mother may bleed heavily after birth. Get help so that someone can care for the baby while you care for the mother.

Torn womb

If the mother has a torn womb, her contractions will stop and she may or may not feel severe, constant pain (see p. 245).The baby's heartbeat will get very slow and then stop. If you think the womb may have torn, treat the mother for shock (see p. 243). **Take her to the hospital immediately, even if it is far away.**

Torn cervix

If the mother began pushing before the cervix was completely open, it might have torn. If there is unexplained bleeding in stage 2, but all else is well, you can go ahead with the birth at home. Follow the instructions for hemorrhage after birth (see p. 278), and ask the mother to keep her legs tightly crossed. The bleeding may continue after the placenta is born. A trained person should examine the mother's cervix for tears after the birth.

3. Waters are brown, yellow, or green

See p. 237 to learn what causes brown, yellow, or green waters and why this is dangerous for the baby.

If you see brown, yellow, or green waters and can get to the hospital in time for the birth, take the mother now. The hospital may have special equipment to wash stool out of the baby's lungs.

If you cannot get to a hospital, vigorously suction the baby's nose, mouth, and throat as soon as the head appears. Make sure you suction correctly (see p. 189). If you do it wrong, you can force stool into the baby's lungs. Try to get all the stool out before the baby begins to breathe. If you do not have suction equipment, wrap a bit of clean cloth around your finger and clean out the mouth as best you can.

After the birth, hold the baby with the head down, so fluid and stool can drain out. Continue to suction or clean out the mouth until you have gotten out as much stool as you can. Be prepared to give special attention to the baby; it may be weak and have trouble getting started.

Caution! If the baby is born limp or unconscious, get the stool out of the mouth, throat, and nose **before** you start trying to get the baby to breathe. Do not give rescue breathing (see p. 280) until you have cleared out as much stool as you can.

---

4. Cord wraps tightly around the baby's neck

Sometimes the cord is wrapped is 1 or 2 times around the baby's neck. Usually you can just loosen the cord and slip it over the baby's head or over the baby's shoulder as it is born. If the cord is wrapped 2 or more times, you may be able to slip one loop over the baby's head and the other over the shoulder.

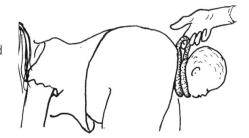

If the cord is wrapped 2 or more times, or is very tight and seems to be holding the baby back, you may have to clamp and cut the cord. Medical *hemostats* and blunt tipped scissors are good for clamping and cutting the cord in this situation. If you do not have them, use something else like clean string and a new or sterilized razor. Be careful not to cut the baby's neck—or the mother.

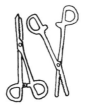
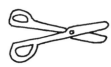

Medical
hemostats

Blunt tipped
scissors

> **Caution!** Never cut the cord before the birth unless it is clearly holding the baby back. Once the cord is cut, the baby must breathe to get air. The baby must now be born quickly.

5. Baby's heartbeat is more than 160 or less than 90 beats per minute

See p. 249 to learn about what may be happening to the baby, and what you can do to help. In addition, have the mother stop pushing for a few contractions so that the baby can rest. Be prepared for a cord around the baby's neck. Try to deliver the baby as soon as possible.

6. Baby gets stuck at the shoulders

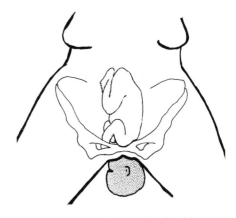

Stuck shoulders are more common when the baby is very big, or the mother's pelvis is very small. Sometimes you can tell that the shoulders will get stuck by the way the head is born. The head may take lots of hard pushing to be born, instead of coming out smoothly after it crowns. Sometimes the baby's chin does not quite come out. Sometimes it looks as if the baby's head is being pulled back into the mother, almost like a turtle pulling its head into its shell.

As soon as the head is born, it will seem to be pulled tight against the mother's skin. The neck will not be loose. Often the baby will not turn to face the mother's thigh. Even hard pushing will not bring the shoulders out.

The baby is in danger! The pressure of the mother's vagina on the baby's body forces too much blood into the baby's head. The head turns blue, and then purple. After a few minutes, the blood vessels in the baby's brain may begin to break and bleed from the pressure. This can cause brain damage, or it can kill the baby.

What to do

You may have to do things which cause pain to the mother, but these are necessary to save the baby's life and prevent brain damage. You must work quickly. Do not panic!

Here are 4 methods for helping the shoulders to come out. Try method 1 first; if it does not work, try method 2. If method 2 does not work, try method 3, if method 3 does not work, try method 4.

Method 1

1. Bring the mother to the edge of the bed. (If she is on the floor, put something under her hips to raise them off the ground.) You will need some space for the baby's head when you pull down.

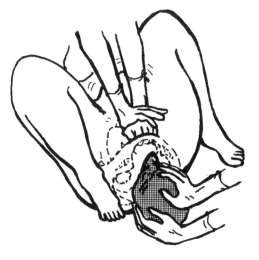

2. Have the mother spread her legs and pull them back as far as she can towards her sides.

3. Ask your assistant or any other person in the room to press hard just above the mother's pubic bone—**not** on the mother's belly. The assistant should push towards the mother's back.

4. Ask the mother to push as hard as she can.

5. Cup your hands around the baby's head (do not hold the baby's neck) and pull downward towards the rectum while counting to 30. When you see the shoulder appear, pull up and deliver normally.

If this does not work, try method 2.

Method 2

1. Put the mother in the hands-and-knees position. Make sure the mother's head is higher than her hips.

2. Cup your hands around the baby's head (just like in method #1) and pull downwards towards the mother's belly while counting to 30. When you see the shoulder, pull up and deliver normally.

If this does not work, try method 3.

Method 3

1. With the mother still in the hands-and-knees position, put your hand inside the vagina along the baby's back. Position your fingers on the back part of the shoulder which is nearest the mother's back.

2. Try to push the shoulder forward until it moves to the side.

3. Try to deliver the baby in the usual way, pulling downward while counting to 30.

If this does not work, try method 4:

Method 4

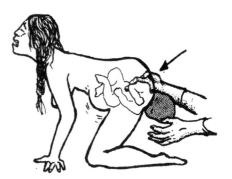

1. Put your hand inside the vagina and up along the baby's back.

2. Move your hand around the baby's body, bend the baby's arm, grasp its hand, and bring it across its chest to pull the hand out of the birth opening. This is often difficult to do.

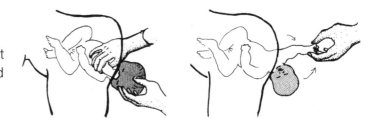

3. The baby can now be born fairly easily. Grasp the baby by the body (not the arm) for the birth.

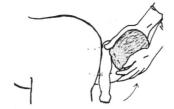

If none of these methods work, it is better to break the baby's collar bone to help it out than to let it die. Reach in with your finger, hook the baby's collar bone, pull up toward the baby's head, and break it. This will require a lot of pressure.

> **Caution!** If you use these methods, be careful not to pull or jerk on the baby's neck, or bend it too far. You could tear the baby's nerves and harm it for life. However, you may need to pull harder if the body does not come out after trying several of these methods. Be prepared to help the baby breathe. The baby may need to be taken to the hospital if it remains limp and weak.

7. Baby is breech

There are 3 kinds of breech:

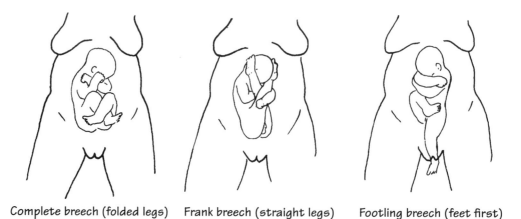

Complete breech (folded legs)   Frank breech (straight legs)   Footling breech (feet first)

Babies are more likely to be breech if:

- The mother's pelvic bones are not formed right.

- The mother has had other breech babies.

- The mother has growths in the womb.

- There are a lot of waters.

- There is placenta previa.

- The baby is small or early.

- The baby or baby's head is unusually large.

- There are twins.

Dangers of breech births

Breech births sometimes go fine, but they can be dangerous for the baby. They are especially dangerous for a first baby, because it is unknown if the mother's pelvic bones are big enough for the birth. A *frank breech* is considered the easiest kind of breech to deliver.

We suggest that breech babies be born in the hospital if at all possible, especially if it is a *footling breech*. If it is not possible, try to have a very skilled person at the birth. If this is not possible, or if you are suddenly surprised by a butt at the mother's birth opening, you can try to deliver the baby at home if the hospital is too far away.

Be aware of these dangers in delivering any breech baby:

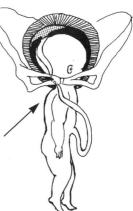

- The cord may prolapse when the water breaks (see p. 250).

- The baby's head can get stuck at the cervix. This can happen if the baby's body (which is usually smaller than the head) comes through the cervix before it is fully open.

- The baby's head may get stuck at the mother's pelvic bones (after its body has slipped through). If the cord gets pinched between the baby's head and the mother's bones, the baby can die or be brain damaged from lack of air.

Note: The danger of breech birth is mostly to the baby, not to the mother. The mother's life is always more important. Remember this when you are thinking about what to do.

Delivering a *complete* or frank breech

1. Have the mother push hard until the baby's bottom is born. The bottom will be pointing upwards to the mother's stomach. Usually the belly is born in the same contraction.

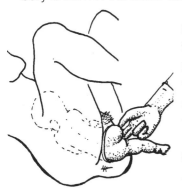

2. The legs usually fall out but you may need to put your fingers inside the mother to bring out the baby's legs.

3. Gently loosen the cord a little so it does not get pulled tight later. If the cord is still under the mother's pubic bone, move the cord to the side where the flesh is softer.

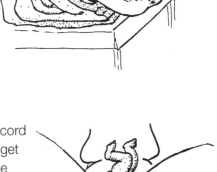

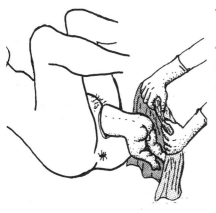

4. Wrap the baby in a clean towel or blanket, so you can hold the baby better. This will help you grip it. Also, cold air on the baby may make it try to breathe inside the mother and its lungs will get full of fluid. (In the rest of the pictures, we will not draw the towel. This is so that you can see better. But in real life, keep the baby wrapped and warm while you deliver it.)

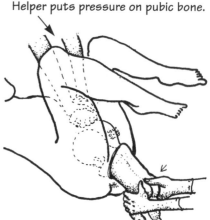

Helper puts pressure on pubic bone.

5. Have a helper put pressure on the mother's pubic bone (not her belly). This is to keep the baby's head tucked in, not to push the baby out. Carefully guide the baby's body down to deliver the top shoulder. **Hold the baby by the hips or below. Be careful! Pressure on the baby's back or belly can injure its insides!**

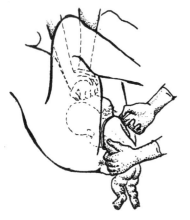

6. You may need to put your fingers inside the mother to bring the arms out. Try to grasp the arms by following them down from the shoulder. Draw the arm across the chest by gently pulling on the elbow. Deliver the top shoulder.

7. Carefully lift the baby to deliver the back shoulder.

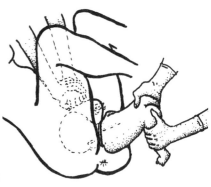

8. The baby now needs to turn so it faces down towards the mother's bottom. You may wish to support its body with your arm, placing your finger in the baby's mouth to help the head stay tucked. You will want the baby's chin to stay tucked to its chest in order to pass easily from the bones.

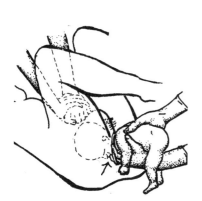

9. Lower the baby until you can see the hairline on the back of the neck. Do not pull too hard! Do not bend the neck or it may break!

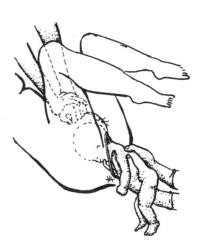

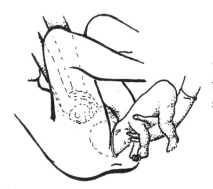

10. Keep the baby's head tucked in while you raise the body to deliver the face. Let the back of the head stay inside the mother.

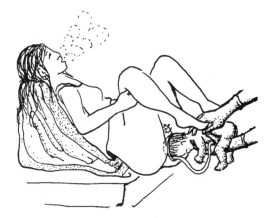

11. The mother should relax, stop pushing, and "breathe" the baby out. **The back of the head should be born slowly. If it comes too fast, the baby could bleed in the brain and die (or be crippled).**

Delivering a footling breech

A footling breech is more dangerous than the frank or complete breech because there is a much greater chance of a prolapsed cord, or of the head getting caught after the legs have been born.

Unless the birth is happening very quickly, it is always better to deliver a footling breech in the hospital. Try to slow the labor (see p. 188, 322). Put the mother in a knee-chest position for the journey.

If you cannot get to a hospital, try to keep the mother from pushing until you are sure that the cervix is fully open (see p. 389). If the mother stays lying down, the cord may be less likely to prolapse. Use the instructions above for a complete or frank breech if you must deliver at home.

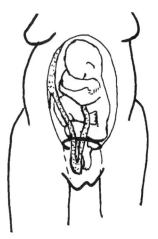

8. Unexpected twins appear

Dangers of twin births

Twin births may go well, but they can be more difficult or dangerous than a single birth. Twins are more than 3 times as likely to die than other babies, for these reasons:

- Twins are more likely to be born early, and to be small and weak.

- The cord (especially of the second twin) is more likely to come down in front of the baby.

- The placenta of the second twin may start coming off the wall of the womb after the first twin is born. This can cause bleeding.

- The mother is more likely to bleed heavily after the birth for 2 reasons: 1) her womb gets overstretched, and 2) the place where the placentas were attached to the womb is very big. This will cause a large open wound after the placentas separate.

- If the second twin is not born soon, the womb may get infected. The second twin may also be infected.

- One or both twins are more likely to be in a difficult or impossible to deliver position. Or the twins may get in each other's way, making it impossible for them to be born. For example:

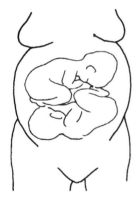 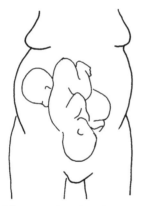 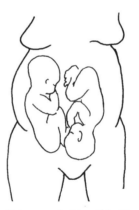 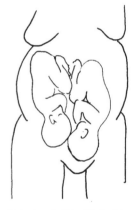

When both babies are sideways, they cannot be born through the vagina. It is very dangerous to try to deliver them at home.	When one head is down, it is a little less dangerous to deliver at home. If the head-down baby is born first, the other baby may turn.	It is even better if both babies are up and down. But a breech twin will have the same dangers as all breech babies.	It is best if both babies are head down, but it is still more dangerous than a single birth.

For these reasons, we suggest that all twins be born in a hospital. If the journey is very difficult, feel the mother's belly to determine the position of the babies. This will help you know how many problems to expect at the birth.

If you have to deliver twins at home, make sure there are at least 2 very skilled people at the birth.

What to do when delivering twins at home

1. Deliver the first baby as you would any single baby.

2. When you cut the first baby's cord, tightly clamp or tie the end that is coming out of the mother. Twin babies sometimes share a placenta, and the second baby could bleed through the cord of the first.

3. After the first baby is born, feel for the position of the second baby. If it is lying sideways, see p. 268.

4. The second baby should be born within 15 to 20 minutes. Deliver it as you would any other baby.

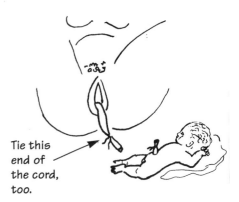

Tie this end of the cord, too.

Possible problems when delivering twins

These are some of the problems that may occur when delivering twins:

Mother does not start to have contractions within 15 minutes of the birth of the first twin

Try to get the labor going again by letting the first baby breast feed. You can also use nipple stimulation (see p. 378). If the baby is head or butt down, try breaking the waters with a sterile clamp (hemostat). See p. 420. But do not break the waters if the second baby is sideways (see p. 268).

If you wait longer than 15 minutes, the placenta may start coming off the womb, the cervix may start to close or, if you wait for a few hours, the second baby and the womb may get infected.

If these methods do not work, seek medical help as soon as you can. Do not give injections to get labor started again.

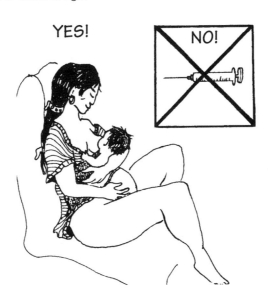

YES!   NO!

The second baby is sideways

If possible go to the hospital. If it is too far away, try to find a skilled person to turn the baby. If you are alone try the following:

1. Try to turn the baby's head down by massaging the mother's belly (see p. 409). It is best if a very skilled person does this.

2. If you cannot move the baby to a head down position, massage the belly and try to move it to the breech position (see p. 409).

3. If you cannot move the baby to either of these positions, go to the hospital. The baby will need to be born by operation.

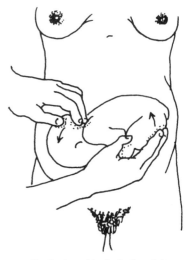

Try to turn the baby head down.

The mother bleeds before the second twin is born (or the first placenta is born before the second twin)

Bleeding after the birth of one twin and before the other means that there may be early separation of the placenta (see p. 257). The mother and second baby may bleed heavily. Get the second baby out as fast as you can.

Caution! If you put your hand inside the mother to help the birth, or if she bleeds a lot, the mother is in great danger of getting an infection. If it is not possible to get medical help, give the same antibiotics that you would give for an infection after birth (see p. 299).

---

9. Baby is very small or more than 5 weeks early

Babies that are born early or small may have special problems:

- The small or *early baby* often has a softer, more delicate skull. It is more likely to be injured in the vagina than a regular baby.

- A small or early baby is more likely to be in a difficult or impossible birth position (like a sideways position).

- A small or early baby may have more trouble keeping itself warm after the birth, and may have more trouble breathing and breast feeding.

For these reasons, it is usually best for small or early babies to be born in the hospital. If they are born at home, it is important that they get medical care as soon as possible (see p. 424–425).

If you must deliver small or early babies at home, take these extra precautions:

- You may want to cut the mother's vaginal opening to make it larger (an *episiotomy*). Do this only if you have been trained, if you have the proper sterile equipment, and if you are permitted to do so in your area (see p. 393–395). This will lessen the pressure on the baby's head during the birth. This may prevent injury or brain damage.

- Have many warm blankets ready for the baby as soon as it is born. Wrap the baby and put it in its mother's arms (since the mother's body is exactly the right temperature for the baby). If you use a hot water bottle, always wrap the hot water bottle and the baby in cloths. Never put a hot water bottle next to a baby's skin.

- See p. 292–293 for how to care for babies that are early or small once they are born.

Complications in stage 3

Chapter 17 contents

Risks signs for the mother

1. Heavy or constant bleeding *before* the placenta comes out

When the placenta separates from the womb, there is usually a small gush of blood. This is normal. But heavy or constant bleeding while the placenta is still inside is not normal. There are 3 ways a woman can lose too much blood after childbirth:

- **A big, fast hemorrhage.** The mother may lose a lot of blood at once, or blood may flow heavily for a while. Often she will quickly feel faint and weak. **This is a severe emergency.**

- **A slow trickle.** This kind of bleeding is easier to miss. Remember that any steady bleeding, even if it is just a trickle, means the mother is in danger.

- *Hidden bleeding.* This bleeding cannot be seen because blood collects in the womb or vagina (which is still large from the baby). This is also extremely dangerous and is easy to miss.

This bleeding can have different causes:

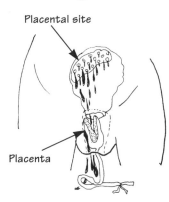

Sometimes the placenta has left the womb and is sitting in the vagina waiting to come out. But the womb may fail to squeeze down because it is tired or for other reasons.

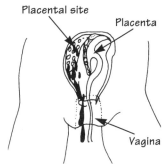

If the placenta comes off the womb wall but stays inside, the placenta holds the womb open. The womb cannot squeeze down and stop the bleeding at the placental site.

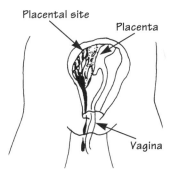

If the placenta only comes part way off the womb wall, the womb cannot squeeze down and stop the bleeding at the placental site.

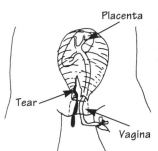

Sometimes bleeding comes from a torn cervix or vagina, or a torn womb.

You may be able to tell where the bleeding comes from by the kind of bleeding that occurs:

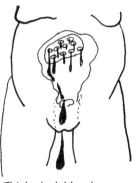

- Bleeding that comes in spurts is more likely to be from the womb. The blood collects in the womb and then, when there is a contraction, some of it spurts out. This blood is usually dark red and thick.

Thick, dark blood comes from the womb.

- Bleeding that comes in a constant trickle or flow may be from a tear in the cervix or vagina. But if the mother is lying on her back, the blood may pool inside and only come out when she sits or moves. This blood is usually fresh, bright red, and thin.

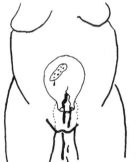

Thin, bright red blood comes from a tear.

Keep in mind that a woman has more risk of bleeding when:

- she is anemic or has been ill in pregnancy.
- she has had a very long or hard labor.
- her baby is very big.
- she has just given birth to twins.
- she has had bleeding problems at past births.
- her bladder is over full.

What to do

Try to get the placenta out by normal methods (see p. 197–199). If the placenta does come out, be ready for more bleeding.

If you cannot get the placenta out by normal methods, check the mother's bleeding again. If she has stopped bleeding and seems strong, it may be OK to wait a little and then try to deliver the placenta again. Keep your hand lightly but firmly on top of the womb. If it grows larger or gets softer, the womb is probably filling with blood.

If you cannot get the placenta out and the mother is still bleeding, or if she feels faint or weak or shows other signs of shock (see p. 243), she is in great danger. If the hospital is close by, take the mother right away. Before you leave, give an IM injection of 10 to 20 units oxytocin. On the way to the hospital, treat the mother for shock (see p. 243).

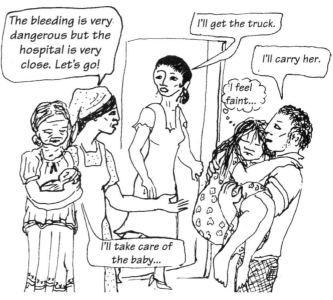

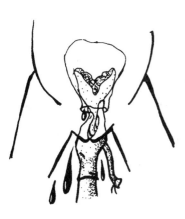

Taking out the placenta by hand

If you think the woman will bleed to death before you can get to the hospital, you may need to put your hand inside the mother's womb to loosen the placenta and take it out.

> **WARNING!** Taking out the placenta by hand is a very dangerous procedure. Putting your hand inside the womb can cause life-threatening infections, tear the cervix or womb, or tear a placenta that is still partially stuck on the womb wall. Do not do this procedure unless you feel that is the **only** way to save the mother's life. It is best to try this procedure only if someone has already taught you how to do it.

1. Quickly scrub your hands and arms up to the elbows with disinfectant soap and boiled water—or use alcohol, if you have it (see p. 159). Put on long sterile gloves. Once your hands have been scrubbed, do not touch anything except the inside of the mother.

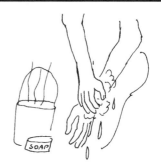

Scrub up to the elbows!

2. Carefully feel up along the cord, inside the mother. The placenta may be just sitting in the vagina or in the bottom of the womb, waiting to be taken out. If so, take the placenta out, massage the womb until it is hard, and give an IM injection of oxytocin 10 to 20 units, or **Methergine** (ergonovine) 0.2 mg or **ergometrine** 0.5 mg. Do not give Methergine or ergometrine if the mother has high blood pressure. If you have the equipment and are trained, start an IV and put 20 units of oxytocin in the IV.

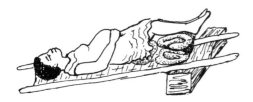

3. If the placenta is still partly stuck to the wall of the womb, you may need to reach inside and peel the placenta off the womb wall with your fingers.

Keeping your hand in a cone shape, gently follow the cord up into the womb. Once your hand is in the womb, a helper can give the mother an injection of oxytocin. (Medicine can make the cervix close up, so do not give it before your hand is in the womb.)

Carefully feel for the edge of the placenta with your fingers. This may be very painful to the mother. Have someone hold her and breathe with her to help her relax while you work.

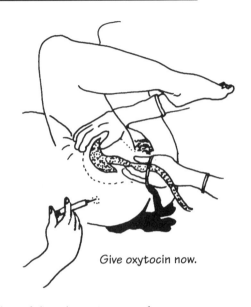

Give oxytocin now.

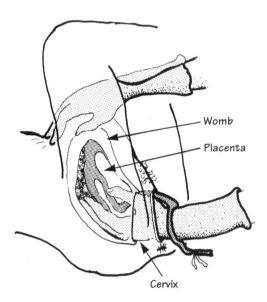

Hand scoops placenta off the womb wall.

Pry the edge of the placenta away from the womb wall using the side of your little finger. Then carefully peel the rest of the placenta off by working your fingers between the placenta and the womb. (It is a little like peeling the skin off an orange or other thick-skinned fruit.) Bring the placenta out in the palm of your hand. Be careful not to leave any pieces or clots inside.

4. After removing the placenta, start an IV (if you can and have not already). Add 20 units of Pitocin or Syntocinon to this IV or give an IM injection of 10 units oxytocin or 0.2 mg–0.5 mg ergometrine or Methergine. Be ready to firmly rub the womb or to use ***two-handed pressure*** (see p. 277), if necessary, to stop the bleeding.

5. Go to the hospital as soon as possible. If the mother has signs of shock, keep her head down, and her hips and legs up. If the mother has lost a lot of blood, she may need a transfusion (blood given by IV) to save her life. She is also in great danger of getting an infection. If it will take more than one hour to get to the hospital, give one dose of the same antibiotic you would give for an infection after birth (see p. 299).

2. Mother has signs of shock

If you do not see heavy or constant bleeding, but the mother has signs of shock (see p. 243), she may be bleeding inside. Put the mother's legs and hips above the level of her head, start an IV if possible, and then follow the instructions above for getting the placenta out (see p. 271–274).

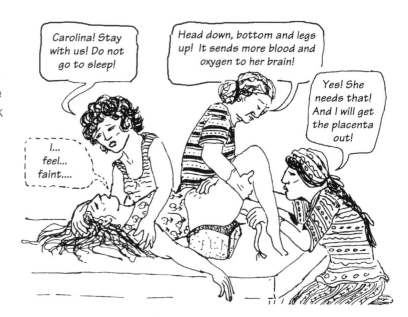

3. There is no sign that the placenta has separated after $1/2$ hour, or the placenta has not come out after one hour

If there are no signs that the placenta is separating from the womb wall (see p. 196) **and there is not heavy bleeding**, try putting the baby to breast. If this does not work, or if the baby does not suck well, try nipple stimulation (see p. 378). Encourage the mother to push the placenta out. Have her squat to push. If the mother is afraid, remind her that the placenta is soft and much smaller than the baby. Explain that she will feel more comfortable when it is out.

Sometimes the placenta separates without any signs of separation. The placenta may be sitting in the vagina or bottom of the womb, or trapped in the womb by the cervix. To check if the placenta has separated, gently try to remove the placenta by the cord-guiding method (see p. 198).

If the cord-guiding method does not work, and there are no signs of separation or bleeding, it is best to wait. Do not give injections or drugs. There is no emergency and you should be careful not to create one.

> Note: The amount of time to wait before going to the hospital will vary from area to area. Check with other midwives or local health workers about when to go to the hospital if the placenta does not come out and there is no bleeding.

4. Heavy or constant bleeding *after* the placenta comes out

Womb stays soft

The most common cause of serious bleeding after the placenta comes out is a soft womb that will not contract properly. The womb often stays soft because of a long, hard labor; a large baby; or because a piece of the placenta or membranes is still inside.

What to do

If you have already tried vigorously massaging the womb (see p. 209) and the bleeding has not stopped, try the following:

1. Have the mother breast feed her baby. If she cannot, have someone else suck or try nipple stimulation (see p. 378) if this is done in her culture. Nipple stimulation causes the womb to contract and become firm.

2. Check the placenta again for missing pieces. If a piece is still in the womb, you may have to remove it for the bleeding to stop (see p. 278).

3. If the placenta is whole and massaging the womb does not stop the bleeding, or if bleeding is very heavy, give one of these medicines:

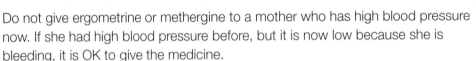

- oxytocin 10 to 20 units IM (or in IV fluids)

- ergometrine 0.25 mg to 0.5 mg IM

- Methergine (ergonovine) 0.2 mg IM

Do not give ergometrine or methergine to a mother who has high blood pressure now. If she had high blood pressure before, but it is now low because she is bleeding, it is OK to give the medicine.

If you do not have **injectable** medicine, you can give ergometrine or methergine pills by mouth. Medicines given by mouth do not work as fast as medicines that are injected, but they still can help.

If you do not have modern medicines (or if you do not want to use modern medicines), there may be herbs growing in your area that help stop heavy bleeding. These herbs should be drunk as a tea.

Traditional midwives may also use other methods besides herbs that work very well. We encourage you to learn about them and then decide whether it is a good idea to use them (see chapter 2). Do not put any herbs or teas in the vagina. This can cause infection.

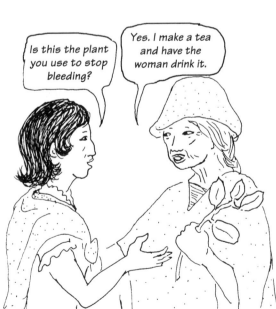

Is this the plant you use to stop bleeding?

Yes. I make a tea and have the woman drink it.

4. Use two-handed pressure. In an emergency—if bleeding is heavy, or if you are waiting for medicine to work, or if you do not have medicine—you can also use two-handed pressure to stop bleeding and save the mother's life. See the sections below for two kinds of two-handed pressure. Try the outside method first.

Outside method: two-handed pressure with hands outside the mother's body

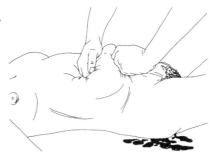

- Massage the belly until you can feel the womb get hard.

- Lift the womb with one hand and with the other hand massage the lower end of the womb.

- As soon as the womb gets firm and bleeding stops, stop your massage. Check the womb every few minutes. You may need to repeat this several times.

- If the womb gets soft again after you have massaged it 4 or 5 times, you may have to try the next technique.

Scoop up the womb, fold it forward, and squeeze it as hard as you can. Or: Press down on the belly and squeeze the womb against the mother's back bones.

If outside pressure does not work, and you are afraid that the woman may die before getting medical help, you may have to try the inside method.

Inside method: two-handed pressure with one hand inside the body

> **Caution!** Putting your hand inside the mother can cause infection. Do not put your hand inside the mother unless the mother's life is in danger and other methods do not work!

- Scrub your hands and put on sterile gloves.

- Explain to the mother and any others at the birth why you need to do this procedure and what will be happening.

- Put your hand into the vagina and move it up under the womb. The vagina is still quite open, so your hand will go in easily (but it may be painful for the mother). Work slowly and gently.

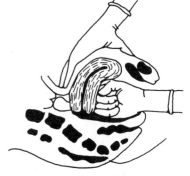

- Make a fist of the hand inside the mother's body, lift the womb upwards. With your other hand, grab the womb from the stomach side. Rub your hands together around the womb, with a slight downward squeezing motion. You should begin to feel the womb harden.

- When the womb feels hard, slowly take your hand outside of the vagina. Try to drag clots of blood out with your hand.

Put one hand inside the mother's vagina. Make a fist. With the other hand, press forward and down as hard as you can, with the womb between your hands.

- If you have the equipment and have been trained, start an IV and give the mother IV fluids.

Keep the womb squeezed down until the bleeding stops. If the womb stays firm, you may decide to keep the mother at home. But if she shows any signs of shock, treat her for shock and get her to the hospital immediately (see p. 243). If you used two-handed pressure with a hand inside the mother and you cannot get to the hospital, give the mother the same antibiotics you would give for an infection after birth (see p. 299).

Torn womb

If the mother's womb is torn (see p. 245), you must treat her for shock (see p. 243) and get her to the hospital immediately.

Torn cervix or vagina

If the mother is bleeding heavily and the womb is hard, the bleeding may be from a tear in the mother's skin. See p. 395 for how to examine the mother for tears.

If the mother is bleeding heavily from a tear and you do not know how to sew it closed, put cloths against the mother's bottom, have the mother cross her legs, and start an IV (if you have been trained to do so). Then take the mother to the hospital immediately. If you have been trained to sew tears closed, see p. 395–405.

A piece of the placenta seems to be missing

If a piece of the placenta or of the membranes seems to be missing, it could still be in the womb. This can cause a problem with bleeding or infection.

If the woman is not bleeding and there are no signs of shock, put the baby to breast and have the mother squat and push. If the woman is bleeding but not too heavily, try giving her an IM injection of 10 units oxytocin. Then get medical help.

If the woman is bleeding so much that she may die before getting help, try taking out the extra pieces yourself:

1. Scrub and put on sterile gloves (see p. 159).

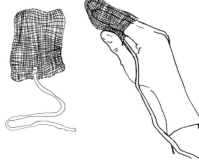

2. Fold a piece of strong, sterile gauze over your fingers. The gauze will help you to scrape up small pieces inside the womb. (Be sure to use strong material that will not shred and leave pieces inside the mother. Or, even better, keep a special sterile packet containing strong gauze with a string attached in your kit. The string will stay outside the mother so that you can get the gauze out if you lose it.)

3. Wet the gauze with *sterile saline* or sterile water, if you have it.

4. Reach inside the mother and try to clean out the missing pieces. This will be very painful to the mother. Someone should hold her and help her breathe and relax while you are working. If you cannot get the extra piece out, give the mother an IM injection of 10 units oxytocin and get medical help. If it will take more than one hour to get to the hospital, give one dose of the same antibiotic you would give for an infection after birth (see p. 299).

> **Caution!** Once the extra piece of placenta is out, the mother still needs to get medical help. If she has lost a lot of blood, she may need a transfusion. She is also in danger of getting an infection and should be given antibiotics. Be sure to tell a doctor what procedures you have done, what medicines you gave, and at what time.

5. Womb comes out with the placenta

Sometimes the womb turns inside out and follows the placenta out of the mother's body. This can occur if someone pulls too hard on the cord before the placenta has separated from the womb wall, or if someone pushes on the womb to get the placenta out. It can also happen by itself—even if no one does anything wrong. Sometimes the womb only comes part way out.

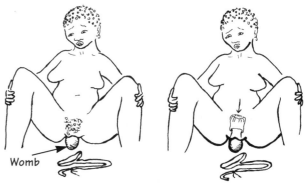

Womb

When you see this,   the womb has turned inside out.

What to do

1. Scrub your hands and arms up to the elbows (see p. 159). Put on sterile gloves and gently but firmly put the womb back where it belongs. You may be able to just push it back up, or you may have to roll it up with your fingers.

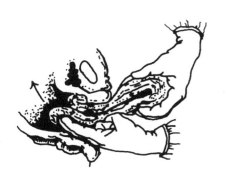
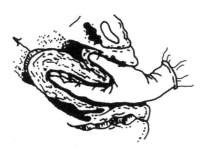
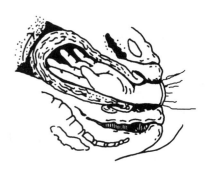

2. After the womb is back inside, massage it to make it firm and hard. You may need to use two-handed pressure to stop the bleeding (see p. 277). Even if the mother is not bleeding, give an IM injection of 10 to 20 units oxytocin, or 0.5 mg ergometrine or 0.2 mg Methergine (but do not give either of these medicines to a woman with high blood pressure). If you do not have the injectable kind of medicine, give it by mouth.

3. The mother should stay on her back with her hips up. Take her to the hospital, if possible. Give antibiotics on the way. Give the same kind and dose as you would give for an infection after birth (see p. 299).

Risk signs for the baby

1. Baby does not breathe at all

A baby **must** begin to breathe on its own within 2 or 3 minutes after the cord becomes white or the placenta separates. If the baby does not start to breathe, it will *suffocate*. This can cause serious brain damage or death.

First, clear the baby's mouth and nose, rub the baby gently, and encourage it to breathe. If these steps do not work, check the baby's heartbeat. If the heart is beating more than 80 beats per minute, do *rescue breathing*. If the heart is not beating (or is below 80 beats per minute), do rescue breathing and *heart massage* (see p. 281).

How to do rescue breathing (without heart massage)

1. Lay the baby on its back, with its head lower than its feet. It should be on a hard surface, like a table or floor, or on a board you can tilt, or in your arms.

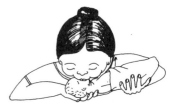

2. Open the baby's throat by tilting its head back slightly, keeping the chin up. Move the tongue away from the back of the throat. Do not tilt the head too far, or the throat will close again.

Chest and belly rise .

3. Put your hand (or a rolled up cloth) under the baby's shoulder, so that the chin is off the chest and the head is slightly to one side. This way, any fluid that comes up will pool in the baby's cheek, not its throat.

4. Put your mouth over the baby's nose and mouth. Gently blow little puffs of air into the baby. Do this at the rate of 30 puffs per minute (which is a little faster than you breathe yourself while resting). Let the baby breathe out between puffs.

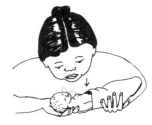

Chest and belly fall between puffs.

The baby's belly and chest will rise and fall with each breath. If the belly stays up, it means that air is going into the baby's stomach, not its lungs. Try changing the angle of the head. Make sure nothing is blocking the throat.

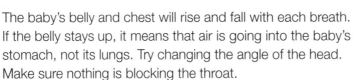

> **Caution!** The new baby's lungs are very delicate. Do not blow too hard or you will break them. Blow little puffs of air **from your cheeks**, not from your chest. Do not force in more air than the baby can take.

5. Keep doing rescue breathing until the baby starts to breathe by itself, or until you are too tired to continue. Sometimes 1 or 2 breaths are enough. Sometimes you need to do rescue breathing for a long time. If the baby's heart is beating, the baby will probably be OK when it starts breathing by itself. If the baby's heart stops, see p. 281.

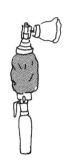

Oxygen tanks and *oxygen bag* masks are useful for rescue breathing. If you have them and are trained to use them, we recommend them. *Oxygen masks* also help prevent disease. If the mother had a contagious disease like syphilis, hepatitis, or active herpes, there is a chance you will get the disease from the baby. This may happen if you get blood, mucus, or waters in your mouth while doing rescue breathing. The danger is greater if you have a cut or sore in your mouth.

Note: Rescue breathing is not difficult. It is easiest to learn when someone teaches you. Practice rescue breathing on a doll, so you will be ready for an emergency.

2. Baby has no heartbeat, or heartbeat is less than 80 beats per minute

A baby with no heartbeat may still be alive! If you know the baby was alive during labor, the baby may just be too weak to have a heartbeat now. It is also possible that the baby was brain damaged while inside the mother. Unfortunately, there is no way to know this for sure.

If the baby has no heartbeat, or if the heartbeat is less than 80 beats per minute (about $1/2$ as fast as normal), you may be able to help the baby by giving heart massage with rescue breathing.

How to do heart massage with rescue breathing

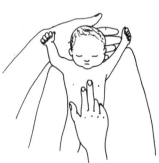

1. Lay the baby on a hard surface or on your arms. Keep it warm.

2. Put 2 fingers on the baby's breast bone (the bone between the baby's nipples).

3. Press down with your fingers about 1 cm (about $1/2$ inch). **Do not use too much pressure!** Press down about 2 times each second. (This is the same rate as the heartbeat inside the womb, and about 2 times as fast as the heartbeat of a resting adult.) If you cannot go quite this fast, do the best you can. It will still help.

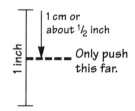

1 cm or about $1/2$ inch

1 inch

Only push this far.

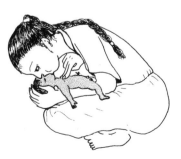

4. Give the baby a puff of air (see p. 280) **after** every 3 pushes. Give the puff just as your fingers are coming up from the baby's chest.

One person can give heart massage and rescue breathing, but it is easier if 2 people do it together. That way, one person can do rescue breathing and one person can do heart massage.

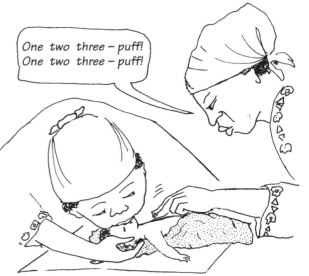

One two three – puff!
One two three – puff!

> **Caution!** Never breathe into the baby while you are pressing on its chest. Give the puff of air **after** you press the chest down. If you breathe and push down at the same time, you can hurt the baby.

5. If the baby is going to live, it will probably get a heartbeat and start breathing on its own within 5 to 10 minutes. If this does not happen, decide how long to keep trying. Think about whether there were any risk signs during the pregnancy and birth, whether you heard the baby's heartbeat shortly before birth, and how long it was between the birth and the start of rescue breathing and heart massage. Use your judgment, knowledge, and intuition to decide whether you can help the baby.

> **Caution!** Do not give heart massage if the baby's heartbeat is more than 80 beats per minute. Count carefully. You could make things much worse if you give heart massage when it is not needed.

3. Baby has trouble breathing

If the baby is having trouble breathing, suction or try to wipe out any mucus, fluids, or stools out of the baby's nose and throat (see p. 189). Also, keep the baby warm. If the baby's temperature is below 36°C or 97°F, or if it feels unusually cool-to-touch, try to warm the baby (see p. 291–293).

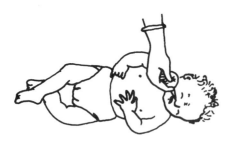

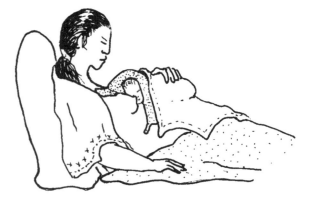

4. Baby is very pale or stays blue after the first few minutes

If the baby's **hands and feet** are blue 5 minutes after birth, it is probably OK. But if the baby's **whole body** is blue or purple for 5 minutes or more after birth, it may be cold, or have heart or breathing problems. If the baby is very pale, it may be cold or anemic (thin, pale blood), or have heart trouble.

If the baby is very pale or its whole body stays blue or purple, check the baby's temperature (see p. 214–215) or touch it to see if it is warm. Give oxygen if you have it. Check the baby's heartbeat and breathing, and follow the directions for giving heart massage and rescue breathing if necessary (see p. 281). Get medical help.

Complications in the first 2 to 6 hours after birth

Chapter 18 contents

Complications in the first 2 to 6 hours after birth

Risk signs for the mother

1. Mother bleeds more than heavy monthly bleeding

The most common reason a mother bleeds heavily in the first hours after the birth is that the womb will not contract. Instead, the womb grows larger and feels soft after the placenta comes out.

If the womb stays soft after the placenta comes out, the womb is not contracting. Let the baby breast feed. If the baby does not suck well yet, try nipple stimulation (see p. 378).

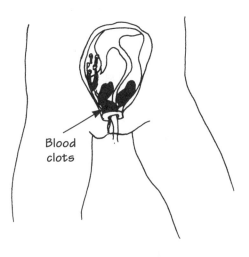

Blood clots

Sometimes the womb stays soft because there is blood or blood clots still in the womb. If the womb does not start to contract after the baby breast feeds or the mother's nipples are stimulated, massage the womb to squeeze out the blood and blood clots. If the mother continues to bleed, try the outside method of two-handed pressure (see p. 277).

Massage should make the womb smaller and harder. If massage does not work, give the mother an intramuscular injection (see p. 383–387) of one of these medicines. (Do not give Methergine or ergometrine to a woman with high blood pressure.)

- 10 units oxytocin

- 0.2 mg Methergine or ergonovine

- 0.5 mg ergometrine

If you do not have IM medications you can give Methergine or ergometrine pills 0.2 mg by mouth every 4–6 hours. They do not work as quickly as the injections.

If the womb continues to stay soft or grows larger, the mother may be bleeding inside. If you see signs of shock, treat for shock (see p. 243). Get the mother to the hospital.

2. Bleeding has stopped, but the mother has lost a lot of blood during the birth

If the mother has been bleeding, consider the following:

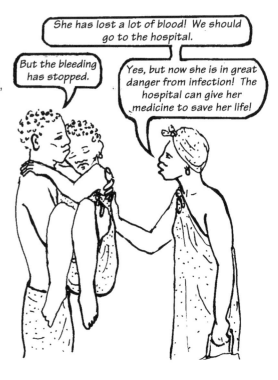

- If she has lost a lot of blood, if she is very weak, or if she has signs of shock (see p. 243), she may need to go to the hospital. Treat the mother for shock on the way (see p. 243).

- If she has lost just a little more blood than usual, or is only a little weak, use your judgment about whether to take her to the hospital or to stay at home. If possible, get medical advice.

If you decide to keep her at home, or if you cannot get medical help, this mother will need:

- complete rest and lots of quiet.

- plenty of fluid to drink in the first few hours. Rehydration drink is best (see p. 172).

- plenty of fluid to drink for the next few weeks.

- plenty of nourishing food, especially foods rich in iron (like meat and green leafy vegetables), or iron pills.

The mother needs all these things to build strong new blood, to feed and care for her baby, and to prevent infection. Be sure to watch her closely for signs of infection (see p. 298–300) for several weeks after birth.

3. Cervix can be seen at the vaginal opening

Sometimes you can see the cervix at the vaginal opening after childbirth. This problem is not really dangerous, and the cervix will usually go back up inside the mother in a few days. Meanwhile, it may help to raise the mother's hips so that they are higher than her head.

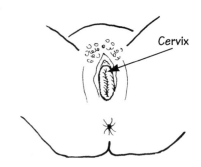

Cervix

However, this mother may be more likely to get infections. She should be very careful to keep her genitals clean, and should be watched carefully for signs of infection during the next 2 weeks (see p. 298–300). If the cervix stays at the vaginal opening for 2 weeks or more, the mother should get medical advice.

4. Mother has pain in the birth area or a growing blood blister (hematoma) in the vagina

Sometimes the womb gets tight and hard and there does not seem to be much bleeding, yet the mother still feels dizzy and weak. If this happens, she may have a hematoma (bleeding under the skin) in her vagina. The skin in this area is often dark in color, tender, and soft.

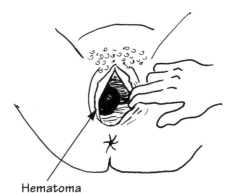
Hematoma

Although a hematoma is painful, it is usually not serious unless it is getting very large. This means that the woman is bleeding heavily into the hematoma. If it is getting very large, apply pressure to the area (if possible). If the mother has signs of shock, treat for shock (see p. 243), and go to the hospital so that the blister can be opened and the trapped blood can come out.

5. Mother feels ill, is hot-to-touch, or her temperature is above 38°C or 100.4°F; her pulse is fast and her womb is tender

A new mother's temperature is often a little higher than normal, especially on a hot day. But if she is very hot-to-touch, she has a fever. This might be a sign of infection.

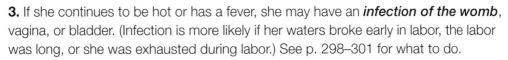

What to do

1. Check to see if she is dehydrated (see p. 171).

2. Give her some fluids and check her skin (or take her temperature) again.

3. If she continues to be hot or has a fever, she may have an *infection of the womb*, vagina, or bladder. (Infection is more likely if her waters broke early in labor, the labor was long, or she was exhausted during labor.) See p. 298–301 for what to do.

6. Mother cannot urinate after 4 hours

If the mother cannot urinate (pee) after 4 hours, there is a danger of bleeding and other problems.

What to do

1. Check her bladder. If it is not full, she may need fluids.

2. If the bladder is full or over full, try different things to help her urinate (see p. 391).

3. If she still cannot urinate, she may need to be *catheterized* (see p. 391–392). If you have not been trained to do this procedure, get medical help.

7. Mother cannot (or will not) eat or drink after 2 or 3 hours

A mother may not eat or drink for several reasons. Each of these reasons requires a different treatment:

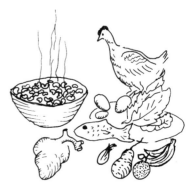

- The mother may have harmful beliefs which make her afraid to eat well or drink nourishing drinks. You can explain the importance of good food for getting her strength back, resisting infection, and making milk for the baby.

- The mother may be ill. You can check for blood loss (see p. 210), fever (see p. 298–301), and other signs of illness that may be taking away her appetite.

- The mother may be depressed (sad, angry, or very unhappy). The midwife can encourage the mother to talk about her feelings and needs.

8. Mother is not interested in the baby

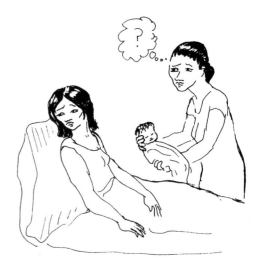

It may take a while for a mother to feel good about a new baby—especially if the mother is very tired, if she has many babies already, or if she did not want to have this baby. But a complete lack of interest can also mean that the mother is ill, that she is bleeding (or has bled) a lot, or that she is very depressed or afraid.

What to do

1. Check the mother for signs of blood loss or infection (see p. 210, 298).

2. If you do not find anything wrong, you may want to talk to the mother about her feelings. Or you may feel it is better to leave her alone, and watch and wait.

3. If the mother is depressed, or if you know that she was seriously depressed after a past birth, talk to the family about giving her extra attention and support in the next weeks. Usually this depression passes by itself in a while. but sometimes it takes a few weeks or even months.

4. If the baby wants to eat, but the mother will not feed it, you may need to find another mother *(**wet nurse**)* who can breast feed the baby and care for it until she is feeling better.

5. If you are very uneasy about the mother's lack of interest, get medical advice.

9. Mother cannot (or will not) breast feed

If the mother cannot (or will not) breast feed the baby:

- It will take longer for her womb to go back to its normal size.

- The baby is more likely to get diarrhea and other illnesses.

- The mother may have less money for good food for her family (since it is more expensive to bottle feed a baby).

- She will miss the pleasure of breast feeding.

"Breast is best" for both the mother and baby. If she does not want to breast feed for a long time, perhaps she would be willing to do it for the first few weeks or even months. If the mother will not breast feed, the family will need to find a wet nurse who will be willing to breast feed the baby.

10. Mother has convulsions (fits) or had signs of pre-eclampsia before delivery

See the sections on pre-eclampsia during pregnancy (p. 112) and labor (p. 246). If the mother had any risk signs of pre-eclampsia then, she still has a risk of convulsions for a full day and night (24 hours) after the birth.

If you are near the hospital you may want to go now, or consult with your local health officer about remaining at home. If you decide to stay at home:

- Keep the mother in a dark room.

- Make sure she is calm and relaxed. Avoid excitement.

- Give her lots of fluid to drink.

- Consider giving the medications for high blood pressure and convulsions (see p. 246–247).

Risk signs for the baby

1. Baby has trouble breathing, or takes more than 60 breaths per minute

Babies normally breathe faster than adults. If a baby has trouble breathing, or if it takes more than 60 breaths per minute, it is a risk sign. It could mean that the baby has an infection, stool in its lungs, drugs in its blood from the mother, or other problems.

What to do

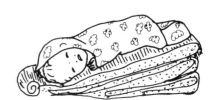

1. Keep the baby warm.

2. Check for signs of infection (see p. 292, 307).

3. Lay the baby with its head lower than its bottom to help fluids drain. Suction the baby (see p. 189)—especially if you think it might have breathed stool into its nose and throat.

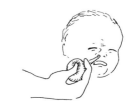

4. Encourage the baby to nurse.

5. Get medical help if you can.

2. Baby is limp, weak, or cannot seem to wake up

Many babies are very sleepy the first few days after birth They should awaken from time to time to breast feed. Some babies will breast feed as soon as they are born. Others will not start breast feeding for several hours.

When awake, the baby should respond to noise and touch. If the baby does not respond, or it seems unusually weak, slow, or limp in the first few hours, it may have one of these problems:

- The baby may not be breathing well (see p. 282).

- The baby may have an infection (see p. 292, 307).

- The baby may be sleepy from drugs or herbs given to the mother during labor.

- The baby may have other problems. If you are not sure what is wrong, get medical help.

Note: Any drug that makes the mother slow or sleepy during labor can make breathing after birth difficult for the baby. **Narcotic drugs** (like heroin, opium, and morphine) and drugs like valium go through the placenta to the baby, and can make it slow and weak. Alcohol and some plant medicines can affect the baby, too.

3. Baby is still blue, yellow, pale, or red one hour after birth

If a baby does not turn a normal color soon after birth, several different things may be wrong. Note the baby's color and which parts of its body are affected:

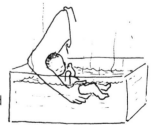

- If the baby is breathing and its hands or feet are still blue $\frac{1}{2}$ hour after birth, the baby may be cold. See #4 below for how to warm the baby.

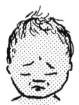

- If the baby's lips or face are still blue one hour after birth, the baby may have a problem with its heart or lungs. It may also need oxygen. Go to the hospital now.

- If the baby seems yellow, it may have a blood problem or an infection. See p. 303 and 306, and get medical help now.

- If the baby is very pale and limp, it may be anemic (thin, pale blood) or have other problems. Get medical help now.

- If the baby is very red, it may be OK. Watch it carefully for a week for signs of **yellow jaundice** (see p. 303). Get medical help as soon as possible if the baby becomes yellow, starts breathing fast, or has trouble breast feeding.

4. Baby is limp, cold-to-touch (or its armpit temperature is less than 36°C or 97°F) $\frac{1}{2}$ hour after birth

If the baby's temperature is still low $\frac{1}{2}$ hour after the birth, try to bring its temperature up to normal as quickly as possible by warming the baby. Here are some ways to warm the baby:

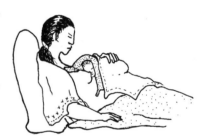

- Put the baby on the mother's skin and cover it with blankets. The mother is exactly the right temperature for the baby (unless she is ill).

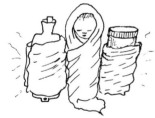

- Fill **hot water bottles** with hot water, wrap them in cloths (so you do not burn the baby) and put the bottles around the baby's body.

- Heat a bath of clean (boiled) water for the baby. Make sure the tub is very clean, too. The water temperature should be a little cooler than you would like for bathing. Warmer water will be too hot.

The baby should become more active soon after it is in the bath. When the bath is over, dry the baby carefully and check its temperature. Wrap the baby to keep it warm.

If the baby still feels cold-to-touch, or if its temperature is still low and it seems weak, get medical help.

5. Baby makes a strange, high-pitched cry

Many babies are tense and upset after birth. But a very nervous baby, or one with a strange, high-pitched cry, may need more sugar in its blood. This is especially likely if the baby is very big or very small, if the birth was unusually hard or long, or if the mother has diabetes (see p. 88).

What to do

1. Breast feed the baby (there is sugar in breast milk).

2. Give the baby sugar water in addition to breast milk. Put 1 teaspoon (about 5 grams or 1 cube) of sugar in 100 cc (about $1/_2$ cup) of boiled water. Let it cool, and give by eye dropper or spoon. The eye dropper or spoon must be very clean; it is better if it is boiled (see p. 154).

If the baby does not seem less nervous or does not stop its high-pitched crying in $1/_2$ day, get medical help.

6. Baby shows signs of infection: baby takes more than 60 breaths per minute $1/_2$ hour after birth; baby is cold-to-touch (or armpit temperature stays below 36°C or 97°F); baby seems ill, sucks poorly, and has a weak, fast heartbeat

If the baby shows any of these signs of infection, get medical help. If the nearest medical help is more than 2 hours away, give the baby antibiotics on the way. See p. 307 for the kind and amount of medicine to give.

7. Baby weighs less than 2.5 kilograms or 5.5 pounds

Very small babies have a greater risk of infection, breathing problems, and jaundice (see p. 303). The smaller the baby, the greater the risk. Small babies also may have trouble breast feeding because the mother's nipple is too big, and the milk comes too fast for them. These babies may have trouble digesting their food.

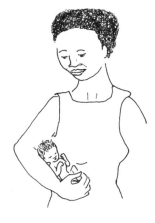

It is best for very small babies to be cared for in the hospital. But if you are going to care for this baby at home, there are some things you can do to help the baby stay healthy.

What to do

1. Keep the baby warm. It takes a lot of energy for a very small baby to stay warm. You can help a baby by **packing** it against its mother's body. If she is well, her body is exactly the right temperature for the baby:

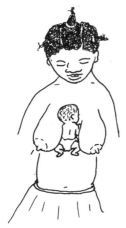

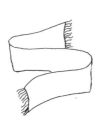

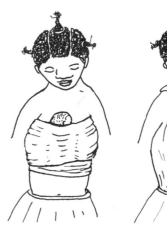

Place the naked baby between the mother's breasts, right on her skin.

Wrap the baby to her with a cloth or shawl. Make the baby snug and comfortable.

The baby stays against the mother's skin all day and all night. The mother can wear her dress or blouse over the baby.

The mother may have to change the baby's position to breast feed. If she needs to bathe, another person can **wear the baby** against her skin until the mother is done.

2. Give breast milk. Breast is best for all babies, but it is even more important if the baby is very small. Breast milk is easier for the baby to digest, it gives the best nourishment, and it protects the baby from some illnesses.

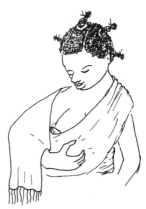

If the baby is too small to breast feed, the mother should remove milk from her breasts herself (see p. 337). The baby can then be fed with an eye dropper or a spoon until it is strong enough to breast feed. Give the baby as much as it will take. Remember to boil the container used to hold the milk, and the eye dropper or spoon, before you use them (see p. 154).

> Note: If the mother cannot breast feed for some reason, it is best for another woman to breast feed this baby.

3. Watch the baby carefullly for risk signs—especially signs of jaundice, breathing problems, and infection.

Try to visit the baby every day for the first few weeks, so that you can check for risk signs. Be sure you and the mother are familiar with signs of jaundice (see p. 303), breathing problems (see p. 290), and infection (see p. 292, 306, and 307). If the baby develops any risk signs, get medical help.

8. Baby weighs over 4 kilograms or 9 pounds

Very big babies are more likely than other babies to have breathing problems. If the mother had diabetes (see p. 88), they may also be more likely to have problems with the amount of sugar in their blood.

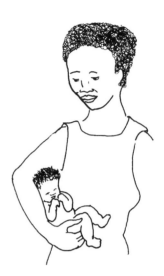

Watch big babies carefully for risk signs. Big baby problems are most likely to start during the first 2 days after birth. Check the baby several times a day during this time. If the baby shows no signs of risk, it is probably healthy and in no more danger than any other baby. If the baby appears to be cold or a little weak, you may give some boiled water with sugar after breast feeding (see p. 292). Keep this baby warm (see p. 293).

9. Baby has birth defects

A baby can be born with many kinds of birth defects. Some birth defects are more serious than others. Most of these children can still have happy, useful lives, if they get the right kind of care and help.

If a baby is born with some kind of defect, we recommend the following:

1. Seek medical advice to find out if anything will cure or reduce the problem.

2. Learn about the special needs this child has.

3. Learn what kind of things this child **will** be able to do. For example, a child who cannot walk because the legs are not formed right may have very strong arms and hands and be able to do many useful things with them. The same child may also be very smart and able to do useful things with its mind.

A very good resource book is *Disabled Village Children* by David Werner (available through Hesperian Foundation). The Foundation's address is on p. 2.

4. Help the mother to accept the child by showing that you care for her and her baby.

Babies with cleft lip *(harelip)* and cleft palate

A ***cleft lip*** is an opening or gap on the baby's upper lip, often connecting to the nostril. A ***cleft palate*** is a split in the roof of the baby's mouth. These problems can be fixed by an operation when the baby is older. Cleft lip is often repaired when the baby is 4 to 6 months old. Cleft palate is often repaired when the baby is about 18 months old.

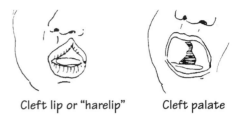

Cleft lip or "harelip"   Cleft palate

Babies with cleft lip or cleft palate may need some special help breast feeding. For babies with cleft lip, the nipple should go deep into the baby's mouth, so the nipple fills up the cleft. It there is still a hole, the mother can put her finger over it. For babies with cleft palate, the nipple should go as far back into the baby's mouth as possible. Point the nipple to the side of the cleft. The baby should eat with its head up so that milk does not go into its nose. If the baby cannot breast feed, the mother can milk her breasts herself and feed the baby with an eye dropper or spoon.

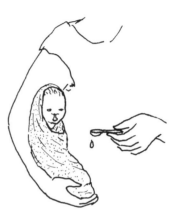

Babies with cleft lip or cleft palate may also have more ear infections and other health problems as they get older. Be sure the mother knows this. Also, a baby with a cleft lip may look very strange, and sometimes parents may feel uncomfortable with the child. It is important to remember that this baby needs and deserves the same love and attention as any other baby.

Complications in the first 2 weeks after birth

Chapter 19 contents

Complications in the first 2 weeks after birth

Risk signs for the mother

1. Womb does not stay round and hard, and it does not get slowly smaller

If the womb keeps getting soft after the first few hours:

- Have the baby breast feed more. If that doesn't work, try nipple stimulation (see p. 378).

- Massage the womb (see p. 209). If a lot of blood comes out when the womb contracts, it means that the mother is bleeding inside when the womb gets soft. If the mother does not have high blood pressure, you can give 0.2 mg ergometrine or ergonervine pills every 6 hours (or 4 times a day) for 4 to 7 days. Or there may be plant medicines that midwives in your area use to stop bleeding.

  If very little blood comes out when you massage the womb, there is probably no need for medicines. Just continue to massage from time to time and teach the mother how to do it herself.

- Watch for signs of infection (see p. 287).

- Watch for heavy bleeding.

2. Mother bleeds a lot

If the mother soaks more than about 2 pads per hour in the first day after birth, or if she soaks more than 1 pad per hour after that, she may be bleeding too much.

Use the same methods described above to make the womb contract. If the mother has been very active, ask her to rest more. If these methods do not work, try IM injections of Methergine or oxytocin (see p. 276). If the bleeding continues, get the mother to medical help. Watch for signs of shock and treat for shock (see p. 243).

3. Mother has signs of shock

If the mother shows signs of shock (see p. 243), she may be bleeding inside or she may have an infection. Treat for shock (see p. 243); see #2 above and #4 below.

4. Mother has signs of *womb infection*: bleeding starts again or gets worse; blood or discharge smells bad or has an unusual color, mother feels ill, is hot-to-touch (or has a temperature above 38°C or 100.4°F), or has chills or pain in the belly

If the mother has any one of these signs, she may have an infection of the womb. These infections are **very** dangerous. The mother could die unless she gets antibiotic medicine.

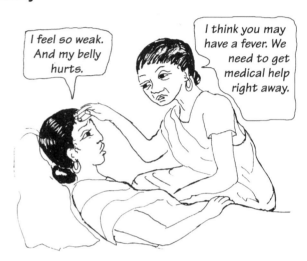

I feel so weak. And my belly hurts.

I think you may have a fever. We need to get medical help right away.

There are many different kinds of infections. Different kinds of antibiotics cure different kinds of infections. It is best for the mother to go to the hospital for special laboratory tests to decide what kind of infection she has and which antibiotic will work best. The hospital can also give her the antibiotics in IV fluids, which means the antibiotic will work better and faster.

Giving antibiotics at home

If the hospital is many hours or days away, you also can give antibiotics at home by mouth or by injection. Since you will not know exactly what kind of infection she has, you will need to give an antibiotic that covers a number of problems. But you should still try to get the mother to a hospital as soon as possible.

Injectable antibiotics work better than antibiotics given by mouth (pills or liquid). Give the injectable medicines every day until the fever has been gone for 2 days. Then, if the antibiotic can also be given by mouth, give the antibiotic by mouth for the next 7 days.

If you do not have any injectable antibiotics, give the antibiotic by mouth from the beginning. Continue giving the antibiotic until the fever has been gone for 10 days.

If you are treating at home and the fever does not go to normal after 2 days (or the mother does not feel better), get the mother to the hospital. She may need other medications (see p. 453–458).

Antibiotics for a womb infection after birth

If the infection begins in the first week after birth, give one of the medicines from the list below. Amoxicillin is the best antibiotic to use, if you have it:

Antibiotic	Dose	How to give	When to give
amoxicillin	1 gram	mouth only	3 times a day
ampicillin	1–2 grams	injection or mouth	4 times a day
cefazolin	1 gram	injection only	4 times a day
cefoxitin	2 grams	injection only	4 times a day
penicillin VK	1 gram	mouth only	6 times a day
penicillin G	2 million units	injection only	4 times a day

If the infection started one week after birth or later, give this medicine in addition to one of the antibiotics above:

metronidazole (Flagyl)	500 mg	mouth only	3 times a day

5. Mother has signs of vaginal infection: pain "down below"; pus; a swollen, hard, red lump in the vagina

Sometimes there is an infection of a tear or wound in the vagina. This is dangerous, but it is not as much of an emergency as an infection of the womb.

You can usually see a red, swollen area in the mother's vagina or feel a hard lump underneath the skin. This means there is probably pus (white or yellow fluid filled with germs) trapped inside (an *abscess*). Or the tear or wound may be open and the pus is draining out.

If you see pus, check carefully to see where it is coming from. If the pus comes from **above** the red or swollen area in the vagina, the pus may really be coming from the womb. This may mean the mother has an infection of the vagina **and** an infection of the womb. (For an infection of the womb, see p. 298.)

If pus gets into the mother's blood, it can cause a *blood infection* that goes to every part of her body and can kill her. Get medical help. If help is not available, try to drain the pus out yourself.

What to do

1. If the wound or tear is open, you can help draw the pus out:

- Apply sterile cloths dipped in very warm water to the infected area. (Boil the water first and let it cool just enough so it will not burn the mother.)

- Use plant medicines (herbs) from your area that draw pus and poison out of a wound. Wrap the herbs in a piece of clean cloth or gauze. Tie the cloth so bits of the herb cannot fall out. Boil this cloth before using, cool it slightly, and then apply it to the infected area.

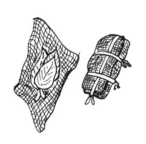
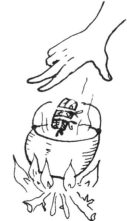

2. If the pus is trapped under the skin, the wound must be opened to let it out. You may need to go to the hospital or contact a skilled health worker in your area. Or, if you are trained and permitted to do so, you may do the following now:

- If the mother has stitches near the abscess, cut the stitches open.

- If there are no stitches to cut, pierce the abscess with a very sharp knife or razor blade. Be sure the knife or razor blade is sterile (see p. 154–156).

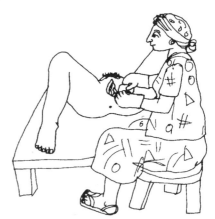

Then follow the instructions above for drawing out the pus.

3. If the mother has a hematoma or blood blister (see p. 287), use warm packs as above. Take the mother to the hospital if she shows signs of shock (see p. 243).

6. Mother's breasts are painful, red, or swollen

See p. 333–334 for the signs and treatment of *breast infection*.

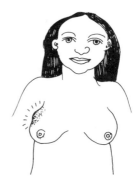

7. Mother feels severe depression (sadness), anger, fear, or craziness

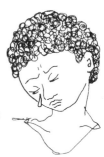

Many women feel very emotional after giving birth. Some get sad or worried or irritable for a few days, weeks, or (in some cases) months. When this happens, you can help by explaining that these feelings are common, and that they will go away after a while.

In rare cases women may get severely depressed or go crazy at some time in the first few months after childbirth. A woman who has felt this way after a past birth is more likely to feel it again after another birth. Although these emotions usually pass after a while, the woman may suffer a lot.

What to do

If the emotions are not severe, it may help for the mother to talk with someone, and to have help with the new baby and with any other work or children. If the emotions are severe, it may help to have someone stay with the mother and baby for a few days or weeks. The mother may also need to be protected so that she does not hurt herself or the baby.

Traditional remedies and rituals may also be very helpful—especially if the mother wants them or believes in them. There are also modern medicines that can help her feel better, but they can cause other problems, too. These medicines should be taken only in extreme cases.

8. Mother's legs are red, hard, and swollen

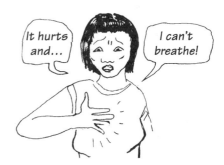

After a birth, a **blood clot** can form in a blood vessel deep in the mother's leg. This clot is very dangerous. If a bit of the clot breaks free and goes into the mother's blood, it can travel to her lungs, get stuck there, and cause her to have difficulty breathing.

You may or may not feel a hard lump in the leg. But the area will usually be painful and red. The leg often hurts when squeezed or when the mother walks. Sometimes one foot and leg will be swollen while the other leg is not. Often one leg will feel hotter than the other leg.

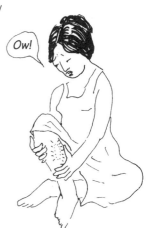

If you see one of these signs, go to the hospital at once. The mother may need special medicines to thin the blood. These medicines should only be given in a hospital, in IV fluids.

On the way to the hospital (or if you cannot go to the hospital right away), you can:

- raise the mother's legs above her hips.

- have the mother stay in bed.

- place warm packs on the swelling.

- use local remedies that you know are helpful for "thinning the blood."

9. Mother's urine or stool seems to leak out of the vagina

Sometimes the pressure of the baby's head inside the mother's vagina can cause a hole to form between the vagina and one of the tubes bringing urine (pee) or stool (shit) to the outside of her body. This is more likely if the pushing stage was long and difficult, especially after the baby's head crowned, or if scars from past surgery or injuries held the baby's head back when it was almost out.

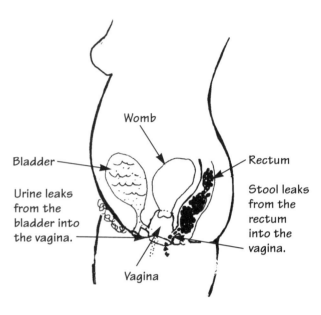

Urine or stool will drip from this hole into the vagina and then come out the vaginal opening. This is unpleasant for the mother, but it is not usually an emergency. The mother can wait 1 or 2 weeks until she has her strength back, and then see a doctor. Sometimes an operation will be able to fix the problem, but not always.

If the mother has signs of infection (see p. 298), or if she has heavy bleeding when she moves her bowels, she should get medical help as soon as possible.

Risk signs for the baby

1. Baby does not have a bowel movement within 24 hours after birth

Most babies move their bowels (shit) during or soon after birth, but some wait a few hours. The first breast milk will help the baby clean out its bowels, so the mother should be encouraged to nurse soon after birth. If the baby does not have a bowel movement within 24 hours, it may be a sign that the baby's intestines (tubes that the stool moves through) are blocked. If this is not fixed, the baby may die. Go to the hospital immediately.

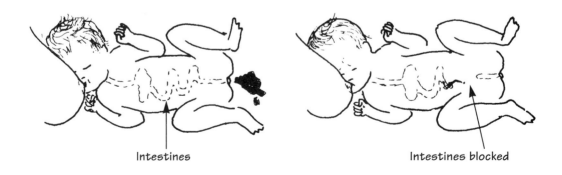

Intestines   Intestines blocked

2. Baby does not urinate within 24 hours after birth

If the baby does not urinate within 24 hours, its urine tube may be blocked. Get medical help immediately.

3. Baby gets yellow *(jaundice)*

Many babies get a little yellow after birth. This is caused by a chemical called **bilirubin** in the baby's blood. This yellow color is very dangerous if it appears in the first day of the baby's life or after the 5th day of the baby's life. It can be life threatening if the baby was born more than one month too early. These babies should go to the hospital immediately to prevent brain damage.

If the yellow color appears between 2 and 5 days after birth, it is probably OK. To keep the yellow color from getting worse, try the following:

- Let the baby breast feed a lot. You also can give boiled water (or rehydration drink—see p. 172) with a clean cup and spoon. (Do not replace breast milk with water. Give water **after** breast feeding, not before.) These fluids help wash the yellow chemical out of the baby's body.

- Let the baby sit in the sun. Sunlight helps the baby get rid of the yellow chemical and helps lessen the jaundice. However, the sun can give the baby severe burns—especially if you live in a tropical or hot climate.

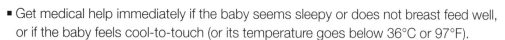

  Be careful not to sunburn the baby! It is best if the sun is coming through a clear glass window, the room is warm (not hot), and the baby is naked. Use a thin, loosely woven cloth to protect the baby's skin. Watch the time closely: 5 minutes of sun on each side (10 minutes total) every 1 to 2 hours is enough.

- Get medical help immediately if the baby seems sleepy or does not breast feed well, or if the baby feels cool-to-touch (or its temperature goes below 36°C or 97°F).

4. Vomit "shoots" out when the baby spits up

Most babies *spit up* (vomit a small amount) often. Usually the vomit just dribbles from the baby's mouth, especially after eating.

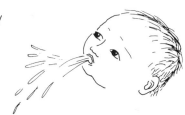

If **vomit shoots out** of the baby's mouth with some force every time it eats—and if the baby is not urinating or having a bowel movement—there may be a problem. Get medical advice.

5. Baby does not gain weight normally, or appears thin and stays small

If this happens, the baby may have one of these problems:

- infection (see p. 306)

- blocked intestines (see p. 302)

- lack of milk

- loose stools

- serious medical problems

If you suspect that the problem is infection or blocked intestines, turn to the pages listed. If you suspect that the baby is not getting enough milk, check the following:

- How often and how long the baby breast feeds. The mother should nurse the baby every 2–3 hours for at least 20 minutes, or until her breasts feel empty.

- The mother's health and diet. If the mother is ill or poorly nourished, her body may not be able to make enough milk. The family may need someone else to nurse the baby.

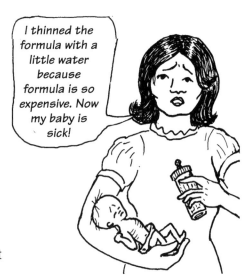

I thinned the formula with a little water because formula is so expensive. Now my baby is sick!

- How the mother prepares *formula* (if she is not breast feeding the baby). Make sure she is mixing the correct amount of powder or milk with the water. If she uses too much water (or too little milk or powder) to make the formula, her baby will become weak or ill. Remember: a baby that is bottle fed has a greater chance of getting loose stools or parasites.

If you cannot find the cause of the problem and correct it, get medical advice.

6. Baby has signs of dehydration

If the baby is not breast feeding very much, if it has diarrhea, if the weather is very hot, or if the baby has a fever, the baby can become dehydrated (not enough water in its body). Dehydration is very dangerous, and the baby might die.

These are the signs of dehydration:

- dry mouth with cracked lips

- sunken soft spot and eyes

- less urine (wets less than 4 times a day)

- dark urine

- eyes without tears

- sudden weight loss

- fast, weak pulse

- fast breathing

- loss of elasticity or stretchiness of the skin

Sunken soft spot on top of head

Sunken eyes

To check for loss of elasticity, pinch the skin on your own arm and release it. See how quickly it returns to normal. Then pinch the skin on the baby's belly and release it. If the skin returns to normal slowly, it may be getting too dry.

Pinched skin   goes down slowly.

What to do

- Have the mother breast feed often and give the baby a lot of rehydration drink in between breast feedings (see p. 172). It is best to boil the water for rehydration drink first. Give the drink with a spoon or an eye dropper. Give a few drops every minute for several hours until the baby is better.

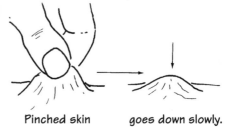

- If you do not have rehydration drink and cannot get the salt or sugar you need to make it, give plain boiled water.

- Get medical help if the baby does not get better in 4 hours.

- If the baby seems ill or stops breast feeding well, look for signs of infection (see p. 306).

7. Baby has signs of infection

A baby can get an infection when germs enter its body through the cord, skin, mouth, or eyes during labor or after birth. These infections are very dangerous and can kill the baby.

A baby has signs of infection when it:

- stops nursing.

- has a weak suck, weak reflexes, and weak cry (see p. 203).

- seems very sleepy or is not active.

- feels hot or cold-to-touch (or has a temperature above 38°C or 100.4°F, or below 36°C or 97°F).

- has diarrhea.

- has convulsions.

> **Caution!** A baby has a greater risk of infection if any of these things happened during labor: the mother's waters broke more than 24 hours before birth; the waters smelled bad, or looked dark or cloudy; or the mother had a temperature above 38°C or 100.4°F during labor. This baby may get an infection sometime in the next few days, even if it does not seem ill now. Check the baby every day for 2 weeks. It is also best if the baby can be in or near the hospital.

The baby may also show other signs of illness, depending on the kind of infection it has:

- **Lung infection** *(pneumonia)*. The baby will take more than 50 breaths per minute or appear to be breathing very fast. It will grunt when breathing, suck in the skin between the ribs with each breath, and have blue skin. Suctioning does not help.

- **Brain infection** *(meningitis)*. The baby will have a stiff neck and lie with its head and neck bent back. It may vomit, the soft spot on its head will bulge, and it may become unconscious. These signs may appear quickly—in a few hours or days—or slowly over several weeks. Without treatment most babies die, become brain damaged, or are disabled.

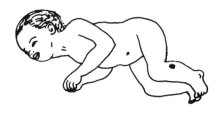

- **Cord infection.** The baby's cord stump will be hot and red, smell bad, and drain pus. When the cord falls off, the mucus underneath will be white or yellow, and smell bad.

- **Blood infection.** The baby will seem very sleepy, have yellow skin or eyes, and vomit or have diarrhea.

What to do

If you see signs of infection:

1. Take the baby to the hospital or health center immediately!
Do not try to treat the baby at home.

2. If you have antibiotics, and are trained and permitted to give them, inject the antiobiotic on the way to the hospital if you will be traveling for more than 2 hours. If the journey will take more than 12 hours or one full day, you may give a second dose of the same antibiotic. Be sure to tell the hospital what medications you gave and when.

The antibiotics listed below can be used to treat any infection. You may need to check with your local health officer about which medications you may use or carry with you. Some areas may use something other than those listed below. Once the baby is at the hospital or health center, it will need to be given antibiotics for 7 to 10 days. For more information about antibiotics, see the Green Pages at the back of this book.

Antibiotics for infection (dosage depends on the baby's weight)			
Give one of the following:			
Antibiotic	**If the baby is 2 kilograms (4 pounds) or less**	**If the baby is between 2 and 4 kilograms (4 to 8 pounds)**	**If the baby is 4 kilograms (8 pounds) or more**
ampicillin OR	200 mg	300 mg	400 mg
gentamicin OR	5 mg	7.5 mg	10 mg
kanamycin OR	15 mg	24 mg	32 mg
penicillin G	200,000 units	300,000 units	400,000 units

Give the antibiotic IM into the top of the baby's thigh (see p. 386).

8. Baby has signs of tetanus (lockjaw)

New babies get tetanus when a germ that lives in dirt and the stools of people or animals gets into its body through the cord. Even with the best hospital care, most new babies with tetanus will die. **It is very important to vaccinate all babies at birth to prevent this serious disease. See p. 229.**

The danger of a baby getting tetanus through its cord is greatest when:

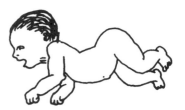

Baby's head and neck
are bent back.

- The mother has not been vaccinated against tetanus during the last 5 years.

- The cord was cut with an instrument that was not completely clean.

- The cord was not kept clean and dry.

- The cord was not cut close to the baby's body (see p. 191).

Signs of tetanus:

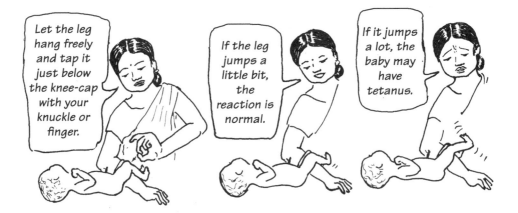

Let the leg hang freely and tap it just below the knee-cap with your knuckle or finger.

If the leg jumps a little bit, the reaction is normal.

If it jumps a lot, the baby may have tetanus.

What to do

Take the baby to the hospital immediately for special medications. If the hospital is more than 2 hours away, inject 100,000 units of penicillin G.

SECTION E

For healthier families

Introduction

Although a midwife will probably spend most of her time with individual women, her work can affect the health of the entire family. She may work with the family directly (for example, when she teaches a pregnant woman's family and friends about labor and birth), or she may affect the family in a less direct way (for example, by explaining family planning methods to a woman after birth).

The following chapters will talk about the different ways a midwife can help families become more healthy:

- Teaching people about birth (chapter 20)

- Breast is best (chapter 21)

- Family planning (chapter 22)

- Sexually transmitted diseases (chapter 23)

Teaching people about birth

Chapter 20 contents

Teaching people about birth

In this chapter we will talk about teaching women, and their families and friends, about birth. We feel this is very important because when people know what is going on and what to do, birth is often safer and easier. Knowing what to expect can help a mother be less afraid and more relaxed during labor. It also can help family members or friends work with the mother and, if necessary, the midwife during the birth.

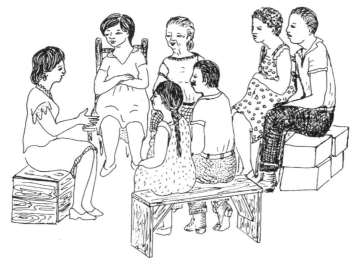

Teaching and learning about birth can happen anywhere. Here are just a few ways it can be done:

- teaching weekly classes

- holding a 1 day or ½ day workshop

- teaching a little at each prenatal checkup

- teaching many women on a **prenatal day** (when many women come for their checkups on the same day)

- going to the woman's home before birth

- training a helper to go to a woman's home before birth

We suggest that you teach everything that is listed in the chapter contents (see the previous page), in that order. Since many of these topics are covered in detail in other parts of the book, we will discuss them briefly here and ask you to turn to other chapters for more information. In addition, review p. 12 for general rules about good teaching.

Two of these topics have not been covered in other parts of the book, so we will discuss them in more detail here. These topics are: *How to have an easier, safer, and shorter birth* and *What to do if the baby comes so fast that the midwife or doctor is not there.*

How the body works

See chapters 3 and 8 to review what is inside the body, and what happens during labor and birth. Mark those sections that you think are important to teach others about. You will probably want to include signs that labor is near, what happens in the body during each stage of labor, and what happens in the body immediately after the birth.

To teach about how the body works, it helps to use pictures and models. The *Teaching materials* section at the end of this book explains how to make many useful things for teaching, and how to use them to demonstrate what the body is doing.

It will also help to tell stories about good labors and births you have seen. Show pictures, photos, films, or videotapes if you can get them. Also, show the equipment in your kit and explain what each piece of equipment is for. Explain any **procedures**—like cutting the cord or putting medicine in the baby's eyes—that occur during a birth.

How to prepare the house and equipment for the birth

Review chapter 9 on how to prepare the house and equipment for the birth. Pay special attention to p. 148, which lists things the mother may want to have ready.

What you decide to teach will depend partly on local customs and partly on what is possible in your area. But 2 important things that should always be emphasized are: 1) keeping the birth area clean, and 2) arranging transportation for an emergency.

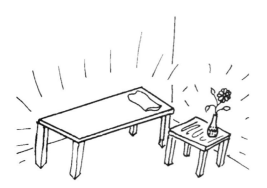
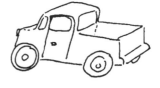

How to have an easier, shorter, and safer birth

Most women have some pain in labor but, in normal birth, no woman needs to suffer *agony*. In normal births, the real suffering usually comes if the mother is fearful or fights her labor, or if people around her do not give her kind and respectful support.

In this section we talk about having a **labor partner** to give good labor support. Then we describe some of the methods a woman can use to relax and work with her body. Most of these methods can be learned during pregnancy. In labor, people can try them out and use the ones that work best.

1. The labor partner

It is best for the woman to have at least one other person with her during labor and birth. We call this person the labor partner. Labor partners should be people who care about the mother and are willing to help her. Most important, they should be people the mother wants to have at the birth.

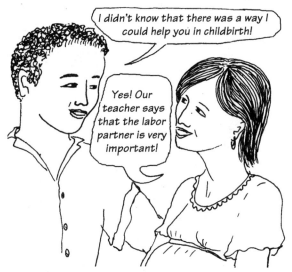

I didn't know that there was a way I could help you in childbirth!

Yes! Our teacher says that the labor partner is very important!

In some places, women are the only people who can be with a woman when she is in labor. In other cultures, it has become the custom for the husband or boyfriend to be the labor partner. In some places, the husband or boyfriend must deliver the baby because there is no one else. In the sections below, we will refer to the labor partner as "she," but we are referring to anyone—either a man or a woman—who helps the woman during labor.

In some cultures it is not OK for friends or family to attend births. The midwife or her helper then needs to act as a labor partner.

2. Relaxation exercises

The way that a woman responds to her labor contractions can make a big difference in how easy or difficult the labor seems. When a woman fights her labor, she gets tense and the pain can seem worse and the labor can seem longer. When a woman relaxes her body and her mind, knowing that strong contractions are good because they help open the cervix, she can sometimes help speed up her labor.

There are 2 kinds of relaxation: **body relaxation** and **emotional relaxation**. If a woman can relax her body during labor, it will usually (though not always) help her relax emotionally.

Body relaxation

Here is an exercise that teaches a woman how to control the tension in her body. You can do it with her, but it is even better to teach her labor partner how to lead the exercise. The mother should practice this exercise every day.

1. Have the mother sit or lie down in a comfortable position. The partner should sit facing her.

2. Explain that you are going to ask the mother to tighten each part of her body, one part at a time, until the whole body is tight. Then you will ask her to relax each part, one part at a time, until the whole body is relaxed.

Explain to the partner that when you ask a woman to relax a part of her body, she should gently but firmly touch the woman there to see if she is relaxed.

3. After leading the women and their partners through this exercise, teach the partners how to lead it without your help. They can give the commands to her, like this:

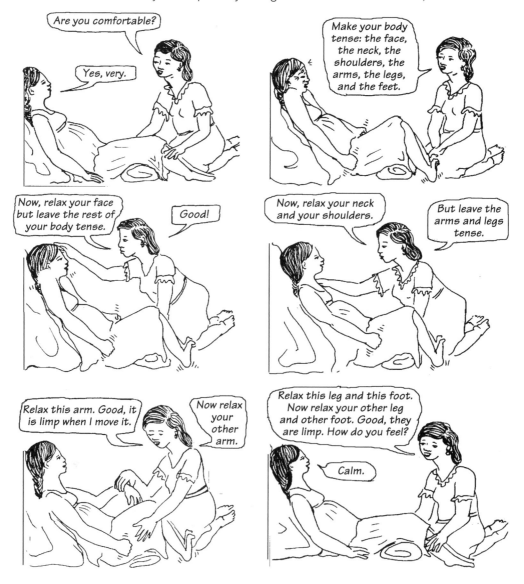

This exercise is helpful in late pregnancy and labor. If a woman in late pregnancy cannot sleep because she is tense or uncomfortable, this exercise may help her relax and rest. During labor, the partner can watch for signs of tension. Then he or she can remind the mother to relax by touching the tense place and saying *Relax your shoulders...* (or whatever is needed).

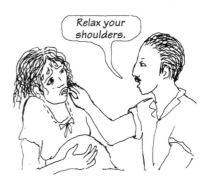

Relax your shoulders.

Emotional relaxation

The most important kind of relaxation is emotional relaxation. A woman can be quiet and keep the body relaxed but still be very nervous or afraid on the inside. The labor partner can help by talking with the mother about her fears, letting her cry for a while, cuddling with her, or letting her get up and move around. She needs to be encouraged and reminded that many women have had babies before her. She can do it, too.

Here is an exercise that can help to calm a pregnant woman's mind. It is called a **visualization exercise**. This exercise is very helpful to some women and useless to others, especially if they get tense when lying still.

1. Ask the mother to stand, sit, or lie quite still—with her eyes closed.

2. Slowly and quietly describe a peaceful image—maybe a favorite image of hers. You might ask her to imagine that her body is made of light, or that she is a stream flowing downhill in the sun, or that she is floating on air. Or, she could imagine that each contraction is a flower opening.

Here are some other things that can help:

- Tell stories about women who have had easier labors because they were relaxed.

- Remind the woman to welcome the contractions.

- If she is a strong, hard worker, ask her to think of labor as work, a job that she must do.

- If she needs to pay more attention to what is going on, ask her to picture the cervix or the womb opening up and letting the baby out.

Oooh! That was a BAD one!

No! It was a GOOD one! Strong contractions are good! You must try to welcome labor. The more you fight it, the longer it will be!

- Ask each labor partner to remind a mother that strong contractions are normal and help bring the baby faster.

- Remind each labor partner that even when a woman is very relaxed, labor can still be long and hard. Never make a woman feel guilty if her labor is long or hard. Encourage her. Do not blame her.

Note: If a woman is very religious she may wish to ask God or the Spiritual World for help during labor. Praying for strength and wisdom during labor can help a woman feel calm and safe.

3. Touch

Touch can be very important in labor, but it is important to find out what kind of touch makes the mother feel best. The best way to teach good touch is simply to touch the mothers and labor partners and let them see how it feels.

Here are some examples of touch that many women find helpful:

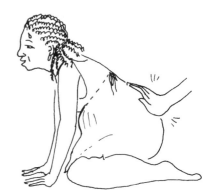

- A firm, calm touch on the body, or pressure against the lower back, during a contraction. A few women also seem to like having the belly gently stroked.

- Massage between contractions.

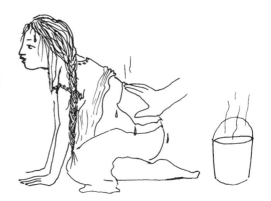

- Hot or cold cloths on the woman's lower back or belly. If the mother is hot and sweating, a cool, wet cloth on the forehead usually feels good.

4. Different positions and movement

There are many good positions in labor. Some women need to lie very still and relax during contractions. Others need to walk, stand, sit, sway the hips, rock back and forth, or even dance during labor. Women should do whatever helps them feel relaxed. The only position that is not good is lying flat on the back.

When teaching, show women and their partners the different positions that may work. Let them practice getting into different positions. Encourage labor partners to find a way to physically support women in these positions. For example, if a woman needs to walk during labor, the partner can go with her and hold her up during contractions.

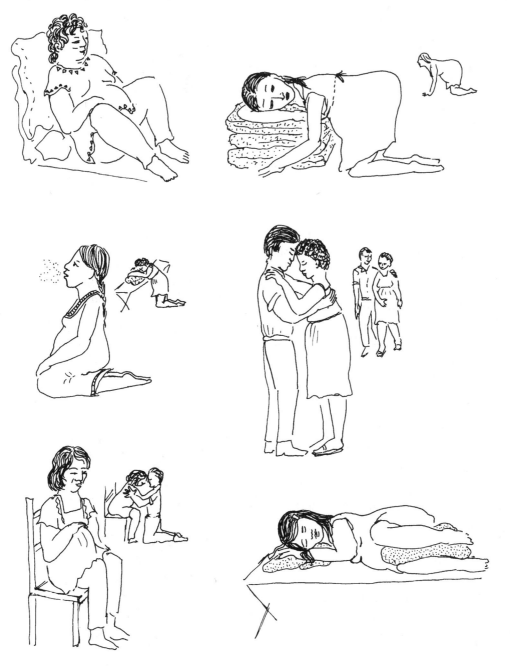

5. Breathing exercises

The purpose of **breathing exercises** is to help a woman relax and say *yes* to her labor. Breathing exercises will help keep her mind on the exercise, not on her fear or worry. This way she can work with her body, not against it.

There are many different breathing methods. It is useful to teach several so that women can use whichever method helps most. Some women even invent their own in labor.

Slow breathing

Slow breathing is one of the most effective breathing methods because it helps women stay calm and peaceful. Slow breathing may also bring more air to the baby.

Here are 2 kinds of slow breathing.

- *Candle breathing.* In this method, a woman breathes in through her nose, then gently and slowly breathes out through her mouth. She breathes out just enough to bend a candle flame, not to put it out.

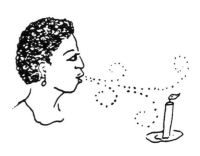

- *Deep slow breathing.* In this method a woman breathes in deep, slow breaths that expand her chest and belly.

To teach people these methods, first demonstrate them yourself. Then let them practice like this:

1. The woman and her partner should sit or lie down in a comfortable position.

2. Talk the woman and her partner through a pretend contraction. Make it as long as a real contraction. Say something like this:

The contraction is beginning. Take a deep breath, let it out, then begin candle breathing. Breathe in through the nose, out through the mouth. Slow and easy. The contraction is getting stronger... stronger... stronger. Now it is getting milder... weaker... and it is over.

3. While the woman breathes, the labor partner should hold her hand or touch her in some way, look into her eyes if this is done in her culture, and breathe with her. If a woman does not have a labor partner, she can look at something in the room that is beautiful or interesting, and practice by herself.

Encourage mothers to practice this breathing at home a few times every day. In late pregnancy, the mother can use her practice contractions (see p. 137) to practice slow breathing, even though these contractions are not painful.

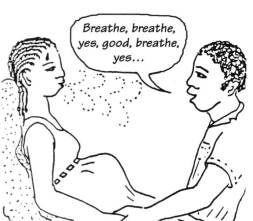

Breathe, breathe, yes, good, breathe, yes...

Other kinds of breathing

A woman may use slow breathing all through labor. If it is working, she should not change. Other women find that when labor gets strong, slow breathing does not hold their attention. A woman may start to feel lost and begin to panic. If this happens, it is time to use another method:

- *Hee breathing.* In this method, a woman makes a sound like a strong but soft *hee, hee, hee....*

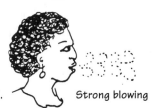

Hee, hee, hee, hee, hee, hee...

- *Light panting.* In this method, a woman takes quick, shallow breaths into the chest, but not into the belly.

- *Pant-and-blow.* In this method, a woman takes shallow, quick breaths into her chest and then blows out, in this pattern: *pant pant, blow blow, pant pant, blow blow.*

- *Strong blowing.* In this method, a woman blows out hard and fast.

Strong blowing

When using any of these methods, the woman should start with slow breathing at the beginning of the contraction and then use fast breathing only during the strongest part. When the contraction begins to pass, the mother should slow her breathing again.

To teach people these methods, first demonstrate them yourself. Then let people practice like this:

1. The mother and labor partner face each other in a comfortable position.

2. Talk the mother and her partner through a pretend contraction. Say something like this:

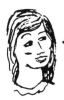

The contraction is beginning. Take a deep breath, let it out, then begin slow breathing. Now the contraction is getting stronger, very fast! Slow breathing does not work anymore. Start pant-and-blow breathing. Pant pant, blow blow, pant pant! Good! The contraction is still strong. It is getting weaker. Slow the breathing down. Slower. Slower. Let it go. The contraction is over. Take a deep breath and relax.

3. If it is OK in their culture, encourage the mother and her partner to look into each other's eyes (unless the mother wants to close her eyes) and breathe together. (During labor, the labor partner may get dizzy when trying to breathe with the mother. The mother does not get dizzy because she is working hard and needs a lot of air. If the partner gets dizzy, she can move her lips **as if** breathing. Or she can gently tap the rhythm of the breathing on the mother's leg, or chant in time with the mother's breathing.)

The labor partner can also look for signs of tension as the mother breathes: Does the mother hunch her shoulders? Make a bad face? Squeeze her knees together? If she does, the partner can help by putting a hand on the tense place and reminding the mother to relax.

6. The voice

Some women find it helpful to make noise in labor. This is perfectly acceptable in some places, and women feel free to do it. In other places, people believe women should be quiet in labor.

We have found that some noise is helpful and some is not. We encourage women to try the following when using the voice in labor:

- Sounds should be low and full, not high and squeaky. Powerful sounds or musical sounds, like *aah, uuuh, oooh* can help a woman feel strong and her body open.

- Screaming, complaining sounds, like *EEEE, Aiii, and OOeee* are usually not helpful. They can make a woman feel closed and tight.

- The sounds can be as loud as the woman wants.

- Labor partners should make sounds with the mother. If the mother begins to whine or squeak, the partner can remind her to keep her sounds low and open.

Here are some examples of helpful sounds:

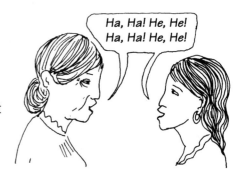

Ha, Ha! He, He! Ha, Ha! He, He!

- **Singing and chanting.** This chant often works well: *Ha, Ha! He, He! Ha, Ha! He, He!* If a woman is having a lot of trouble accepting her contractions, it sometimes helps to have her chant *Yes! Yes! Yes!* during the strongest ones. Or sometimes singing a simple musical *Aaaaaaaaa* during contractions is very good.

- **Moaning and other sounds.** This moan is often useful: *Aaaaaaaaaauuuuuuuuunnnnnnh.* Or women may make up useful sounds of their own.

To practice, do a pretend contraction that starts with breathing and then go into a chant or other sound. Many people may feel silly and laugh when you ask them to practice this. But since using the voice can be very useful in labor, it is good to know it.

7. Pushing

Once the cervix is open, the mother needs to push the baby out. Use pictures or models (see p. 447) to show how this works. Talk about the urge to push that many women feel, and that pushing often feels good.

Pushing methods

There are 3 helpful pushing methods that women should know:

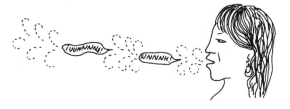

- **Pant pushing.** The mother pants like she would in pant breathing, then pushes whenever she wants to.

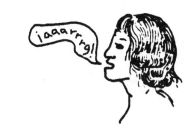

- **Moan or growl pushing.** The mother takes a deep breath and lets it out. Then she takes another deep breath and pushes. While pushing, she lets her mouth go loose, her jaw go forward, and she moans or growls (or gives any low, open sound).

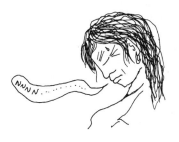

- **Hold-the-breath pushing.** The mother takes a deep breath and lets it out. Then she takes another deep breath and fills her chest completely. She holds this breath for a little bit and then drops her chin to her chest and pushes as long and hard as she can. When she needs to breathe, she takes 2 deep breaths, holds the second breath, and then pushes as long and hard as she can again.

In teaching, show the mother and her partner these methods. The mother can practice if she wants to, but she should practice pushing very gently. Remind her that she will be pushing much harder in labor.

Pushing positions

A woman can also push better if she is in one of these good pushing positions:

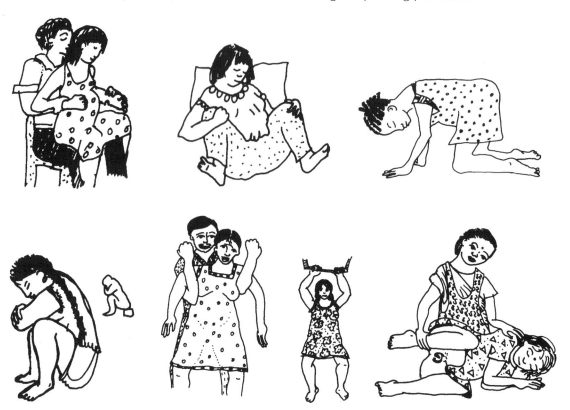

Mothers and labor partners can practice different positions before birth. Labor partners can practice holding the women up and encouraging them to push.

How to stop pushing

When the baby's head crowns (see p. 187–188, 141–142), you may want the mother to stop pushing so that the head can come out slowly. Her womb will keep pushing by itself, but the pushing will be more gentle without her help. The easiest way for the mother to stop pushing is for her to blow very hard and fast when she breathes out.

To practice, explain to the mother and her partner that it may be very hard for her to stop pushing just because the midwife asks her to. To help them understand how blowing hard can help, have the mother blow hard while trying to push with her stomach muscles. It is hard to do! Ask the labor partner to help by holding the mother's hands, looking into her eyes (if this is OK in her culture), and chanting: *blow, blow, blow* with each breath. Or the partner can tap the rhythm on the mother's leg.

Here is a story that shows how the methods described above can help make labor safer and easier:

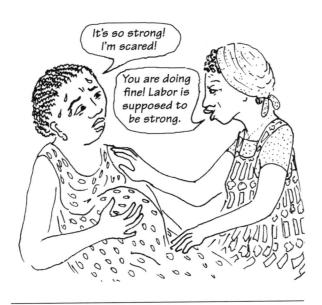

Teresa's Birth
(based on a true story)

Teresa was having her first baby. She was young and did not yet have a lot of experience in life. When her midwife, Adelina, came to her house that morning, things seemed to be going well. The contractions were regular and slow, but getting stronger.

Teresa labored all day. By midday the labor was very strong. Teresa's contractions were hard and long, and came closer and closer together. "This is going to be an easy one," thought Adelina. "The baby will probably be born before sunset." But after a while the labor seemed to slow down and get stuck. By evening Adelina realized that Teresa was laboring and laboring but making no progress. In fact, things seemed to have gone backwards. Her contractions were weaker and further apart than they were before. But there were no other risk signs. It seemed to Adelina that Teresa was resisting her labor. She did not know what to do about it, so she sent for another midwife, Dolores, and asked for help.

When Doña Dolores arrived, she found Teresa lying down in a dark room with 3 friends. Every time she had a contraction, she would make a terrible face, throw her arm over her eyes, turn her face to the wall, and make a miserable moaning sound. Her friends just sat there looking very serious and grim. Sometimes Teresa would sit up suddenly in a panic and cry, "I have to shit! I have to shit!" and run outside to relieve herself. Of course she did not really have to move her bowels; she was just feeling the pressure of the baby's head. Then she would cry, "NO! NO!" and run back to her cot and lie down.

Dolores watched for a little while, and then decided what to do. First, she made a cup of relaxing herbal tea for Teresa to drink. Then she opened up all the windows (it was a warm, beautiful night) and lit the lamps. She sat down on Teresa's bed and had a serious talk with her:

"Teresa," she said, "do you want to go to the hospital?"

"What will they do for me if I go there?" asked Teresa.

"Well, they might give you medicine to make the labor stronger and faster. They also might use forceps or do an operation."

"Do I have to go?" asked Teresa.

"No, not yet," said Dolores. "There are no signs of risk except that your labor is stuck. If you like, we can stay home a little longer."

"I want to stay here," said Teresa, "but I don't know what to do. It hurts so much."

"First, you must stop fighting your labor," said Dolores. "If you welcome your contractions, labor will be faster. Remember, it has to get strong to bring the baby."

Adelina said, "Yes. When you started this labor you were still a young girl, but now you must become a woman."

At that moment, Teresa had another contraction. She closed her eyes and started to panic, but Dolores took her hands, and said, "Teresa! Sit up! Look into my eyes and breathe with me! Breathe! Breathe! Relax your shoulders! Breathe! Breathe! Good!" Soon they were working together breathing and relaxing. Dolores encouraged her, and also kept her so busy breathing and relaxing during contractions that she did not have time to be afraid. Between contractions she gave Teresa some fruit to eat and water to drink, and talked some more about welcoming the contractions. The labor began to come alive again. She began to make progress. Teresa's friends watched and soon learned how they could cheerfully and firmly support her during contractions.

When the contractions got stronger and stronger, Teresa began to panic again. "Teresa!" said Dolores, "Let's chant with these strong ones! Ha HA! He HE! Ha HA! He HE!" Her friends held her hands and chanted with her. This helped a lot and Teresa continued to progress. The birth was getting near. Labor kept getting stronger. After a while the contractions got so strong that she would forget to chant and start to panic again. "Teresa!" said Dolores, "You are strong. You are doing beautifully. Let's pant and blow! Pant Pant! Blow Blow!" Together they panted and blew through several more contractions, and then Teresa was ready to give birth. She got up onto her hands and knees, and gave birth to a healthy baby girl.

After the birth, when they were sure that all was well, Adelina said to Dolores, "Thank you. I did not know what to do for her." Dolores answered, "That is because you are always so strong. When you had your babies you were never afraid. That is the way you are. But I am a lot more like Teresa. With my first birth I started every contraction with the word "No". My labor was very long! When I had my next baby, I had someone who knew how to help me relax. The birth was much shorter and easier, so I learned how to help other women relax." "In the future, I will know what to do, too." said Adelina.

What to do if the baby comes so fast that the midwife or doctor is not there

You may want to teach the labor partner what to do if the baby comes before the midwife or doctor can be there. This is especially important if the family lives far away from medical help.

Review chapters 11 and 12 on what happens during and immediately after the birth. These are the important things to include in your teaching:

- how to keep everything clean (see p. 5)
- how to clear the baby's mouth and nose to help it breathe (see p. 189)
- when to have the baby breast feed (see p. 204)
- how to deliver the placenta (see p. 197)
- how to cut the cord after the placenta is out (see p. 191)
- how to test if the womb is firm after birth (see p. 209)
- how to massage the mother's womb if the mother bleeds heavily (see p. 209–210)
- how to treat the mother for shock if she loses a lot of blood (see p. 243)

What to do if things go wrong during labor and birth

Review chapters 15 through 17 on the complications of labor and birth. The mother and family should know what the most common complications are and what can be done about them. This way, if something goes wrong they will be less afraid.

But remember to emphasize that most births are normal. People should expect things to go well, but they should be prepared in case they do not.

What happens after birth

Review chapters 13, 14, and 18 about what happens after birth. Here is a list of things you may want to cover in your teaching:

- risk signs in the first 2 weeks after birth (see p. 226)
- why breast is best (see chapter 21)
- immunizations (vaccinations) for the new baby (see p. 228–229)
- child spacing and family planning (see chapter 22)
- eating good foods after childbirth (see chapter 4)

Massaging a soft womb

One of the most common risk signs after birth is a soft womb that does not contract. To show women how to massage a soft womb, try the following:

1. Ask 2 women to help. One woman with a soft belly lies down and lets the other women feel her belly. This is how a soft womb will feel. The women can practice massaging the soft womb.

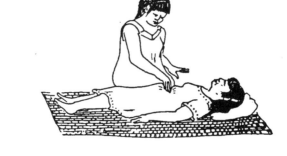

2. Then ask the second woman to lie down. Place a coconut or hard gourd on her stomach, and cover it with soft cloth at least 2 centimeters or $3/4$ inch thick. Then let the women feel it; this is what the womb should feel like after birth. After a real birth they should massage the womb until it feels like this.

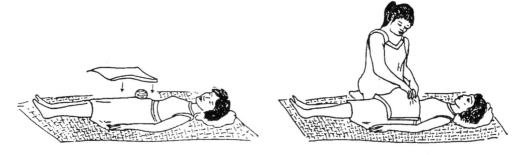

Other things you may want to cover

These things are not covered in this book, but you may want to talk about them if you are experienced in these areas:

- sex after birth
- older children and the new baby
- checkups and clinic visits for the new baby and young child
- healthy diets for young children

Breast is best!

Chapter 21 contents

Breast is best!

Why breast is best

Breast milk is the perfect food for a baby:

- It has all the *nutrients* the baby needs.

- It is easy for the baby to digest.

- It gives the baby important protection from infections.

- It is always fresh, clean, and ready to eat.

Breast feeding also has advantages for the mother and her family:

- It slows the mother's bleeding after birth.

- It helps prevent the mother from getting pregnant again too soon (see p. 343).

- It does not cost a lot of money.

Baby *formula* or milk from other animals has several problems:

- It can be less nutritious, especially if it is not made correctly or is watered down *(diluted)*.

- It is harder for the baby to digest.

- It will not help prevent infections.

- It can cause infections and illness in the baby if it is not made or stored correctly (if it "goes bad").

- It can be expensive and hard to get.

- It can cause diarrhea (loose stools) or even death if the water is dirty.

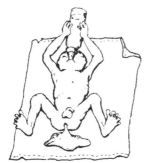

Bottle-fed babies are more likely
to get sick and die.

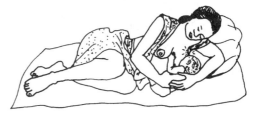

Breast-fed babies are healthier.

Who should not breast feed

For the reasons listed above, it is important for all mothers—whenever possible—to breast feed their babies. However, there are 2 situations in which a mother should **not** breast feed **if a safe alternative is available**:

- The mother is seriously ill or dehydrated (see p. 171). Breast feeding could make the mother's health worse.

- The mother has AIDS or HIV infection. The disease can be passed to the baby through breast milk.

These women should be helped to find another way to feed their babies—if possible (see p. 337–338). If there is no safe alternative, then the mother should breast feed.

How to have enough milk

Breast milk is the best and only food the baby needs for the first 6 months. In order to produce enough milk, the mother needs to be healthy herself. She needs to drink plenty of liquids, eat plenty of nutritious foods, and get enough rest.

The amount of breast milk is also affected by how much and how long the baby sucks at the breast. (New babies usually breast feed every 2 or 3 hours.) Normally, the breasts make as much milk as the baby needs. If the baby empties the breasts, they begin to make more. If the baby does not empty them, they will soon make less milk.

Note: If a mother gives a baby formula, water, or other foods, the baby will suck at the breasts less. This will cause the breasts to make less milk. Start breast feeding within 2 hours of the baby's birth. Even though the mother's milk does not come in right away, the baby needs the colostrum (see p. 204) that comes in before the milk.

The mother will know that the baby is getting enough breast milk if the baby wets more than 7 times a day, and if the baby seems healthy and gains about 200 grams or 7 ounces a week.

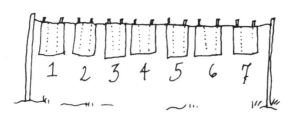

This baby gets enough milk! It has 7 wet nappies (diapers) in a day!

Care of the breasts

A mother must keep her hands and nipples clean to prevent dirt and germs from getting into the baby's mouth. This also helps prevent sore nipples and **breast infections**.

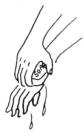

A mother should wash her hands with soap and water before touching her nipples and before breast feeding. She should also wash her hands after she urinates (pees), has a bowel movement (shits), or touches something dirty.

She should also try to clean her breasts with clean water once a day. She should not put any cream, oil, or alcohol on the nipples.

CLEAN BOILED WATER

Common problems while breast feeding

1. The mother has flat or inverted nipples

If the mother's nipples are flat or **inverted** (sink into the breast), the baby may have problems holding on to the breast while breast feeding.

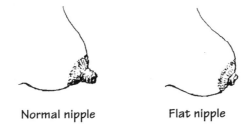

Normal nipple   Flat nipple

It is a good idea to check for flat or inverted nipples during pregnancy. Gently pinching and pulling the nipple several times a day in the last month of pregnancy may help them stand out better.

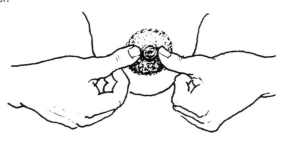

Babies may have the most difficulty sucking on a flat or inverted nipple during the first few days after birth, when the breasts are very full. But most babies can learn to suck well once they learn to get the nipple deep into their mouths. Here are some things the mother can do to help the baby take the breast correctly:

- If the nipple is flat, the mother can pinch the nipple to make it stand out before giving her breast to the baby:

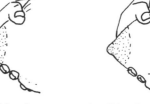

- If the nipple is inverted, the mother can take the breast in her hand and then pull back toward the chest. The nipple will stand up:

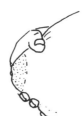

Take the breast like this   **and pull back toward the chest. The nipple will stand up.**

- If the breast is hard, the mother can milk the breast (see p. 337) a little to help soften the nipple and help pull it out.

- The mother can try different positions, like holding the baby in the under arm position or lying down with the baby, so that its mouth does not slip off the breast.

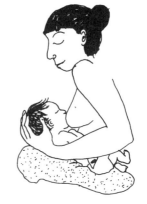

- The mother can put a few drops of milk on the baby's lips to encourage it to suck.

- If the baby is not able to take the nipple correctly after 2 days, the mother can milk her own breasts and give it to the baby by spoon. The mother should keep trying to breast feed the baby during this time. Most babies will learn to take milk from a breast with a flat or inverted nipple with time.

To prevent infection, the mother should also dry an inverted nipple well after each breast feeding.

2. The mother has swollen *(engorged)* breasts

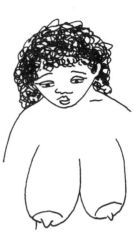

Sometimes a mother's breasts get very full and hard, especially during the first few days and weeks after the birth. This can be painful for the mother and make her more likely to develop a breast infection. It can make it hard for the baby to suck on the nipple. If the mother begins breast feeding the baby very soon after the birth, this may be less of a problem. But if a mother's breasts do get swollen, she can:

- Breast feed the baby more often (every 1 or 2 hours, for at least 10 minutes on each breast).

- Put warm damp cloths on the breasts for a few minutes before breast feeding, and then apply cool cloths after breast feeding.

- Between feedings, let the milk leak freely and support the breasts with a bra or cloth.

- Take paracetamol (acetaminophen) about 20 minutes before breast feeding to lessen the pain.

- If the baby has trouble getting onto the breast because it is swollen, squeeze the milk out until the breast is soft enough for the baby to take.

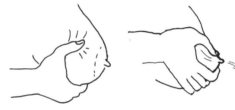

3. The mother has a breast infection *(mastitis, abscess)*

Infection inside the breast can occur if the mother has sore, cracked nipples; full, engorged breasts; wears a very tight bra; or is over tired or in poor health. Preventing these situations will help prevent breast infection.

Signs of breast infection:

- hot, red, sore area or lump on the breast

- hot-to-touch, or has a fever or chills

- body aches and pains

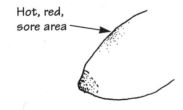

Hot, red, sore area

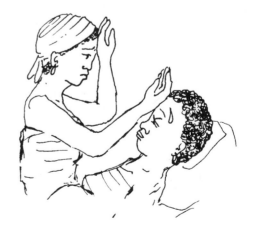

If a mother thinks she may have a breast infection starting, she should:

- keep breast feeding frequently (every 2 hours), giving the baby the sore breast first.

- stay in bed (and keep the baby with her so it can feed often).

- drink lots of liquid.

- place hot, wet, clean cloths on the sore breast for 15 to 20 minutes before and between each feeding.

- gently massage the sore breast.

- take paracetamol (acetaminophen) for pain.

If she is hot-to-touch or has fever and chills, she should do all of the above and:

- Take one of the following antibiotics right away! **Take the antibiotic 4 times per day (every 6 hours) by mouth for a full 10 days. She should not stop taking the medicine until 10 days have passed.** (Dicloxacillin is the best antibiotic to use, if you have it.)

dicloxacillin	500 mg
erythromycin	500 mg
amoxicillin	500 mg
ampicillin	500 mg

A small amount of the antibiotic will pass to the baby through its mother's breast milk. This will not harm the baby.

Caution! If it feels like there is a hard, round ball in the breast that does not go away, or if the infection does not get better after the mother has been on antibiotics for 2 days, get medical help! The mother may have a **breast abscess** (a pocket of pus) and need different treatment. An untreated abscess is very dangerous!

---

4. The baby does not seem satisfied after breast feeding

Many mothers notice times when the baby suddenly seems to want more milk than she has. This is common at 10 to 14 days after birth, at 5 to 6 weeks after birth, and at about 3 months after birth.

This is normal and healthy. It means the baby's appetite is increasing—not that the mother has less milk. It is the baby's way of telling the breast to make more milk.

Do not give the baby anything else to eat or drink. Just let it breast feed more often. After 2 days of extra breast feeding, the mother's milk supply will increase to meet the baby's needs.

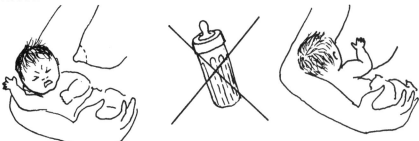

If the baby does not seem satisfied, do not give solid food or a bottle.

Give the breast more.

5. The baby has gas pains *(colic)*

Very young babies often get gas in their stomachs because they swallow air when sucking. When there is gas in the stomach, sucking and swallowing make the gas move in the belly. This makes the baby uncomfortable.

If the baby starts to cry and pull its legs up soon after it starts to suck, the baby probably has gas. Some babies have gas pains at the same time every day (often in the afternoon). Others have gas pains all day. Gas pain usually stops when the baby is about 4 months old.

Here are some things the mother can do if her baby has gas pains:

- **Help the baby burp.** If the baby seems to get gas pains when it starts breast feeding, the mother can take the baby off the nipple and try to help it burp. It may help to lay the baby on its belly across the mother's knees and pat its back. The mother can then try breast feeding again after a few minutes (whether the baby has burped or not). Some babies need to be burped several times during breast feeding.

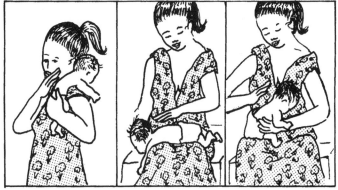

Lay the baby on the shoulder and pat its back. OR Lay the baby across the knees and pat its back. OR Sit the baby up leaning forward and pat its back.

- **Change her diet.** Sometimes a baby seems to get gas pains when the mother eats a certain food, especially if it is a food that gives the mother gas. The mother can try eating that food without spices, or stop eating the food for 2 or 3 days (if she is getting enough nutrition from other foods). There is no particular food that should be avoided, because each baby is different. A food that is fine for most babies may give another baby gas.

Special situations that affect breast feeding

1. The mother has twins

It is best to breast feed twins, just like other babies. To make enough milk for twins, a mother must eat well, drink plenty of liquids, rest as much as she can, breast feed often, and feed the babies nothing but breast milk. Remember: The more a mother breast feeds, the more milk her body will make.

A mother can breast feed both babies at the same time. Or, if she prefers, she can breast feed them separately. Here are some good positions for breast feeding twins together. It may help to put pillows or cloths under the babies.

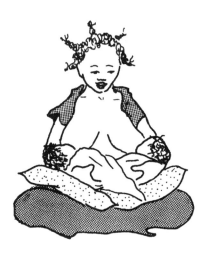
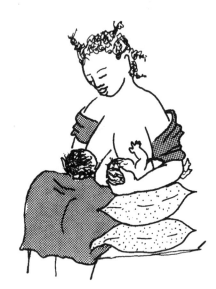

2. The mother works away from home, or the baby cannot drink all of the mother's milk

If the mother works away from home and cannot take her baby with her to work, her breasts at first will get very full and then they will start to make less milk. To keep her breasts producing milk (and to save milk for the baby, if possible), she can try milking her breasts herself during the day.

The mother can also milk her breasts if a baby is sick and unable to drink all the milk she makes. This way her breasts will not stop making milk, and the baby will have enough milk when it can drink more.

To milk the breasts by hand:

Take hold of the breast way back, like this:	Then move your hands forward, squeezing.	Finally, squeeze the milk out of the nipple.

The mother may prefer to milk her breasts with a **breast pump**, if she can get one. This pump needs to be washed after each use and boiled for at least 20 minutes once a day.

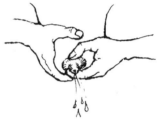

To keep a good milk supply, the mother should empty her breasts as often as possible, but no less than 4 times in a day and night (24 hours). Whenever the mother is with the baby, she should breast feed frequently to keep the milk supply up.

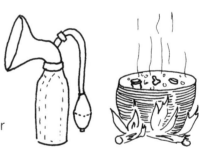

When feeding the milk to the baby, use a very clean eye dropper, cup, spoon, or a feeding bottle and rubber nipple. Either boil them or wash them with boiled water.

Saving milk

Breast milk can be saved in clean, boiled containers. It can sit in a room for 2 to 3 hours before it spoils. It can be stored for up to 2 days in a very cold refrigerator. It can also be kept in a very cold freezer for up to 2 weeks, but once it thaws it should not be frozen again.

Note: If there is no way to save the milk safely, it is better to throw it out. Spoiled breast milk can make a baby very ill.

Alternatives to breast feeding

If the mother cannot breast feed, she should try to find another way for the baby to get breast milk. Where local customs permit, another woman can breast feed the sick mother's baby, along with her own. If custom forbids a woman to breast feed another woman's child, the healthy woman could milk her own breasts, and give the milk to the sick mother's baby with a very clean eye dropper, cup, or spoon.

If there is no way to get breast milk for the baby, the baby may need formula or animal milk.

Basic rules for using animal milk and formula

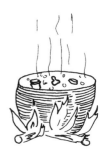

- Keep everything clean. The cup, spoon, eye dropper, bottle, rubber nipples, and any containers used for milk or formula should be washed thoroughly and boiled for 20 minutes before each use. Feeding bottles are hard to keep clean, but germs inside the bottles can cause diarrhea.

- If the mother is using formula, she should make sure it is mixed correctly. If she is using packaged formula, follow the directions exactly. If she is making her own formula, boil the milk and water before mixing. Use the correct amounts of milk, water, and oil or sugar. **Do not thin the formula by adding extra water, or by using less milk or powder. Watering the milk is very dangerous. The baby will become weak and may die.**

- The mother should make sure animal milk or formula is fresh and unspoiled when given to the baby. Formula or animal milk should **never** be left at room temperature for more than 2 hours. It will begin to spoil and could make the baby very ill. Formula can sit in a cold refrigerator for up to 12 hours. If the mother does not have a refrigerator, mix only as much formula as the baby will drink in the next 2 hours.

- Check with local health authorities for formulas that are available in your area, or how to make formula from local products.

When to stop breast feeding

Babies should **only** breast feed (no other foods) for the first 4–6 months. Speak to your local health authorities about when to start other foods and which other foods to add. It is good to breast feed each child for at least 2 years. It is best to breast feed a child for 3 or 4 years, especially if there are no younger children. The baby will be eating other foods and breast feeding.

Most older babies and young children do not need to breast feed as often as young babies. Most mothers prefer to stop breast feeding slowly as the child gets older. Little by little, the breast will become less important.

Family planning

Chapter 22 contents

Family planning

Family planning *(birth control or contraception)* is when parents decide **when** they want to have children and **how many** children they want. Every couple must decide for themselves if and how they want to plan their family. No one can decide for them. However, midwives can help women plan their families by teaching them about ways to prevent unwanted pregnancies.

> **Caution!** Women who have babies very close together (sooner than 2 years) or have more than 4 babies are at greater risk for health problems and even death. Their babies are also in greater danger of becoming ill and dying. Family planning can help mothers and their children have longer, healthier lives.
>
> Even though some family planning methods have some risks that women have heard about, birth control is safer than pregnancy and childbirth. The risk of serious illness or death because of pregnancy is many times greater than the risks of any of the family planning methods discussed in this chapter.

If you are already caring for a pregnant woman, we recommend that you talk with her about family planning a few weeks before the baby is due. Then talk with her again in more detail 1 or 2 weeks after the birth. If she chooses a family planning method, it is a good idea to meet with her again to find out if she has any questions and if the method is working well for her.

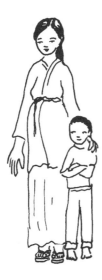

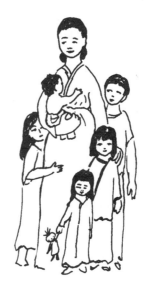

Helping a woman choose a family planning method

On the following pages we describe 13 different family planning methods. Some work better for some women than for others. We recommend that you study these pages and think about what might work best for the women you care for. You will need to think about how well each method prevents pregnancy (how effective it is), how safe it is, how convenient and available it is, and how much it costs. In many areas, there are only a few methods available.

Here is a chart that shows you how effective each method is, as well as how many women have problems with each method:

Of each 20 women using this method...	on the average this many are likely to get pregnant in spite of the method...		and this many must (or should) stop the method because of problems.
Pill	👤		👤
Condom	👤👤		
Diaphragm	👤👤👤		👤
Spermicide	👤👤👤👤		
IUD	👤		👤👤👤👤👤👤
Pulling out	👤👤👤👤👤		
Sterilization			*
Injections			👤👤
Sponge (home)	👤👤👤👤👤👤👤👤		👤👤👤
Rhythm	👤👤👤👤👤👤👤	combined 👤👤👤👤👤	
Mucous	👤👤👤👤👤👤		

* With sterilization, problems occasionally result from surgery but the method is permanent.

Family planning methods that sometimes work

This section describes 5 methods that can help prevent pregnancy. The good thing about these methods is that they are safe, available without medical help, and do not cost anything. The bad thing is that they do not always work well. Even so, these methods are better than using no method at all.

1. No sex

Not having sex at all is the most sure way to prevent pregnancy, but this is very difficult for couples to practice for a long time. It is usually best to use this method in combination with other methods.

2. Breast feeding

Breast feeding can delay the next pregnancy for a while, especially if **all** of the following things are true:

- The baby is less than 6 months old.

- The mother gives only breast milk to the baby.

- The baby does not use dummies *(pacifiers)* to suck on.

- The mother breast feeds the baby whenever it is hungry.

- The mother has not yet started her monthly bleeding again.

However, breast feeding is not a sure protection against pregnancy. Breast feeding women who do not want to get pregnant should use some other method as well, if possible.

3. Pulling out *(withdrawal)*

In this method, a man pulls his penis out of the woman before his sperm (seed) comes.

To use this method correctly, the man should wipe off any fluid at the tip of his penis before he puts it inside the woman. When he feels that the sperm is about to come, he takes his penis out and moves it away from the woman's vagina. This prevents sperm from getting inside the vagina.

Unfortunately, this method does not always work. Some men leak sperm early, and many men do not pull out in time. This means the woman may get pregnant.

4. *Homemade sponge* method

In this method, a woman puts a wet sponge deep in the vagina before having sex. This method will not prevent pregnancy every time, but it may help a woman get pregnant less often. A woman may wish to try it when no other method is available.

To use this method, a woman should:

1. Mix: 2 tablespoons of vinegar in 1 cup of clean, boiled water

OR

1 teaspoon of lemon juice in 1 cup of clean, boiled water

OR

1 spoon of salt in 4 spoons of clean, boiled water

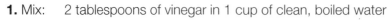
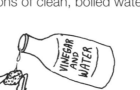

2. Wet a very clean sponge with one of these liquids.

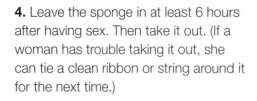

3. Push the sponge deep into the vagina no more than one hour before having sex.

4. Leave the sponge in at least 6 hours after having sex. Then take it out. (If a woman has trouble taking it out, she can tie a clean ribbon or string around it for the next time.)

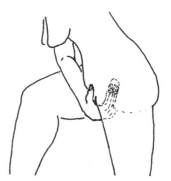

The sponge can be washed, boiled, and used again many times. Keep it in a clean, dry place. The liquid can be made ahead of time and kept in a bottle.

5. Fertility awareness—avoiding sex when a woman is fertile (the *rhythm method* and the *mucous method*)

Most women are able to get pregnant (are **fertile**) for about 8 days a month. These 8 days start 10 days after the beginning of her monthly bleeding (if she has regular 28 day cycles). The rest of the time she cannot get pregnant, even if she has sex.

The rhythm method and the mucous method are both ways to guess when the woman is fertile, so the couple can avoid sex during this time. For either method to work, a woman must have regular monthly bleeding that is always about 4 weeks (28 days) apart. (Count the weeks or days from the beginning of one monthly bleeding to the beginning of the next monthly bleeding.) The rhythm and mucous methods are most effective if they are used together.

The rhythm method

In the rhythm method, a woman counts the days from the beginning of her last monthly bleeding to find out when she is most fertile. To use a calendar to figure out the fertile time, a woman can:

1. Circle the day of the beginning of the last monthly bleeding. This is day number 1.

2. Count forward 10 days from day number 1. This is day number 10.

3. Put a line under day number 10 and under the next 7 days (8 days in all). These are her fertile days. She should not have sex during this time.

In this example, this woman's monthly bleeding started on June 5. Her fertile days are June 14 to 21. This woman can begin having sex again on June 22.

Day number 10: fertile time begins.

Day number 1: monthly bleeding begins.

SUN.	MON.	TUE.	WED.	THU.	FRI.	SAT
		1	2	3	4	(5)
6	7	8	9	10	11	12
13	14	15	16	17	18	19
20	21	22	23	24	25	26
27	28	29	30	31		

This woman should not have sex from June 14 to June 21.

If a woman does not use a calendar but can count, she can count 10 days after the first day of her monthly bleeding. She should then avoid sex for the next 8 days.

To be even safer, a woman can stop having sex as soon as her monthly bleeding is over. She then waits until her fertile period is over to have sex again.

Monthly bleeding ends.

Day number 1: monthly bleeding begins.

SUN.	MON.	TUE.	WED.	THU.	FRI.	SAT
		1	2	3	4	(5)
6	7	8	9	10	11	12
13	14	15	16	17	18	19
20	21	22	23	24	25	26
27	28	29	30	31		

This woman's monthly bleeding stopped on June 10. She should not have sex between June 10 and June 21.

The mucous method

In the mucous method, a woman examines mucus from inside the vagina. Since the mucus looks and feels different during a woman's fertile period, she can tell when to avoid having sex. (This method does not work well if the woman has a vaginal infection with a lot of discharge. She should see a trained person first to make sure she does not have a vaginal infection.)

To use this method, the woman takes a little mucus out of the vagina with a very clean finger every day. She then checks to see if the mucus will stretch between her thumb and forefinger. As long as the mucus is sticky like paste and it will not stretch between her fingers, she probably is not fertile.

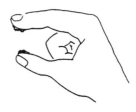

The mucus is sticky and will not stretch between the fingers.

When the mucus begins to get slippery or slimy (like a raw egg), or if the amount increases, it will stretch part way between her fingers. She may now be able to get pregnant.

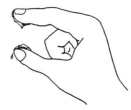

The mucus starts to get slippery.

When she can stretch the mucus between her fingers, she is probably fertile. She should not have sex until 3 or 4 days after it becomes sticky again.

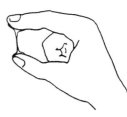

The mucus stretches into a string between the fingers.

Using the rhythm method and mucous method together

To use these methods together, a woman can check the mucus with her calendar. The mucus should stretch between the fingers during the fertile period marked on the calendar.

These methods do not always work, since an emotional upset or illness may cause a woman's body to be fertile at different times. For this reason it is best to combine both these methods with other methods like the condom.

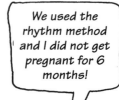

We used the rhythm method and I did not get pregnant for 6 months!

We combine rhythm and mucus and we also always use condoms.

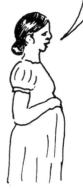

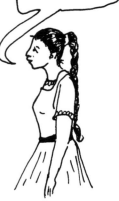

Family planning methods that often work well

The main advantage of the methods described below is that they work well to prevent pregnancy. The disadvantages are that they may cost something, they may require a medical visit, and they may have certain health risks. Make sure you know both the good and bad things about each method before you recommend any of them. Make sure the woman understands the good and bad things about each method, too.

1. Condoms (rubbers or prophylactics)

A *condom* is a narrow bag of thin rubber that the man wears on his penis while having sex. The bag traps the man's sperm (seed) so that it cannot get into the woman's womb. A condom must be used each time a couple has sex. A new condom should be used each time.

Condoms work well to prevent pregnancy. They work even better when used with foam or cream that helps prevent pregnancy (*spermicide*—see the section below). Condoms also help prevent diseases spread by having sex, including AIDS, but they are not a complete safeguard. You can buy condoms at pharmacies; some health clinics give them away free.

How to use a condom

1. Condoms are usually rolled up into a ring. A new condom should be inside a small tin foil or plastic packet that has not been opened. Be careful as you take the condom out of the packet so that it does not tear. (If a new condom is stiff, hard, or feels sticky, throw it away. It will not work.)

2. Put on the condom when the penis is hard (erect), but before it touches the vagina.

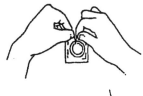

3. Make sure the rim of the condom is on the outside, away from the penis. This makes it easier to roll down.

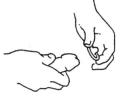

4. Place the rolled condom over the end of the hard penis. Leave a space at the end to collect the sperm.

5. Squeeze the air out of this space with your thumb and first finger. This will help to stop the condom from breaking.

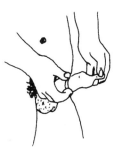

---

6. Then slowly unroll the condom down over the penis until the penis is covered. (If you want to use some water-based lubrication like K-Y jelly, now is a good time to rub it on the sides of the condom after it is on the hard penis.)

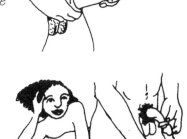

7. Right after the man cums (ejaculates), he should pull his penis out of the vagina before his penis goes soft. While he takes it out, he should hold onto the condom around the base of his penis to keep the condom from slipping off. This will help to stop any sperm from getting into the vagina and making a woman pregnant. It also helps stop the man from passing any infection to the woman.

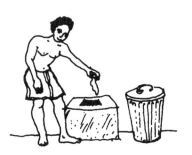

8. Look at the condom before throwing it away. If it is broken, or if it came off in the vagina, try to put contraceptive foam or jelly that contains Nonoxynol-9 in the vagina right away. This will help to kill any germs that could cause an STD. (Make sure you throw the used condom into a latrine, or bury it, out of the reach of children.)

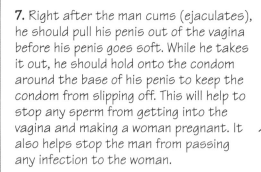

2. Spermicides *(contraceptive foam, jelly, cream; or suppositories)*

A spermicide is a chemical that kills the man's sperm, so it cannot make a woman pregnant. The woman puts the spermicide in her vagina. Foam or jelly is put in with a special applicator; suppositories (tablets) are put deep in the vagina with the fingers.

Spermicides should be put in the vagina no more than $1/2$ hour before having sex and should be left in for at least 6 hours afterwards. A woman needs a new dose of spermicide each time she has sex, even if it is several times in one night.

Spermicides are a fairly good method when used alone, and are a very good method when used with a condom or diaphragm (see the section below).

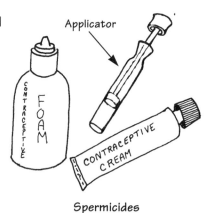

Applicator

Spermicides

Note: Not all foam, jelly, or suppositories have spermicide in them. Be sure it says either *contraceptive* or *spermicide* on the label.

3. Diaphragms and cervical caps

The *diaphragm* and the *cervical cap* help keep the man's sperm from getting up into the womb. To work well, contraceptive jelly or cream should be put in the diaphragm or cervical cap to kill any sperm that get past it. The diaphragm is a soft, shallow cup made of rubber. The woman wears it in her vagina (over her cervix) while having sex.

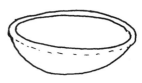

A health worker or midwife should help fit a diaphragm because different women need different sizes. If diaphragms are used in your area, we recommend you get training in how to fit them.

To use the diaphragm, a woman should first wash her hands and then put the contraceptive jelly or cream in the diaphragm. Then she puts the diaphragm deep into her vagina, right over the cervix.

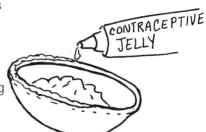

She should put in the diaphragm up to 6 hours before having sex. If she has sex more than once in the same night, she should put some more spermicide into the vagina. (She should **not** remove the diaphragm.) The diaphragm should stay inside her body for 6 to 8 hours after the last time she has sex. It should not stay in longer than 24 hours.

To work well, contraceptive jelly or cream should be put in the cup of the diaphragm.

A woman should take out her diaphragm and wash it in clean, boiled water and dry it carefully. She should also check it regularly for holes by holding it up to the light. If she finds a hole, she needs a new diaphragm right away. It is best to get a new diaphragm every 2–3 years, even if there are no holes.

A diaphragm is a safe, effective method when used with spermicide.

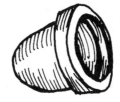

The cervical cap is smaller than the diaphragm. It can be used with spermicide again and again, just like a diaphragm. It also needs to be fitted by a health worker, and the woman needs to be taught how to put it in correctly.

4. Contraceptive sponges

In some areas, *contraceptive sponges* may be available. This method works like a diaphragm: it fits over the cervix and prevents sperm from entering the womb.

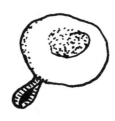

The contraceptive sponge is a special sponge that is full of spermicide. It works fairly well but has to be thrown away after one use (so it gets expensive).

5. *Intrauterine devices (IUDs)*

The IUD is a plastic device that a trained person puts inside the womb. Here are some of the different kinds and shapes of IUDs:

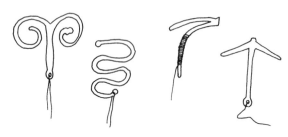

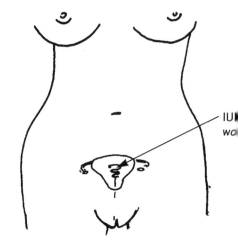

IUD
wo

Once the IUD is put in, it stays inside the womb until it is taken out by a trained person. Some IUDs should be replaced every year; others can stay in the womb 5 or more years.

The main advantages of the IUD are that a woman does not have to remember to do anything before having sex, she cannot feel the IUD inside the womb, and the IUD is effective for a long time. Some of the disadvantages or risks of the IUD are:

- The IUD can make monthly bleeding painful, or heavier (which can cause anemia).

- The IUD can make infections in the womb worse, which can make it hard to get pregnant later.

- The IUD can cause miscarriage (see p. 82), serious infection (see p. 363), or tubal pregnancy (see p. 100) if a woman gets pregnant while using an IUD.

For these reasons, it is best if only women who live close to health centers use IUDs. Women who have infections (vaginal or womb infections, or AIDS or HIV infections), or who are at risk of getting infections because they have many sexual partners or their husbands have many sexual partners, should not use an IUD. Also, if a woman bleeds easily or is anemic, she may want to use another family planning method.

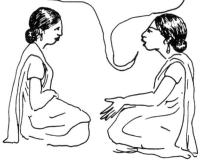

You had 2 infections of the womb this year, and the clinic is very far away. I don't think that the IUD is the best birth control for you.

Caution! A woman with an IUD should get medical help if any of these danger signs appear:

- Late monthly bleeding (pregnancy), or unusual spotting or bleeding. A woman who gets pregnant while using an IUD must have the IUD taken out right away.

- Pain in the belly that does not go away, or pain during sex.

- Signs of infection: unusual discharge from the vagina, fever, chills, feeling ill.

- IUD string gets shorter or longer, is missing, or the IUD can be felt in the vagina.

- Heavy bleeding.

6. Birth control pills (oral contraceptives or "the pill")

Birth control pills are made of chemicals (*hormones*) that are normally in a woman's body. These pills make the woman's body think that she is already pregnant, so her eggs do not come down into her womb. This means she does not have a fertile time and cannot get pregnant.

When a woman remembers to take a birth control pill every day, this method is one of the most effective ways to avoid pregnancy. But if she misses her pill for any reason, there is a risk she can get pregnant. For this reason it is good for a woman using the pill to have another family planning method on hand—just in case she does forget to take the pill once in a while.

Note: It is important for a woman to take one pill every day—even if she is taking other medicine, eating special foods, or is ill.

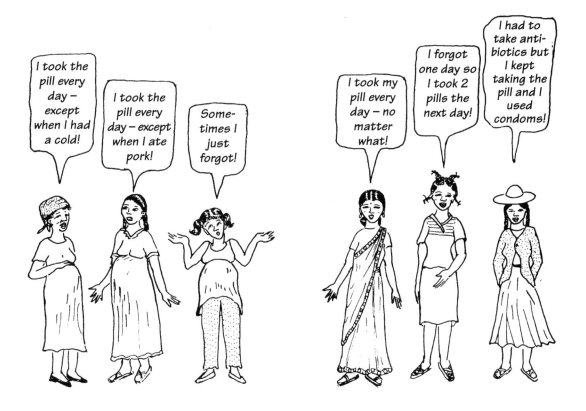

How to take birth control pills

Most pills come in packets of 21 or 28 tablets. We recommend you give a woman 7 packets to start.

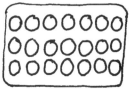

Packet of 21 pills

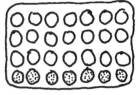

Packet of 28 pills

She should take the pills in order—the first pill in the first row first, then the second pill in the first row, and so on. If the pills are in a spiral or circle, she should also take them in order. It is best to take the pill at about the same time every day. Many women prefer to take the pill with food, especially if they feel some nausea during the first few months on the pill.

How to take the packet of 21 pills

A woman should count the first day of her monthly bleeding as day 1. She then begins taking the first pill on day 5. She takes one pill every day until the packet is finished (21 days).

1st pill
2nd pill
3rd pill   TAKE:
—— This row first
—— This row next
—— This row last
Last pil'

Packet of 21 pills

After finishing the packet, **she waits 7 days before taking any more pills**. Normally her monthly bleeding will be during this time. Then she begins taking the pills from a new packet—one pill every day. She should begin taking the new packet of pills even if her monthly bleeding does not come.

How to take the packet of 28 pills

A woman should count the first day of her monthly bleeding as day 1. She then begins taking the first pill on day 5. She takes one pill every day until the packet is finished (28 days). The last 7 pills are usually a different color. Normally her monthly bleeding will occur during this time. As soon as she is finished with one packet, she starts using another packet. This way she never stops taking the pills.

During the first month on pills the woman should use condoms, or another "backup" method.

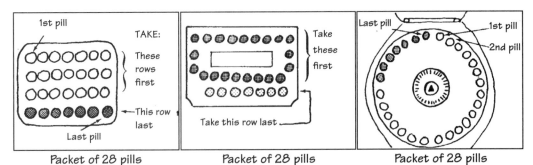

Packet of 28 pills   Packet of 28 pills   Packet of 28 pills

What if a woman forgets to take her pill?

If a woman forgets to take her pill for 12 hours or less, she should take the forgotten pill right away. Then she should continue taking the rest of the pills as before, even if she takes 2 pills in one day.

If a woman forgets to take her pill for more than 12 hours (but within 2 days), she should take the forgotten pill right away. Then she should take the next pill the next day at the regular time and continue taking one pill every day. It is a good idea to use another family planning method for the next 14 days.

If a woman forgets to take her pill for 2 days or more in a row, she should take 2 pills right away. Then she should take her pills for the rest of the month and throw away any forgotten pills. **She should also use another family planning method or not have sex until she gets her monthly bleeding—she may get pregnant.**

Note: If a woman is breast feeding, the pill will not harm the baby. Regular birth control pills sometimes cause a breast feeding woman to make a little less milk. If a woman has just given birth, it may be better to wait until the milk has come in and the baby is nursing well before starting the pill.

Problems with the pill

Common problems that usually go away

Women often have some of these problems when they first begin taking the pill: weight gain, breast tenderness, nausea, and unusual bleeding (spotting or bleeding at odd times, or the monthly bleeding stops).These problems usually go away in 3 months. It is a good idea to plan a visit with a woman 3 to 6 months after she begins taking the pill, so you can talk with her about problems that do not go away. She may need to change to a different kind of pill.

More serious problems

Like all medicines, birth control pills can cause serious problems in some people (see section below). The most serious problems are blood clots in the heart, lungs, or brain. **However, the chance of getting dangerous clots is even higher when women get pregnant than when they take the pill.**

Death related to taking the pill is very rare. **On the average, pregnancy and childbirth are many times more dangerous than taking the pill.**

Of 15,000 women who become pregnant, this many are likely to die from problems of pregnancy or childbirth.

Of 15,000 women who take birth control pills, only 1 is likely to die from problems related to having taken the pills. This woman might also have died from the same problem if she had become pregnant.

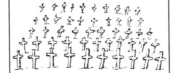

Conclusion: It is much safer to take the pill than to become pregnant.

Women who should not take the pill

For most women, the pill is much safer than getting pregnant. However, for some women both pregnancy and birth control pills are dangerous. It is best for these women to use other family planning methods to avoid pregnancy.

A woman who has any of the following signs should **not** take birth control pills (or use family planning methods that are injected). If a woman develops one of these signs after starting the pill, she should stop and use some other family planning method:

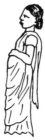

- A woman who thinks she may be pregnant.

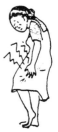

- A woman who has deep or steady pain in one leg or hip. This may be caused by a vein that is tender, sore, and red *(inflamed)* or by a blood clot in the leg. Big blue veins (varicose veins) are not a problem if they are not inflamed.

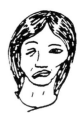

- A woman who has had any signs of a blood clot or bleeding in the brain *(stroke)*. In a stroke, a woman may suddenly fall down and lose consciousness. She may be unconscious for hours or days. Afterwards, she usually has difficulty speaking, thinking, seeing, or moving one side of her face or body. In strokes that are less severe, the woman may not lose consciousness.

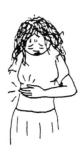

- A woman who has liver disease (hepatitis, *cirrhosis*, and so on). Hepatitis is a serious illness in which the white part of the eyes turns yellow and the stools may turn white. Cirrhosis happens to people who drink too much alcohol. If a woman's eyes got yellow during pregnancy or if she has had hepatitis, she should not take the pill for one year.

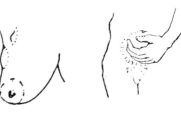

- A woman who has **cancer** (especially of the breast or womb), or who thinks she may have cancer. Birth control pills do not cause cancer, but if cancer already exists the pill can make it much worse. Ask a woman to examine her breasts carefully for lumps before taking birth control pills. If available, she should also get a **pap smear** to check for cancer of the cervix.

Women who should get medical advice before taking the pill

If a woman has any of these problems, she should see a doctor or experienced health worker before using the pill:

- severe headaches (migraines)

- blood pressure above 140/90 now or during pregnancy

- diabetes

- chest pain or heart disease

- difficulty breathing (asthma)

- seizures *(epilepsy)*

In addition, women who smoke or are over 40—especially those with high blood pressure or heart problems—should see a doctor before starting the pill.

Caution! If a woman taking the pill develops any of these signs, she should get medical advice right away:

- abdominal pain

- chest pain, shortness of breath or coughing up blood

- headaches

- any trouble seeing, blurred vision, flashing lights, not able to see

- leg pain

---

7. Injections and implants

Injections

In this method, a woman is given an injection every 2 or 3 months to keep her from getting pregnant.

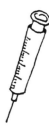

The advantage to this method is that a woman does not have to remember to do anything before having sex. Injections usually work very well, and pregnancy is rare if a woman gets the injections on time. No one can see where she has the injection and no one but the woman knows she is using contraception.

The disadvantages are similar to those for birth control pills—weight gain, breast tenderness, nausea, and unusual bleeding (spotting or bleeding at odd times, or the monthly bleeding stops).

When a woman stops getting injections, it may take longer than usual (as much as a year or more) for her to get pregnant. (A woman should always be told this before getting an injection.) For this reason, injections are best for women who are sure they do not want to get pregnant in the next year or more.

Implants (Norplant)

In this method, a trained health worker puts 6 small, soft tubes (of the same medicine that is in the injections) under the skin of a woman's arm. The *implant* then prevents pregnancy for about 5 years. After 5 years the woman needs to have a new implant. If she wants to get pregnant before the 5 years are over, the implant can be removed by a health worker.

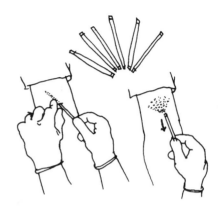

The advantage of implants is that women do not have to remember to do anything before having sex. Implants are comfortable and almost invisible. They work very well in all women (though very fat women may have more chance of getting pregnant). Monthly bleeding is usually lighter, and anemia may get somewhat better.

The disadvantages are similar to those for birth control pills and injections. Most women notice that their monthly bleeding is very irregular, with spotting and bleeding between periods. This usually does not get better until the 2nd or 3rd year. Women who live in areas where culture or religion restricts them from housework, caring for children, or religious activities when they are bleeding may not want to use implants because of this irregular and frequent bleeding. If a woman using implants has any of the following serious problems, she should get medical help immediately:

- Severe pain in the lower belly.

- Heavy bleeding from the vagina.

- Arm pain near the implant.

- Signs of infection: pus, redness, or bleeding around the implant.

- Implant comes out.

- Monthly bleeding stops after being regular for a long while.

- Severe headaches or difficulty seeing.

Another disadvantage is that the woman cannot remove the implants herself. They can only be removed by a trained health worker. Women must know this before the implants are put in.

8. Sterilization

When a man or woman is sterilized, they can never make a baby again. Sterilization is a fairly safe, simple operation. In some countries these operations are free.

Sterilization for men

This operation is called a **vasectomy**. Small cuts in the man's scrotum (balls) are made so that the tube carrying the man's sperm can be cut.

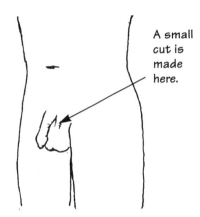

A small cut is made here.

This operation is safe and simple if done correctly, and can be done in a doctor's office or a health center. After the operation the man should still use a condom for the first 10 times he has sex because some sperm may be left in his tubes. In some countries a sperm count is done after 2 to 6 weeks to make sure there are no sperm left.

This operation has no effect on the man's sexual ability or his pleasure. His fluid comes just the same but has no sperm in it. The operation may even make sex more pleasant since he no longer needs to worry about making a baby.

Vasectomy is almost always completely effective. A doctor can try to undo a vasectomy, but this operation is expensive and often does not work.

Sterilization for women

This operation is called a **tubal ligation**. Small cuts are made in the belly so that the tubes carrying the egg to the womb are cut or tied closed. This way the egg cannot reach the womb where it meets the man's sperm.

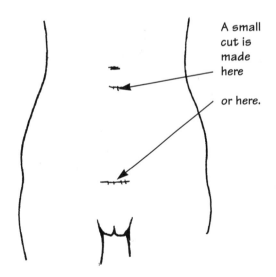

A small cut is made here

or here.

This operation can usually be done in a doctor's office or health center, and in some areas professional midwives also do these operations. The woman may or may not be put to sleep. But tubal ligation is more serious than the man's operation because the cut is made in the belly and the risk of infection is greater. After the operation a woman may have some pain or soreness for a few days.

This operation has no effect on the woman's monthly bleeding, or on her sexual ability or pleasure. It may even make sex more pleasant because she does not have to worry about getting pregnant any more. Tubal ligation is almost always completely effective. A doctor can try to undo a tubal ligation, but this operation is expensive and often does not work.

Ending a pregnancy on purpose (planned abortion)

There are 2 kinds of abortions: spontaneous abortions and planned abortions. In this book we use the word *miscarriage* to mean a spontaneous abortion (see p. 82). We use the word *abortion* to mean a planned abortion.

A planned abortion is when a woman purposely ends a pregnancy before a live baby can be born (usually in early pregnancy). This is often a difficult decision. Most women will need to talk about their plans, and to receive warm and caring support before, during, and after an abortion.

When abortions are done correctly in a hospital or clinic by a trained health worker, they are fairly safe.But they still have more risk than other family planning methods. It is always better to prevent pregnancy in the first place, if possible. Women need to be checked after any abortion for infection, heavy bleeding, and depression.

Note: In some areas it may be possible to get an **abortion pill** called RU 486 (mifepristone). This pill causes miscarriage or early labor, and should only be given by a trained person.

When abortions are done at home, or by untrained persons (including experienced traditional midwives and abortionists), they can be **very** dangerous. In some places home abortions are a major cause of death for women 12 to 50 years old. In some countries more women die of home abortions than of any other cause.

WARNING! Home methods for ending a pregnancy—such as putting something in the vagina or through the cervix, squeezing the womb, or giving modern or plant medicines to start a miscarriage—can cause severe bleeding, infection, illness, and death.

Infections of the genitals and sexually transmitted diseases (STDs)

Chapter 23 contents

Infections of the genitals and sexually transmitted diseases

This chapter is taken from a book draft that is being produced by The Women's Health Book Project at the Hesperian Foundation.

What are sexually transmitted diseases?

STDs (*sexually transmitted diseases*, or STDs for short) are diseases that are passed from one person to another during sexual relations. Some common STDs are gonorrhea, chlamydia, trichomonas, syphilis, chancroid, herpes, and AIDS.

STDs can have bad effects on the health of women, men, and on their children. This chapter will tell you how to know when someone has one of these problems, how to treat it, and how to prevent it.

Although STDs can hurt both men and women, **the problems are worse for women**. Women often have no signs and yet they can have a serious infection inside. Here are some problems STDs can cause for women:

- unable to become pregnant (*infertility*)
- baby born too soon, too small, or blind
- baby born dead
- pregnancy in the wrong place
- cancer of the cervix
- death from severe infection

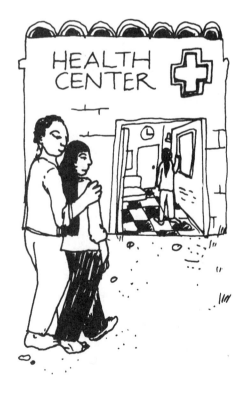

Many of these problems can be prevented if STDs are treated early. Some women do not go for treatment for many reasons. The same fears, guilt, and shame a woman may feel when talking about sex make it hard for her to learn about, and understand how to prevent, STDs.

A woman may fear that she will be treated badly if anyone finds out that she has an STD. She may be treated badly by her husband, her community, or even by the health worker in the clinic where she goes for help. Even if she got the disease from her husband, she may be accused of being unfaithful.

How STDs are spread

STDs are passed from one person to another by close physical contact with someone who is already infected. Usually this is during sex. The contact can be penis to vagina sex, or penis to anus (butthole) sex, or mouth sex (mouth to penis, mouth to vagina). Sometimes it can happen from just rubbing an infected penis or vagina against another person's genitals.

Unborn babies can get infected through their mother's blood (this is common with syphilis, hepatitis B, or HIV infection), and also when the baby passes through the vagina (this is common with gonorrhea, chlamydia, and herpes).

To learn how to prevent STDs, see p. 371.

Discharge from the vagina

It is normal for women to have a small amount of discharge (wetness) that comes from the vagina. It is the way that the vagina cleans itself. The amount of discharge changes during the days of the monthly cycle when a woman is not bleeding.

A change in the amount, color, or smell of the vaginal discharge can mean there is an STD, especially if there are other signs of infection.

1. Gonorrhea (clap, the drip, gono, VD) and chlamydia

Both men and women can have gonorrhea or chlamydia without any signs.
Gonorrhea and chlamydia can have the same signs, though gonorrhea usually starts sooner and is more painful. A woman can have gonorrhea and chlamydia at the same time so it is best to treat for both.

In a man the signs can begin as early as 2 to 5 days after he has sex with an infected person. But **in a woman** the signs may not begin for weeks or even months.

Signs

- yellow or green discharge from the vagina or anus
- pain or burning during urination (peeing)
- pain in the lower belly
- fever
- pain during sex

Treatment

See Chart 1 on p. 373. A woman's sex partner or partners (husband, boyfriend, or anyone she has sex with) should be treated at the same time.

Caution! Penicillin has been used in the past to cure gonorrhea. Now the germ causing gonorrhea is *resistant* to penicillin in many areas. In some areas, co-trimoxazole and thiamphenicol do not work either. Find out which drugs work best against gonorrhea in your community. **Remember that if you must use a more costly drug now it may cure you more quickly and save you a trip to the hospital later.** See Chart 1 on p. 373.

---

2. Infected eyes in newborn babies from gonorrhea and chlamydia (*neonatal conjunctivitis*)

Women who have gonorrhea or chlamydia while they are giving birth can pass them on to their newborn babies. This can cause blindness and serious lung problems. See p. 205 for the prevention of neonatal conjunctivitis.

Treatment

Give the baby erythromycin syrup by mouth, 30 mg 4 times a day for 2 weeks.

3. Pelvic inflammatory disease (PID)

Pelvic inflammatory disease is a serious infection of the female organs. It is caused by germs that travel up from the vagina into the womb, tubes, and ovaries. If not treated quickly, it can cause a dangerous illness right away or months later.

Causes of PID

- untreated gonorrhea or chlamydia
- infection after abortion
- infection after childbirth

Signs

- unusual discharge from the vagina
- pain in the lower belly, sometimes during sex
- high fever (more than 38°C or 100.4°F)
- feeling ill and weak

Treatment

If the woman is very ill with these signs (so ill she cannot walk or is vomiting), get her to a health center or hospital right away. She needs to be treated with intravenous medicines. In the meantime, give her the medicines listed in Chart 2, p. 373.

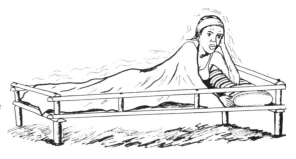

If she has these signs but does not feel very ill, give her the medicines in Chart 1, p. 373. If she is not feeling better after 2 days and 2 nights (48 hours), send her or take her to a health center or hospital.

> **Caution!** A woman can get PID more than once. It can cause:
>
> - a pregnancy in the wrong place (ectopic pregnancy)
> - infertility
> - chronic pain in the lower belly

4. Trichomonas (trich)

This vaginal discharge does not cause PID or infertility but it is very uncomfortable and itchy. There is no pain in the belly and no fever. Men usually do not get any signs of trich but they can carry it in their penis and give it to a woman during sex. So, to get rid of it, **a woman and her partner must both be treated at the same time.**

Will you come with me to the clinic? It is best if we both get treated at the same time.

Signs

- gray or yellow discharge that is sometimes bubbly
- bad smelling genitals
- red and itchy genital area and vagina

Treatment

See Chart 3 on p. 374. Both the woman and her partner should be treated.

To help the woman feel better, she can sit in a pan of clean, warm water for 15 minutes as often as possible. This is soothing to the genitals and will speed healing. She should not have sex until she and her partner are finished with treatment and all the signs are gone.

5. Yeast (candida, white discharge, fungus)

Yeast is **not sexually transmitted**. But it is a very common infection, because it likes to grow in warm wet places like the vagina. It is especially common in pregnant women, women who have diabetes (see p. 88), or women who are taking antibiotics or birth control pills. Men can also get yeast infections.

Signs

- white lumpy, sticky discharge
- bright red skin outside and inside the vagina that sometimes bleeds
- itchy genitals
- burning feeling when urinating
- a smell like mold or baking bread

Treatment

It is best to treat yeast before the birth or the baby can get yeast in its mouth *(thrush)*. See Chart 3 on p. 374.

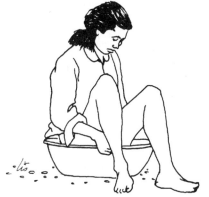

To get relief from the itching, a woman can sit in a pan of warm water. Add 3 tablespoons of vinegar or yogurt for every 1 liter (about 1 quart) of water in the pan. She can sit in this liquid 2 times a day until she feels better. Ask her not to have sex until she feels better.

Sitting in a pan of clean, warm water can help make sore and itching genitals feel better.

Prevention

All women should wear underclothes made of natural fiber (like cotton) that lets air around the genitals. Wash or change the underclothes often (once a day, if possible). Do not put soap in the vagina when bathing. Do not douche.

Sores on the genitals *(genital ulcers)*

Most sores or ulcers on the genitals are caused by having sex with an infected person. A single, painless sore may be a sign of syphilis. But several sores are likely to be a sign of other sexually transmitted diseases such as chancroid or genital herpes.

It is important to keep any sores on the genitals clean until they are healed. If possible, wash them every day with clean water and dry carefully.

> **Caution!** The AIDS virus can easily pass through a sore on the genitals from one person to another during sex. To help prevent the spread of AIDS, a woman should not have sex with anyone when she has sores, or when her sex partner has sores.

1. Syphilis

Syphilis is a common and dangerous disease that is spread from person to person through sexual relations. A pregnant woman with syphilis can also pass the disease to her unborn child.

Signs

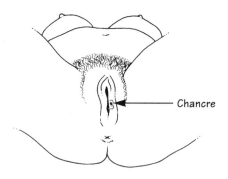

Chancre

- The first sign is a sore, called a **chancre**. It appears 2 to 5 weeks after sexual contact with a person who has syphilis. The chancre may look like a pimple, a blister, or an open sore. It usually appears in the genital area of a woman or man (or less commonly on the lips, fingers, anus, or mouth). This sore is full of germs, which are easily passed on to another person. **The sore is usually painless, and if it is inside the vagina, a woman may not know she has it—but she can still infect others.**

- The sore only lasts a few days or weeks. It then goes away by itself without treatment. **But the disease continues spreading through the body.**

- Weeks or months later there may be a sore throat, mild fever, mouth sores, or swollen joints. Or any of these signs may appear on the skin:

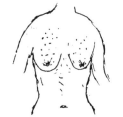
A painful rash or "pimples" all over the body

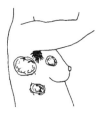
Ring-shaped welts

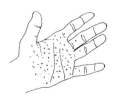
An itchy rash on the palms of the hands or soles of the feet

During this stage the disease can be spread by simple physical contact, like kissing or touching, because the syphilis germs are on the skin.

All of these signs usually go away by themselves, and then the person often thinks she is well. But the disease continues. Without proper treatment, syphilis can invade any part of the body, causing heart disease, paralysis, craziness, and sometimes death.

Note: Because syphilis often looks like many other diseases, it is important to get a blood test to see if a woman really has syphilis.

Treatment

It is best to treat for chancroid and syphilis at the same time because they are hard to tell apart without a blood test. See Chart 4 on p. 374.

2. Chancroid

These sores appear 3 to 5 days after sexual relations with an infected person. Each sore begins as a soft, painful pimple that quickly opens up to become a shallow ulcer with ragged edges. The ulcer is usually red around the outside edges.

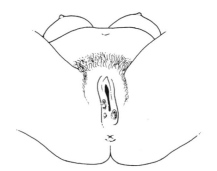

Signs

- soft, painful sores on the genitals or anus

Sores caused by chancroid

- enlarged **lymph nodes (buboes)** in the groin

If chancroid is not treated, it is easier to become infected with the AIDS virus.

Treatment

It is best to treat for syphilis and chancroid at the same time because they are hard to tell apart without a blood test. See Chart 4 on p. 374. Suggest that the woman's partner (or partners) be treated at the same time.

Also, if there are enlarged lymph nodes in the groin, the woman should see a trained person who can drain them for her.

3. Genital herpes

Genital herpes is a painful skin infection caused by a virus and spread from person to person during sex. Small blisters appear on the genitals and sometimes on the mouth (from mouth sex—mouth to vagina or mouth to penis). You can also get herpes sores on the mouth, that are not spread by sex. Children often get them (see Cold Sores in *Where There Is No Doctor*, page 232).

Signs

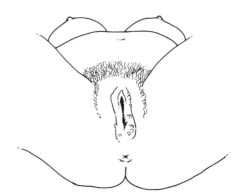

- A tingling, itching, or hurting feeling of the skin in the genital area or thighs.

- One or more small very painful blisters, like drops of water on the skin, appear on the genitals, anus, buttocks or thighs.

- The blisters burst and form small, open sores that are very painful.

- The sores dry up and become scabs.

The first time someone gets herpes sores it can last for 2 weeks or more—with fever, headache, body ache, chills and swollen lymph nodes in the groin. There may be pain when she urinates.

The virus stays in the body after all the signs have gone away. New blisters can appear at any time, from weeks to years later. Usually the new sores appear in the same place. But there are not as many, they are less painful, and they usually heal faster.

People with AIDS can get herpes infections all over their bodies that take much longer to go away.

Treatment

At this time there is no cure for herpes. But here are some things that can be done to help the person feel better:

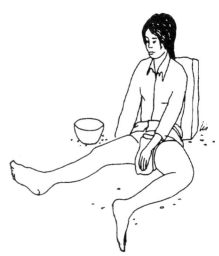

- Pouring cool, clean water over the genitals when peeing. This can help stop the burning.

- Putting ice directly on the sore as soon as the woman feels it. This can either stop it or make it go away sooner.

- Soaking some cloths in cool black tea or clove tea, and putting them on the sore.

- Sitting in a pan or bath of clean, cool water.

Putting a wet cloth on herpes sores and blisters will help them feel better.

- Mixing baking soda or corn starch with water until it makes a paste and putting it on the sore area. Or applying witch hazel, or any local plants or flowers that make the skin dry.

- Taking one or two 500 mg tablets paracetomol or acetaminophen every 4 hours for pain.

- Not having sex until all the sores are healed.

Note: A woman should always wash her hands with soap and water after touching the sores. She should also be careful not to touch her eyes. A herpes infection in the eyes is very dangerous.

Caution! A pregnant woman with herpes can pass the disease on to her baby if she has sores at the time of birth. This can cause dangerous problems for the baby. If a woman has a herpes sore when her labor begins, it is best for her to have an operation to get the baby out, especially if it is the first time she has had an infection.

Other problems

1. AIDS (Acquired Immune Deficiency Syndrome)

AIDS is also a sexually transmitted disease caused by a virus. It is spread when blood, wetness from the vagina, or *semen* (a man's seed) of someone already infected with the AIDS virus gets into the body of another person. It can be spread through:

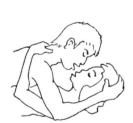 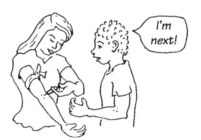 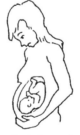 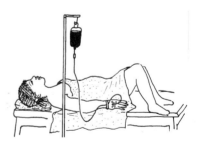

Sex with someone who has the AIDS virus.	Using the same needle of a syringe (or any instrument that cuts the skin) without sterilizing it.	An infected mother to her unborn child.	Blood transfusions – if the blood is not tested to make sure it is free from the AIDS virus.

At the present time there is no cure for AIDS. Women can get AIDS more easily than men during male-female sexual relations. STDs that cause sores can make it easier to get AIDS, because the virus can get into the body through the open sores. **A woman can get AIDS from someone who looks completely healthy.**

Prevention

Teach the women you care for:

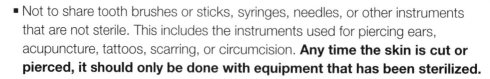

- Not to have sex with an infected person, unless he uses condoms.

- To **use condoms with any new sex partner** (see p. 347). He may have hepatitis or AIDS, without having any of the signs.

- Not to share tooth brushes or sticks, syringes, needles, or other instruments that are not sterile. This includes the instruments used for piercing ears, acupuncture, tattoos, scarring, or circumcision. **Any time the skin is cut or pierced, it should only be done with equipment that has been sterilized.**

2. Hepatitis B (yellow eyes)

Hepatitis B is also a dangerous infection, caused by a virus, that attacks the liver. It spreads very easily from one person to another, especially during sex. Hepatitis B is spread when the blood, spit *(saliva)*, wetness from the vagina, or sperm of someone already infected with the virus gets into the body of another person.

You can get hepatitis B in the same way you get AIDS:

- by having sex with an infected person

- by sharing injection needles or syringes with an infected person

- from an infected mother to her unborn child

- from blood transfusions—if the blood is not tested to make sure it is free from hepatitis

Signs

- fever

- no appetite

- tired and weak feeling

- yellow eyes, and sometimes yellow skin (especially the palms of the hands and soles of the feet)

- pain in the belly

- urine the color of Coca-Cola, and stools (shit) that look whitish

- no signs at all

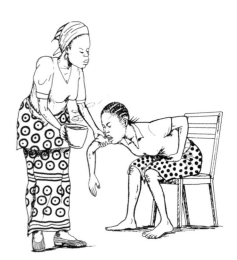

If a woman has some of these signs while she is pregnant, seek medical advice. She may be able to get a vaccination for the baby to prevent it from getting hepatitis B.

If a woman's husband or partner has had some of these signs, she should not have sex with him until he is completely well.

Treatment

There is no medicine that will help. In fact, taking medicine can hurt the liver even more. Most people get better from hepatitis B. Resting, eating foods that are easy to digest, and not having any alcohol will make the person feel better.

Prevention

The same things that help prevent the spread of AIDS will help prevent the spread of hepatitis B.

Teaching women how to prevent STDs

To help prevent the spread of STDs, encourage the women in your community to:

- **Use condoms.** When they are used correctly, condoms can help prevent the spread of sexually transmitted diseases, including AIDS. Condoms used with a contraceptive jelly, cream, or foam that contains Nonoxynol-9 work even better. (See p. 347–348 for how to use condoms.)

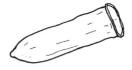

- **Be careful who they have sex with.** It is best to have sex only with one faithful partner.

- **Not have sex with anyone who has many sex partners** or with anyone who injects illegal drugs.

- **Treat STDs early.** This will protect them from more serious problems later on, and will prevent the spread of infection to others. They should not wait until they are very ill.

- **Help their partners to get treated when they do.** Encourage them to take the proper medicine, or to see a health worker.

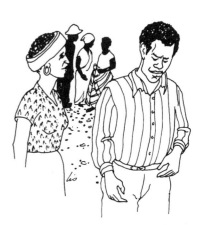

Try to persuade a woman's partner to get treated at the same time.

- **Make sure to take *all* the medicine**, even if the signs start to go away. Remind them that they will not be cured until all the medicine is finished.

- **See a health worker, or go to a clinic or hospital, if they do not feel better soon.**

- **Not have sex with a man who has a rash, sores, or a discharge from his penis, or burning when he urinates**.

- Go to a clinic or hospital to be checked if they have had sex with a man who they think has an STD (even if the women do not have any signs).

If the man will not use condoms, encourage women to:

- Use vaginal spermicide jelly or cream, especially one containing Nonoxynol-9 (see p. 348). This can help prevent infection.

- Use a diaphragm or cervical cap with spermicide.

- Wash the outside of the genitals after sex (but do not douche).

- Urinate right after sex.

- Not have sex during the monthly bleeding, or when they have sores or signs of an infection.

How to help in your community

Here are some ideas to help prevent the spread of sexually transmitted diseases in your community:

- Find out from your local health center, hospital, or Ministry of Health what STDs are the most common in your community and what medicines work best to treat them.

- Find out what medicines you can get in your community to treat STDs, and how much they cost.

- See if it is possible to start a community pharmacy so that it will be easier for people to get medicines and condoms.

- Organize a group to talk about health topics, including STDs and AIDS.

- Support education about sex in your local school. Help parents understand that teaching children about STDs, including AIDS, helps them make safe choices later on when they start having sex.

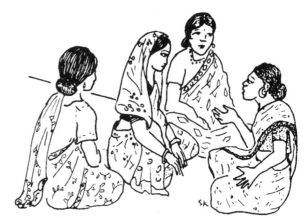

Work together with other women to persuade the men in your community to use condoms.

Medicines for infections of the genitals and STDs during pregnancy

The medicines in the tables below are for infections of the genitals and STDs during pregnancy. There are other drugs that can be used if a woman is not pregnant. See the Green Pages in the back of this book and *Where There Is No Doctor* for more information.

CHART 1: VAGINAL DISCHARGE (NO BELLY PAIN)

Best Treatment: **Take one medicine each for gonorrhea and chlamydia**

GONORRHEA	Medicine	Dose	How to take	Caution
Best treatment: Choose 1	**ceftriaxone** or	250 mg	1 injection only	
	spectinomycin	2 grams	1 injection only	Does not work for gonorrhea of the throat.
Next best:	**co-trimoxazole (Bactrim, Septra)**	80/400 mg	10 tablets by mouth each day for 3 days	**Do not take in the last 3 months of pregnancy.**
CHLAMYDIA	Medicine	Dose	How to take	Caution
Choose 1	**erythromycin** or	500 mg	1 tablet 4 times a day for 7 days	
	sulfafurazole	500 mg	1 tablet 4 times a day for 7 days	**Do not take in the last 3 months of pregnancy.**

CHART 2: VAGINAL DISCHARGE (WITH BELLY PAIN); PID

Treatment: Take **1 medicine for gonorrhea** from Chart 1.

and

Take **1 medicine for chlamydia** from Chart 1

and

Take **metronidazole (Flagyl)** 500 mg, by mouth, 2 times a day for 10 days.

(Do not take metronidazole in the first 3 months of pregnancy, and do not drink alcohol while taking metronidazole.)

If a woman became pregnant with an intrauterine device (IUD) and is infected, she must have the IUD removed. The best time is one day after she starts the medicine. Get medical advice.

CHART 3: DISCHARGE FROM THE VAGINA WITH ITCHING

YEAST	Medicine	Dose	How to take
Effective and cheap	**gentian violet**	1% aqueous (water) solution	Have a health worker paint the inside of the vagina with gentian violet. Or soak a clean strip of cloth in gentian violet. Leave a tail so you can get it out. Put the cloth high in the vagina each night for 3 nights. **Do not use during the first 3 months of pregnancy.**
More expensive: Choose 1	**nystatin vaginal tablet**	100,000 units	Put 2 tablets high into the vagina each night for 14 nights.
	clotrimazole vaginal tablets	500 mg	Put 1 tablet high into the vagina for 1 night only.

TRICHOMONAS	Medicine	Dose	How to take
Best treatment	**metronidazole (Flagyl)**	250 mg **(Do not drink any alcohol while taking metronidazole.)**	Take 8 tablets by mouth all at once. If this does not help, take 2 tablets 2 times a day for 7 days. **(Do not take during the first 3 months of pregnancy.)**

CHART 4: SORES ON THE GENITALS

Best Treatment: **Take one medicine each for syphilis and chancroid**

SYPHILIS	Medicine	Dose	How to take	Caution
Best treatment: Choose 1	**benzathine penicillin** or	2,400,000 units	1 injection only	If possible, divide into 2 injections.
	aqueous procaine penicillin	1,200,000 units	1 injection each day for 10 days	
If allergic to penicillin	**erythromycin**	500 mg	1 tablet 4 times a day for 15 days	If stomach upset, take 250 mg 4 times a day for 30 days.

CHANCROID	Medicine	Dose	How to take	Caution
Best treatment: Choose 1	**ceftriaxone** or	250 mg	1 injection only	
	erythromycin	500 mg	1 tablet 4 times a day for 7 days	If stomach upset, take 250 mg 4 times a day for 14 days.
	co-trimoxazole	80/400 mg	2 tablets 2 times a day for 7 days	**Do not take in the last 3 months of pregnancy.**

If a woman is breast feeding a small baby when she gets an STD, it is best if she does not take sulfa medicines, or thiamphenicol. A small amount can get into the breast milk. But if there are no other medicines available, it will probably do **less harm to the baby than if the mother is not treated. If possible, have another mother nurse the baby. The mother should milk her breasts (see p. 337) to keep her milk supply up, but throw away the milk until she stops taking the medicine.**

SECTION F

Special procedures that midwives can learn

Introduction

The following *special procedures* have been put in a separate section of this book because many midwives will not need to use them. Since most labors and births go well, these procedures will not need to be done very often. Or, if you are close to medical help, a health center, or a hospital, medical people will usually be doing these procedures.

However, sometimes medical help is far away and the mother will die unless the midwife can perform some of these special procedures. If you are far from medical help, check with your local health officer or health authorities about learning these procedures.

If midwives in your area are allowed to do these procedures, try to get a skilled person to teach you. Most of these procedures are very hard to learn from a book—even one with lots of pictures. A skilled teacher can watch you practice and check to make sure you have learned to do them correctly. She can teach you at real births and with real women.

Caution! In some places midwives are forbidden to do some of these procedures. Please check with your local authorities. All procedures have risks as well as benefits. **Most of the procedures in this chapter can be very dangerous if done incorrectly. If you do them wrong, or do them at the wrong time, you can cause more harm than good. Never use a medical procedure unless there is a real medical need.**

This section on special procedures has 2 parts:

- Special procedures that can be used outside the hospital (chapter 24).

- Special procedures that are often used in hospitals (chapter 25).
  This chapter does not teach a midwife how to do hospital procedures, but it explains the different procedures that often happen in a hospital. We include it so that a midwife can help the mother and family know what to expect if the mother goes to the hospital.

Special procedures that can be used outside the hospital

Chapter 24 contents

Special procedures that can be used outside the hospital

Home methods for starting or strengthening a labor

These are some of the times when you may want to start or strengthen a labor:

- The bag of waters has broken, but active labor does not start within 6 hours (see p. 236).

- The bag of waters has broken, and the birth is not near after 12 hours of labor.

- The mother has been in fairly active labor for several hours, but the birth is not near.

- The mother has been in light labor for many hours. The labor is active enough to keep her from resting but it is not strong enough to open the cervix.

There are both home methods and hospital methods for starting or strengthening a labor. The advantage of using home methods is that they are often cheaper, easier to use, safer, and more pleasant than hospital methods.

However, there are also risks to home methods. The greatest risk is that if a home method does not work—and the slow labor was caused by some problem needing medical attention—you may have lost precious time trying to use it. Or there may be other, hidden risks. For example, some plant medicines may strengthen labor but also cause high blood pressure in some women. Some remedies are powerful and effective but can cause contractions that are too strong and therefore dangerous.

> **Caution!** Home methods should not be used if you find any risk signs—especially if the baby is sideways or too big to fit through the mother's pelvic bones, if there is any unusual bleeding, or if the baby's heartbeat is less than 110 beats per minute. Get medical help instead.

1. Home methods that have very little risk

Walking about

Labor often gets stronger if a mother stands or walks around. This is because the baby's head presses downward on the cervix and causes stronger contractions. Some women also get stronger contractions just by changing positions (see p. 317). There is no risk to trying different positions and movements.

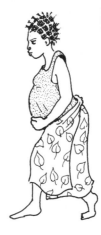

Nipple stimulation

When a baby sucks on a woman's nipples, her body makes the hormone oxytocin. Oxytocin causes stronger contractions.

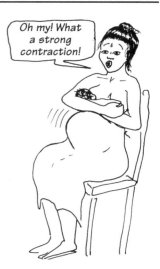

When a woman is in active labor but the contractions are not strong enough to open the cervix, it may help to put a baby (or an adult) to her breast and let them suck. Sometimes it is necessary to have someone sucking on both breasts at the same time. The baby or other people may need to keep sucking until the cervix is all the way open, and the mother is ready to give birth.

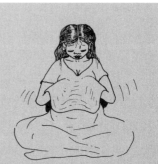

Note: If a woman is uncomfortable having another woman's child or an adult suck on her nipples, she can pull on her nipples herself.

If a woman feels comfortable pulling on her own nipples, she should rub and pull on both nipples until contractions are strong enough to open the cervix and stay strong without nipple stimulation. Clean vegetable oil on her nipples will help protect her skin from getting irritated.

If a woman feels uncomfortable pulling on her own nipples, this method will probably not help. Her discomfort may even slow the labor.

Special massage (acupressure)

Massage pressure on certain parts of the body sometimes helps start a labor or make a weak labor stronger. In this section we talk about one kind of massage called *acupressure*, which is based on an ancient Chinese method of healing. Local midwives and healers in your area may know of other kinds of massage as well.

To give an acupressure massage, do the following:

1. If the woman seems weak or tired, try to build up her energy first. Give her tea, sugar water, rehydration drink, or any liquids (see p. 171–172). Warm her if she is cold. If there is time, help her get some rest.

2. It often helps to give a regular massage before you use acupressure massage. Pay special attention to the mother's feet. Use your thumbs and fingers on the top and bottom of the feet, on the toes, the ankles, and the heels. Also, put a little oil on her lower back and massage it. Use more pressure when you rub downwards. Use less pressure when you rub upwards.

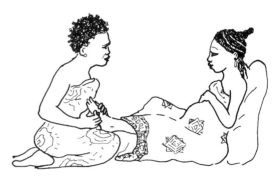

3. Then begin the acupressure massage. Press on the following spots, using your own sense about how long and how often to press, and when to stop:

▪ **The leg above the ankle.** You can find the right spot by putting 4 fingers above the ankle bone, on the inside of the leg, like this:

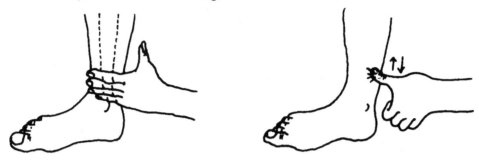

Then press on this spot with your thumb or finger, on the back of the bone. Do both legs at the same time. Press hard and move your fingers in little circles, or up and down. Push and rub extra hard when the mother has a contraction. Relax between contractions.

If the method is working, the woman may feel a tingling sensation or soreness around the point. She may also feel the baby start to move, or she may feel energy or an ache in her lower belly.

▪ **The hand.** Use your thumb like this:

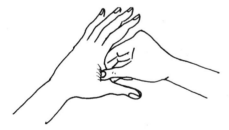

You do not need to press as hard on this spot as you did on the leg above the ankle. Do both hands at the same time, in between working on the leg above the ankle.

▪ **The big toe.** If the first 2 methods (the leg above the ankle and the hand) do not work after about 5 or 10 minutes, or if the mother is especially tense or angry (or if she eats a lot of fat in her diet), try putting pressure near the big toe, like this:

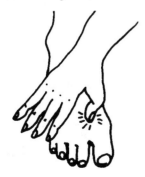

Use the side of your thumb, very close to your fingernail. Press deep for $1/2$ a minute (or count to 30). Stop for 2 minutes, then press again. Keep pressing off and on for 10 minutes. Then stop and do something else or let the woman rest for a while. Try again later. (Do not use this point if the mother is bleeding.)

These are some other spots that sometimes work:

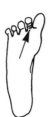

- **The bottom of the second toe.**

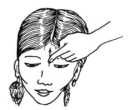

- **Between the eyes.** Gently stroke upwards on the forehead, especially if the mother needs to be more calm.

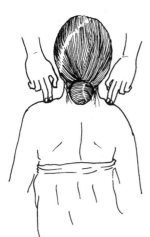

- **The top of the shoulders.** Press hard for about $\frac{1}{2}$ a minute (or count to 30). Then stop for 2 or 3 minutes and press again. Keep trying like this for a while.

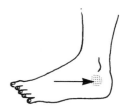

- **Below the ankle bone.** If the mother is in a lot of pain, press here:

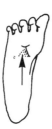

- **The bottom of the foot.** If nothing else works, press in here, **very hard**. It hurts but it sometimes works.

4. Watch the labor closely. If acupressure massage is going to work, you will usually see contractions start or get stronger within the first 10 minutes. As long as you are getting results, keep doing the acupressure massage until the labor stays strong on its own. This may be a few minutes or a few hours.

Enemas

An enema may make a labor stronger by itself, or it may be used as a way of giving plant medicines to make a labor stronger. (Medicines given by enema may work better than medicines given by mouth because the stomach does not use foods and medicines well during labor.) An enema may also relieve some pain in labor if the woman has hard stools (shit) sitting inside her body.

Enemas have some risks. The greatest danger is that the stool washed out of the rectum will get into the vagina and cause an infection after birth. **To avoid causing infection, keep the dirty enema water away from the mother's vagina. Keep everything clean!** Also, an enema may cause labor to become strong very quickly. Be prepared for this to happen.

An enema can be given to the mother by the midwife, or sometimes the mother can do it herself. Page 174 lists the equipment you will need and what to do.

2. Home methods that have more risk

The methods in this section are sometimes more powerful for starting or strengthening labor, but they also have more risk.

Castor oil drink

In some parts of the world, midwives make a drink out of castor oil and fruit juice to start or strengthen a labor. This method can be very useful when the bag of waters has broken and there is no labor after several hours, when the safer home methods have been tried but have not worked, or when medical care is difficult or impossible to get. This method can sometimes start a labor when there have been no contractions at all.

To make castor oil drink, put about 60 ml (2 oz.) castor oil in 1 glass (240 cc or 8 oz.) of fruit juice. Lemonade or orange juice is especially good, but other fruit juice may be used. The mother should drink the whole glass down. If the remedy is going to work, labor should start within 4 hours. **Do not give more than 1 glass.**

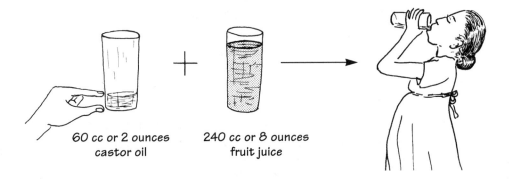

60 cc or 2 ounces
castor oil

240 cc or 8 ounces
fruit juice

Caution! Castor oil drink is often unpleasant to drink and has some risks. It can cause uncomfortable, watery stools and gas. Having such watery stools near the birth opening increases the risk of infection. And sometimes the contractions will be too long or strong.

Plant medicines

Many traditional midwives and healers use various plant medicines to start or strengthen a labor. Different plants are used in different areas. Many of these plants work very well, but some are not very helpful or are dangerous. We suggest that you find out about the plant medicines that are used in your area. We also suggest that local health departments study the local plant medicines to find out more about them.

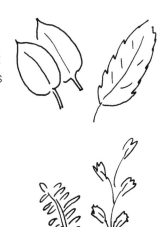

Common **risks** with plant medicines are:

- high blood pressure

- contractions that are too strong

- allergic reactions

Common **problems** with plant medicines are:

- It is difficult to control the dose. The same plant grown in different areas or in different soil, or picked in different seasons, will have different strengths.

- Any medicine given by mouth during labor may be difficult for the body to use. The stomach does not work well during labor.

Caution! These methods are dangerous and should never be used:

- Never put plant medicine into the vagina to start a labor. The medicine might cause an infection after birth.

- Never inject oxytocin or any other medicine to start or strengthen a labor. These medicines will often start contractions that are too strong. In rare cases, the oxytocin injections may cause the womb to break inside the mother. She and the baby may die from bleeding inside (that you never see).

- Never give oxytocin by mouth (buccal pitocin). This method of giving oxytocin can also cause contractions that are too strong.

- Never push on the womb to bring the birth more quickly. This can cause the placenta to come off the wall of the womb too soon. It can cause the womb to break inside the mother.

- Never ask a woman in labor to confess unfaithfulness or sins in order to hurry the birth. These things do not cause long labors. Forcing a woman to confess things can make her upset and make labor even longer.

Procedures that may need to be done in special circumstances

> **Caution!** Please check with local health authorities before using any of these procedures. Try to get training from an experienced person before performing these procedures.

1. Giving injections

In this book we sometimes recommend giving medicines. In the Green Pages there is a list of these medicines; the list tells what each medicine is for, when to use it, how much to give, and what the risks are. Be sure to read this section before giving any medicine.

When you inject a medicine, you put medicine into the body through a needle in the skin. Here are some situations in which a midwife might use an injection to give medicine: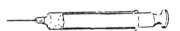

- severe bleeding after birth

- convulsions or very high blood pressure during labor and birth

- infections of the mother or baby after birth

- sewing tears after birth

> **Caution!** Give medicine by injection only when it is necessary to save the mother's life or when medical help is very far away.

Remember these precautions when giving injections:

- Never give an injection if you can get medical help quickly, unless the injection is needed to keep the problem from getting seriously worse on the way.

- Never give an injection if medicine by mouth would work just as well.

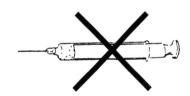

- Never use needles or syringes that are not sterile.

How to give an injection

Preparing the syringe

There are 2 kinds of syringes: those that can be reused and those that are disposable. The reusable ones must be taken apart, cleaned, and boiled before each use. The disposable kind come in sterile packages (see p. 157). If the sterile package is dry and unbroken, the syringe can be used right out of the package (without boiling the syringe first). Sometimes you can use a disposable syringe several times if you take it apart, wash it with soap and water and soak it for 20 minutes in 70% ethanol or in a solution of 1 part bleach to 7 parts water or boil it for 20 minutes just as you would a reusable syringe (see p. 154).

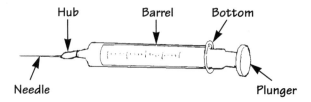

Hub   Barrel   Bottom

Needle   Plunger

> **Caution:** After boiling or soaking in disinfectant never touch the needle with your fingers or anything else that is not sterile! Ony touch the outside of the barrel, the outside of the hub of the needle, or the button of the plunger.

Drawing up medicines for injections

Injectable medicines come in 3 forms:

- in a small, special bottle called an ***ampule*** (a very small glass bottle whose top is broken to get the medicine out)
- as a liquid in a bottle
- as a powder in a bottle to which you add sterile water

If the medicine comes in an ampule, draw up the medicine like this:

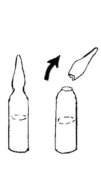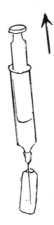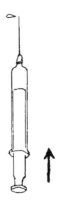

1. Clean the ampule well, then break off the top. Wrap a clean or sterile cloth around the top of the ampule so you do not cut yourself.

2. Put the syringe and needle into the ampule. Be careful that the needle does not touch the outside of the ampule. Draw the medicine up into the syringe by pulling up on the plunger.

3. Hold the syringe with the needle pointing up and slowly push the plunger until a little medicine comes out of the syringe.

If the medicine comes as a liquid in a bottle (with a soft place to stick the needle in and get the medicine out), take the prepared and sterile needle and syringe and then:

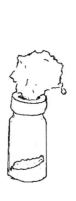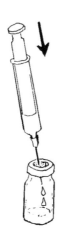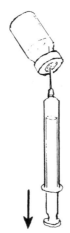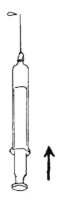

1. Rub the rubber top of the bottle with a small cloth boiled in water or soaked in alcohol, or with a sterile gauze square wet with alcohol or boiled water.

2. Inject a small amount of air (1–3 cc) into the bottle.

3. Turn the bottle over and the liquid will flow into the syringe. Then pull the syringe out of the bottle.

4. Hold the syringe with the needle pointing up and slowly push the plunger until a little medicine comes out of the syringe.

If the medicine comes in a bottle that has powder inside, you will need to add sterile water to it to turn it into a liquid.

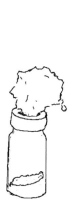 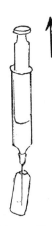 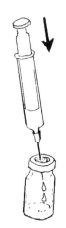 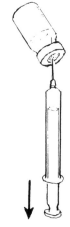 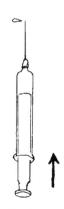

1. Rub the rubber top of the bottle with a clean cloth with the alcohol or boiled water or with a sterile gauze square.

2. Draw up the correct amount of sterile water.

3. Inject the sterile water into the bottle with the powdered medicine inside. Gently shake the bottle to make sure the powder and water mix completely.

4. Turn the bottle over and slowly pull all of the liquid into the syringe. Then pull the syringe out of the bottle.

5. Hold the syringe with the needle pointing up and push out the air until you see a drop of liquid come out of the syringe.

Where to give an injection

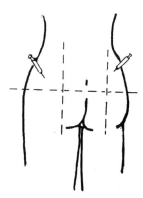

It is best to inject into the muscle of the buttocks in adults—always in the upper, outer quarter.

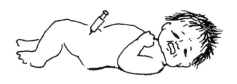

Never inject babies or children under 2 years of age in the buttock. Inject them in the upper, outer part of the thigh.

It is best to practice injecting before you ever go to a birth where an injection may be needed. To practice, use old needles and plain water. Practice injecting into an orange or other soft fruit or vegetable, a pillow, or a piece of foam rubber.

How to inject

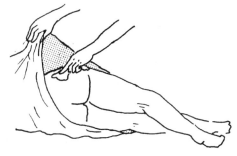

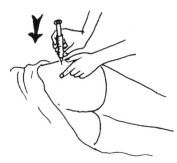

Clean the skin with soap and water. You can also use alcohol—but to prevent severe pain, be sure the alcohol is dry before injecting.

Put the needle straight in, all the way. If it is done with one quick movement, it hurts less.

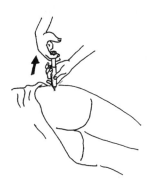

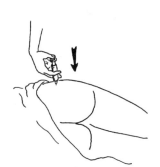

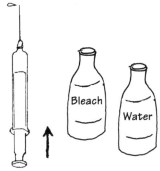

Before injecting the medicine, pull back on the plunger. If blood enters the syringe, it means the needle is in a vein. Take the needle out and put it in somewhere else.

If no blood enters, inject the medicine slowly.

Remove the needle and clean the skin again. Then rinse the syringe and needle at once in water and bleach (use 1 part bleach to 7 parts water). Squirt the water and bleach through the needle and then take the syringe apart and wash it. Boil before using again.

Risks and precautions

There are 2 main risks when injecting medicines:

- Germs (especially HIV) causing infection or illness can enter the body with the needle.

- The medicine may cause an allergic reaction.

Infection or illness from germs entering with the needle

To lower the chance of causing an infection, take care that everything is completely clean. It is very important to take the needle and syringe apart and boil them before you use them. After boiling, do not touch the needle with your fingers or anything else.

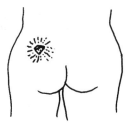

An abscess like this one comes from injecting with a needle that has not been well boiled and is not sterile.

Never use the same needle and syringe to inject more than one person without boiling it again first. Sterilize your needles and syringes at home and keep them in a sterile container (see p. 154) so they will be ready in case of an emergency at a birth.
Remember: A midwife can get an infection or AIDS if she sticks herself with a needle that is dirty from someone's blood.

An allergic reaction caused by the medicine

Before giving an injection, it is important to know what reactions it might cause. It is also important to know that medicines in the same family often cause the same reaction (see p. 90).

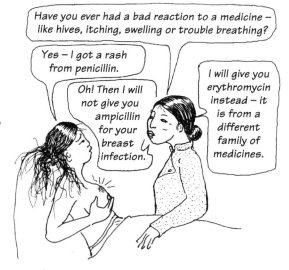

To prevent a serious reaction from an injection, do the following:

1. Before injecting a medicine, always ask the woman if she has had itching or any other bad reaction from a similar medicine in the past. If she says yes, do not use this medicine in any form, or any medicine from the same family.

2. Stay with a woman 30 minutes after giving an injection. During this time, watch for a severe reaction called **allergic shock**. These are the signs of allergic shock:

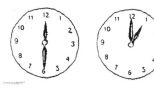

- cool, moist, pale, gray skin (a cold sweat)

- weak, rapid pulse or heartbeat

- difficulty breathing

- loss of consciousness

3. If possible, have ready 2 ampules of epinephrine (adrenaline, p. 458). The ampule should say 1:1000 on it. Also have ready an ampule of antihistamine, like promethazine (phenergan, p. 459) or diphenhydramine (benadryl, p. 459).

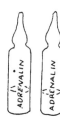

If you see signs of allergic shock, immediately inject .5 cc of adrenaline IM. If symptoms persist, you may give another .5 cc adrenaline IM in 20–30 minutes. Then inject 50 mg of benadryl or phenergan. If you have pills or syrup instead, give the medicine by mouth or by rectum (see p. 248).

2. Giving internal exams

An *internal exam* is when the midwife examines the cervix inside the woman to see whether it is opening up. These exams can be useful because they are the most sure way to know if labor is progressing normally. You can also tell whether the baby is breech or head first by doing an internal exam.

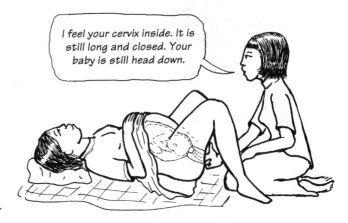

I feel your cervix inside. It is still long and closed. Your baby is still head down.

But there is also a great risk of infection each time your fingers go inside the mother's vagina. For this reason it is best to avoid internal exams if all is going well.

- Do not do an internal exam if the waters broke before labor started and labor is slow (see p. 236).

- Do not do an internal exam any time after the waters break unless there is a real medical need, and you cannot make a decision without the information an internal exam can give (see p. 177).

- Do not do an internal exam if the mother is having **any** unusual bleeding from the vagina (see p. 244).

How to give an internal exam

It is very hard to describe how to do an internal exam in a book. This is partly because you will "see" things with your fingers, not your eyes, when doing the exam. We strongly recommend that midwives get training from a skilled person before trying an internal exam themselves. Midwives should also check with local authorities to see if this procedure is allowed.

1. First explain to the woman what you are going to do and why.

2. Ask the woman to lie on her back, to bend her knees, and to place her legs apart.

3. Always scrub before putting your hands in the mother (see p. 159). Wear sterile gloves. **If you do not have sterile gloves, do not do an internal exam.**

4. Gently put 2 fingers into the mother's vagina. If the woman is having light labor, you will usually have to reach inside almost as far as your fingers will go to find the cervix. If the woman is in late labor, the cervix may be pushed closer to the outside by the baby's head. Your fingers may only have to go inside the woman's body about half way.

5. Feel the cervix to see if it is opening up:

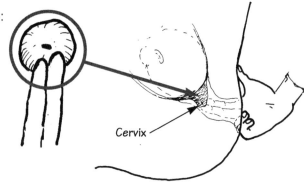

Cervix

- If the cervix is closed, it feels like a wet big toe with a hole in the center.

- As the cervix gets ready to open, it gets more flat and smooth. The baby's head behind the cervix feels something like the bone in your chin under the skin. If you feel something that is soft, not hard, you may be feeling the baby's bottom. This is a breech position.

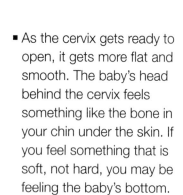

- As the cervix opens slowly during labor, it begins to feel like round lips stretched over a hard, round fruit (the baby's head).

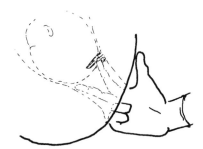

- Sometimes, towards the end of labor, the cervix is almost gone, but there is a "lip" left on one side. It is usually best to wait until the lip is gone before you allow the mother to start pushing.

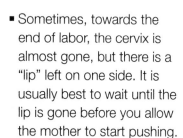

- When the cervix is completely open, this means it is completely gone. All you can find is the wall of the vagina and the baby's head (or whatever part of the baby is being born first). It is now time for the mother to start pushing.

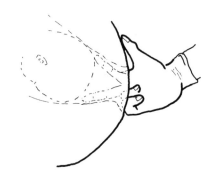

6. If you are worried that the mother's pelvic bones are too small for the baby to come through, feel the shape and size of the pelvic bones now. It is usually not possible to tell for sure if the pelvic bones are too small simply by feeling them. However, if the pelvic bones feel smaller than most women, it is more likely that the baby will get stuck during the birth. The woman may need to give birth in a hospital or maternity center.

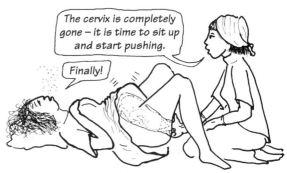

The cervix is completely gone – it is time to sit up and start pushing.

Finally!

3. Using a tube to help the urine (pee) come out (catheterization)

If a woman does not urinate (or urinate enough) for several hours, her bladder may become over full. This can cause many problems.

Sometimes you can see an over full bladder by looking at her belly. Sometimes you cannot see it, but you can feel an extra bulge (like a tight bag full of water) on the lower front of the belly. But remember that it is not always easy to tell if the bladder is over full. We recommend that midwives get training in this.

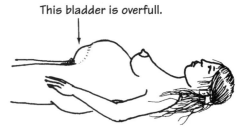

This bladder is overfull.

You can usually prevent a woman from having an over full bladder by reminding her to urinate every 2 hours during labor. If the mother has problems urinating, here are some things you can do for the mother while she tries to urinate:

- Put her hand and wrist in a bowl of warm water.
- Let her hear the sound of running water.
- Put a clean towel or cloth between her legs so she can urinate while lying down.
- Let her sit in a crouching position, or on a pot.
- Let her sit in a tub of warm water and urinate into the water.
- Pour warm, clean water on her genitals.

If a woman is unable to urinate, she may need to have a tube put into her bladder to help the urine come out. This tube is called a *catheter*. The procedure is called *catheterization*.

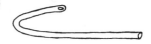

> **Caution!** Using a catheter has serious risks. Even careful use of a catheter can cause infection of the bladder and kidneys. Never use a catheter unless you think the mother will die or become dangerously ill before you can get medical help.

To catheterize a woman, you will need a catheter, *antibiotic cream* or *sterile lubricant* (which makes the tube slide in easily), sterile cloths, sterile gloves, and a bowl or bucket.

How to put a catheter into a woman's body:

1. Boil the catheter for 20 minutes.

2. Wash the mother's belly, thighs, and genitals well with boiled water and disinfectant soap.

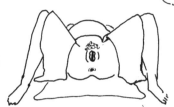

3. Put sterile or very clean cloths under the mother, and over her thighs and belly.

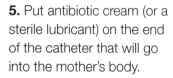

4. Scrub carefully (see p. 159). Wash your hands with alcohol or disinfectant, and put on sterile gloves.

5. Put antibiotic cream (or a sterile lubricant) on the end of the catheter that will go into the mother's body.

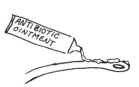

6. Hold the woman's *labia* apart with one gloved hand, so that you can see the woman's urine hole.

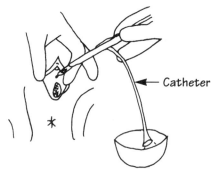

← Catheter

7. With the other hand, gently put the catheter into the woman's urine hole little by little, very carefully. Usually the catheter goes straight in, but if the baby's head is in the birth canal, you need to point the catheter up at first, so it can get over and past the head. Be careful that the catheter never touches anything but the urine opening and your gloved hands. If the catheter gets stuck, roll it gently between your fingers, but **do not force it**. This might injure the mother.

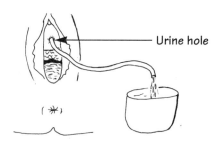

— Urine hole

7. When the tip of the catheter gets to the mother's bladder, urine will start to drip out the other end. You should have a bowl or bucket ready to catch it.

8. Take the catheter out when the urine has stopped dripping. During the next few weeks, watch the mother carefully for signs of bladder infection (see p. 115). Make sure she knows what to look for, too.

4. Making the vaginal opening larger for birth (episiotomy)

An *episiotomy* means cutting the opening of the vagina to make it larger for the baby to come through. It should only be done when it is truly necessary.

It is usually not necessary to make the vagina larger unless 1) the baby is already in the vagina and needs to be born quickly because of some special danger, **and** 2) the outside opening of the vagina seems to be stretching too slowly for a safe birth. Here are some examples of when an episiotomy may be necessary:

- The baby is breech and a first baby.

- The baby's shoulders get stuck, and you need more room to get them out.

- The baby is head down, and the head gets stuck just inside the vagina.

- The baby is about to be born, and there is a gush of blood from the vagina (which probably means the placenta has come off the womb wall). This baby must be born very quickly or it will die.

- The cord can be seen in front of the baby's head.

- The baby is born early (which means its head is very soft). Cutting the vagina will help prevent damage to the baby's head.

- The mother has been circumcised, and heavy scars may prevent the vagina from stretching open for the baby. If you know how, you can cut the circumcision scar (see p. 406). If you do not know how to cut this scar, you may need to do an episiotomy.

How to do an episiotomy

1. Wait until you can see the head inside the vagina during a push, and the vagina is bulging open between pushes. If you cut too early, there will be bleeding. If you cut too late, there is more chance of cutting the baby.

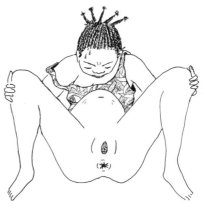

2. Scrub and put on sterile gloves (see p. 159).

3. Inject a *local anesthesic*, if you know how. This numbs the area around the vagina.

4. Put your fingers into the vagina like this. Your fingers will move the skin away from the baby, making it easier to cut without hurting the baby.

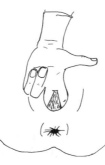

5. Feel with your thumb to find the round muscle around the anus *(rectal sphincter, see p. 395)*. **Never cut through this muscle.**

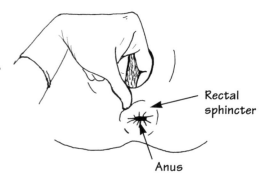

Rectal sphincter

Anus

6. Cut the skin about 2.5 centimeters or 1 inch. It is best to cut the kind of episiotomy that you have been trained to do or have watched someone else do or that is most commonly done in your area. Here are the 2 most common kinds of episiotomy:

■ In a **mediolateral cut**, the midwife begins cutting downward at the bottom center of the vaginal opening, but points the scissors either right or left so that the cut does not go near the anus.

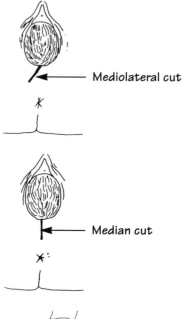

Mediolateral cut

Median cut

■ In a **median cut**, the midwife cuts straight down from the bottom center of the vaginal opening towards the anus. Be careful to hold the scissors so that the tips will not snip the rectal sphincter muscle.

Gently pat the cut with a sterile cloth and feel it with your fingers. Make it larger only if you have to. It is better to make one cut than several small cuts.

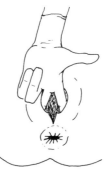

7. Press on the cut with a sterile cloth to slow the bleeding.

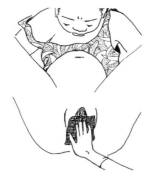

8. After the birth, sew the cut flesh together, if you have been trained to do this. See the next section below on sewing torn flesh and episiotomies (p. 395, #5).

The risks of doing an episiotomy

When you do an episiotomy, there are several risks:

- The cut might get infected.

- The cut may hurt the baby.

- The cut may hurt the rectal sphincter.

- The cut may go through an important blood vessel and cause a lot of bleeding.

- The cut may be painful to the mother afterwards and make healing slower after childbirth.

> **Caution!** Do not do an episiotomy unless it is needed to save the life or health of the mother or baby—especially if you do not have special training in how to sew torn flesh and episiotomies.

5. Sewing a tear or an episiotomy

Most babies will be born without seriously tearing the mother. But sometimes, no matter how careful you and the mother are, her vagina will tear. Some tears and cuts heal better if they are sewn together. It is not hard to sew them, but it is important to learn from a skilled teacher.

How to judge if a tear needs to be stitched

1. Review how things normally look. If you could see under the skin of a woman's bottom, you would find these things:

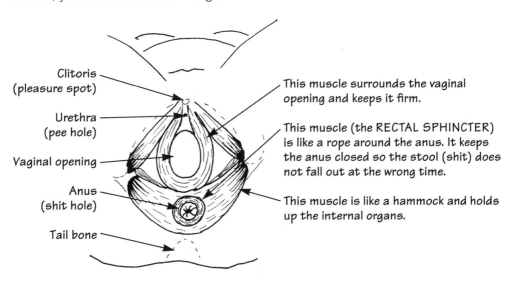

Clitoris (pleasure spot)

Urethra (pee hole)

Vaginal opening

Anus (shit hole)

Tail bone

This muscle surrounds the vaginal opening and keeps it firm.

This muscle (the RECTAL SPHINCTER) is like a rope around the anus. It keeps the anus closed so the stool (shit) does not fall out at the wrong time.

This muscle is like a hammock and holds up the internal organs.

2. Judge **how long** the tear is and how much of the flesh is torn.

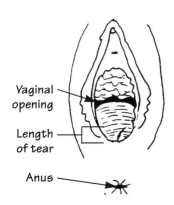
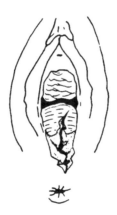
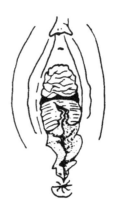
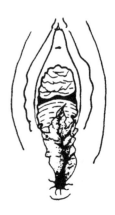

Vaginal opening

Length of tear

Anus

This tear is only in the vagina. Medical people call this a 1st degree tear.

This tear is in the vagina, in the skin of the outside, and in the muscle. This is called a 2nd degree tear.

This tear is in the vagina, in the muscle, in the skin of the outside, and in the muscle around the anus (rectal sphincter). This is called a 3rd degree tear.

This tear is in the vagina, in the muscle, in the skin of the outside, and goes through the rectum. This is a 4th degree tear.

3. Judge **how far inside** the mother the tear goes. If you think that a tear extends inside the mother, scrub and put on sterile gloves. Then use 1 or 2 fingers to stretch the vaginal opening so you can see inside. Then find the end or tip of the tear. Most tears have only 1 tip inside, but some have more.

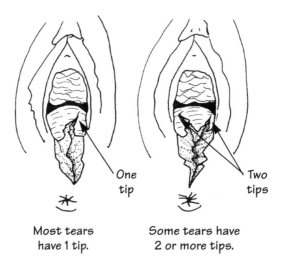

One tip

Two tips

Most tears have 1 tip.

Some tears have 2 or more tips.

4. If you think the muscle around the anus may be torn, do this test:

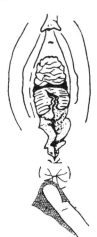

Cover your finger with gauze and lightly brush the anus with your finger. If the anus contracts, the muscle is probably OK.

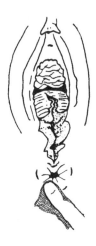

If the muscle does not contract, the muscle may be torn.

5. Decide what needs to be done. First degree tears do not need to be stitched. Second degree tears will heal better if they are sewn (but they may heal OK without sewing). Tears that go deep into the flesh or down to the anus should be sewn, or the mother may have trouble controlling her bowels later on.

It is best to sew tears within the first 12 hours or $1/2$ day. If you sew a tear after 12 hours, it is likely to get infected and will not heal as well. If you cannot sew the tear during this time, leave the tear alone. Instead, clean the tear carefully. Have the mother soak her bottom in very clean warm water. In some places, traditional healers make teas out of plant medicines that help healing. These teas should be boiled before using.

Some basic rules for sewing tears

When you sew a tear, remember to:

- Wait until after the placenta has come out, and you are sure that the mother and baby are doing fine.

- Stay aware of how the mother and baby are doing as you sew.

- Keep everything as clean and sterile as you can.

- Think about what parts should be sewn to each other, and where to put each stitch before you put it in. It is important to sew muscle to muscle, and skin to skin—and to sew the jagged edges so they fit together correctly.

- Take your time. If you have to take out a stitch, that is another injury to the mother's vagina.

- Know your limits. If a tear looks too deep or complicated (see the next section below), get medical help.

Caution! Do not take unnecessary risks. Sewing a tear wrong is often worse than not sewing it all. It is important to get training before sewing. **Remember: Unless a tear is bleeding heavily there is no emergency.**

Equipment for sewing tears

If you decide that a tear needs to be sewn, you will need to have the right equipment to sew it correctly.

Equipment you need to have

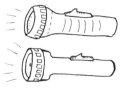

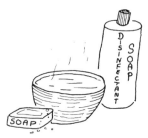

Good, strong light to see the tear.

Sterile scissors

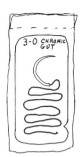

Chromic gut or Vicryl suture for sewing the tear. If possible, use size 000 inside the vagina. Use size 00 for sewing muscles. If you have only one of these sizes, use it throughout.

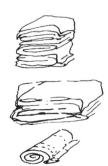

Sterile gauze or rags for cleaning and wiping. Sterile cloth to put under the mother and to lay your instruments on.

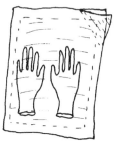

Sterile gloves to protect against infection.

Boiled water and disinfectant for washing. Use soap if you do not have disinfectant.

Chromic gut or Vicryl suture: These are the best kind of **sutures** to use, since they slowly dissolve. You will not have to take the stitches out later. If possible, get the kind of gut which has the thread attached to the end of the needle, not the kind where the thread goes through a needle with a hole in the end. A **curved needle** is better than a straight needle.

If there is no chromic gut or Vicryl suture available, you can use plain cotton thread that has been boiled. But since you will need to take the stitches out later, make only one layer of stitches.

Equipment that is useful to have

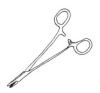

A needle holder makes it easier to grip the needle.

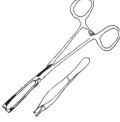

Allis forceps or tissue forceps (toothed tweezers) help grab hold of torn muscle, clots, and so on.

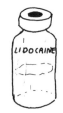

Local anesthetic makes suturing more comfortable for the woman.

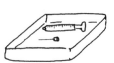

Sterile needle and syringe for giving local anesthetic.

How to get set up

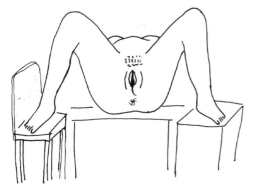

Put the mother in a good position
so you can see the wound.

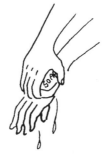

Carefully scrub your hands (see
p. 159). Put on sterile gloves if
you have them. If not, wear clean
plastic bags.

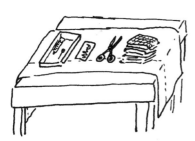

Set your sterile instruments
out on a sterile cloth.

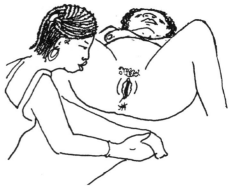

Put a sterile cloth under the woman's bottom

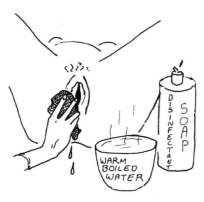

Gently wash the tear with boiled water
and disinfectant soap. If possible, ask
a helper to shine a light on the tear, so
you can see it better.

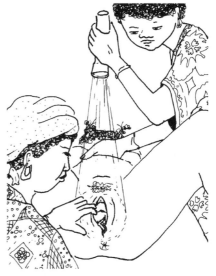

Explore the wound to make sure you know
how deep it is. If possible, show a helper how
to check the womb and make sure it stays
small and hard (see p. 209). She should
check it from time to time while you work.

Injecting medicine to numb the torn area

After birth, the woman's genitals may be numb, so it is possible to sew the tear without using any medicine. However, she may be more comfortable if you use a local anesthetic. This is most important if the tear goes down toward the anus.

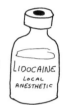

Llidocaine is a ommon local anesthetic. There may be others in your area. (Be sure these do **not** contain epinephrine.) They usually come in liquid form and do not need to be kept cold.

Before you give the anesthetic, ask the mother if she has ever had this medicine. If she has never had a reaction to this medicine, follow the instructions for giving injections on p. 383–386. Withdraw about 10 cc of medicine.

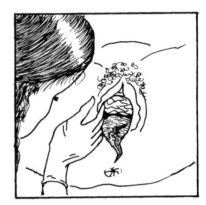

Look carefully at the shape of the tear. Think about what pieces of flesh will be sewn together. This is important because the tear will swell and change shape after you put in the medicine.

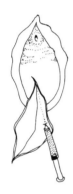
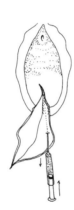
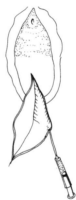
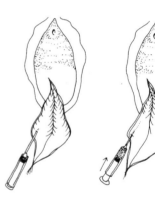

1. Slide the needle under the skin, just inside one side of the tear.

2. Slowly inject medicine as you slowly pull the needle out.

3. You will see the flesh swell up a little with medicine as you put it in.

4. Do the other side of the tear the same way.

Each side should take about 4 cc of medicine. If the tear is very deep, you may need to put in 2 layers of medicine. Use this pattern. (But do not put in more than 10 cc of medicine.)

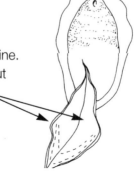

Another way to put in the medicine is to put several small doses along the sides of the tear. Put in a dose at each *x* spot:

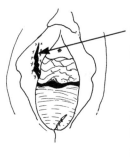

If the tear is in the lips of the genitals, you can put in little doses of medicine around it.

If there is still some medicine left in the syringe, set it down in a sterile place. You may need to use a little more medicine later.

Sewing tears

Some tips for better sewing

- A curved needle can make sewing easier. When you use a curved needle, it works like this:

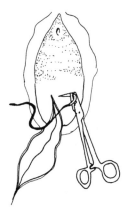

- A *needle holder* also makes sewing easier. If you use a needle holder, grasp the curved needle in the middle, a little towards the base, not the point. Be careful not to clamp the suture where it is stuck to the needle. Hold the needle holder like this when you put the needle in, and use your wrist to move it.

If you want the point to come out in this direction, you have to put the needle in pointing down.

- There are several kinds of stitches used to sew tears and episiotomies. Try to learn from one trained person who has experience sewing tears that don't get infected or fall apart. Use whatever stitch that person can teach you. We recommend *interrupted stitches* for most tears and episiotomies.

An interrupted stitch is a single stitch that is knotted with a 3-layered *knot* (see p. 403) then both sides of the thread are clipped.

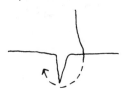 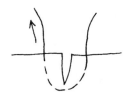

| Put the needle in one side of the cut or tear, about ¹/₂ cm from the edge of the tear. | Bring the needle up on the other side of the tear, ¹/₂ cm from the edge. | Make a three layer knot (see below). |

- The stitches should be tight enough to bring the sides of the tear together snugly, but if they are too tight it can cause problems in healing (and pain when having sex later).

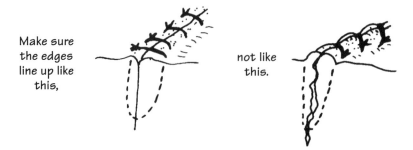

Make sure the edges line up like this,

not like this.

- Try to match the sides of the tear exactly:

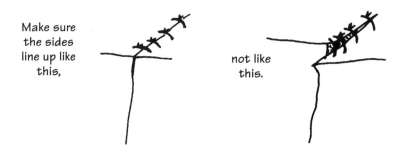

Make sure the sides line up like this,

not like this.

- The thread should come through just **above** the bottom of the tear. If the stitch is too shallow, the space between the bottom of the tear and the thread can fill with blood or pus and get infected. If the stitch goes too deep, you can pierce the rectum. This increases the chance of infection, and of stool leaking into the vagina.

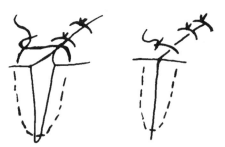

This stitch is done right.

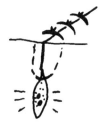

This stitch is too shallow. Blood and pus will collect here.

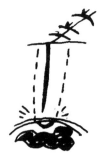

This stitch is too deep. It goes into the rectum where the stool is.

- Stitches are fastened with knots. Here is how to tie a 3-layered knot:

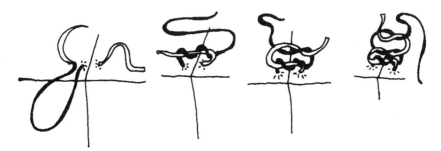

A 3-layered knot (or square knot) is like the knot you tie when you tie the baby's cord. In the drawing we show each end of the thread with a different color to make it easier to see. In real life, it will be all one color. In this picture one end goes OVER, then UNDER, and then OVER the other. This makes a strong knot that won't come untied.

Be sure to test the knot to make sure it holds.

Also remember:

- Do tears that are inside the vagina first.

- Be careful not to sew blood clots or hairs into the tear. These could cause infection.

- Do as few stitches as possible, just enough to hold the tear together. Too many stitches increase the injury to the mother.

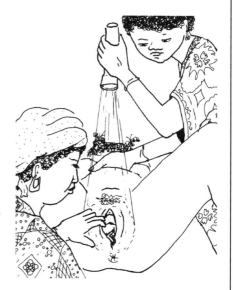

- Have a helper check the mother's womb (to see if it stays hard) from time to time as you sew.

One way of sewing tears inside and around the vagina, or episiotomies

1. It helps to put a sterile gauze in the vagina above the tear to stop blood from leaking and getting in your way. Be sure to take the gauze out when you are done sewing.

2. The inside of the vagina is made of a kind of tissue called ***mucous membrane*** or ***vaginal mucosa***. Under the mucous membrane there is muscle, which is redder and tougher to touch. It is important to sew muscle to muscle and mucous membrane to mucous membrane.

3. Using chromic gut or Vicryl suture, put the first stitch above the inside tip of the tear in the vagina and tie a 3-layered square knot. Clip the stitch with sterile scissors.

4. Continue to make interrupted stitches as shown, through the length of the vagina.

5. Now stitch the muscle layer together. Use interrupted stitches and make as few as possible, just enough to hold the muscle together. Usually 2 or 3 will do. With each interrupted stitch tie a 3-layered knot (see p. 403) and clip the ends with sterile scissors. Do each stitch this way, so that if one stitch comes undone the others will not.

6. Then close the skin over the muscle, using the same type of interrupted stitches and 3-layered knots. Clip the ends with sterile scissors. Be sure that the stitches that close the muscle are covered by the skin.

7. From time to time, push all the pieces of the tear together to make sure things are going together nicely.

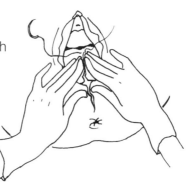

8. Before you quit, put your finger up into the mother's rectum to make sure that no stitches went all the way through. If you feel a stitch in the rectum, you must take her stitches out and do them over again! Be careful not to get any stool on her wound. Wash carefully and sterilize your gloves before you use them to sew again.

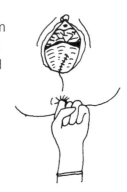

Sewing the rectal sphincter

It is not hard to sew the rectal sphincter, but it is difficult to describe with words and drawings. It is best if a skilled person shows you how to sew this at a real birth.

1. Examine the tear carefully to see if it goes into the rectum. If it does, and you do not know how to sew this tissue, get medical help at once. If the rectum is not torn, but just the sphincter muscle, first sew the vaginal mucosa as above (see p. 404, #2).

Tear goes into the rectum.

2. Using an **allis forceps** or other sterile instrument, pull the end of the muscle out so you can see it.

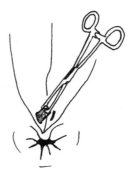

3. If you have 2 clamps or allis forceps, pull both ends of the muscle out before you sew. Hold the muscle so a little sticks out beyond the clamp.

4. Use size 00 chromic gut or Vicryl suture for sewing the sphincter muscle. Insert the needle at one end of the torn muscle. Hook each end of the muscle.

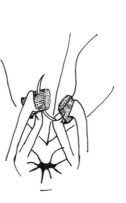

5. It usually takes interrupted stitches to hold the muscle together.

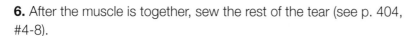

6. After the muscle is together, sew the rest of the tear (see p. 404, #4-8).

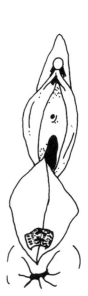

6. Cutting a circumcision scar

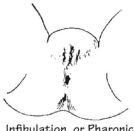

In many parts of the world, especially Northern Africa, South Asia, and some parts of Egypt and Western Africa, many women have been circumcised. Some circumcisions remove only a little bit of skin, but some (*Pharonic circumcision or infibulation*) remove all of the skin around the vagina. All that is left is a tiny hole and a lot of scar tissue.

Infibulation, or Pharonic circumcision

Circumcision can cause health problems—like bleeding, infection, tetanus, and difficulty urinating. It can also cause pain during sex. When it is time for a woman to deliver a baby, circumcision scars can make the second stage of labor longer. These scars can often tear and cause heavy bleeding, pain, and infection to the mother.

If a woman has been circumcised and the scar is preventing the baby from coming out, the scar needs to be cut open. This procedure needs to be done with sterile instruments and sterile gloves, and then sewn with sterile needles and chromic gut or Vicryl suture.

To cut the scar (deinfibulation)

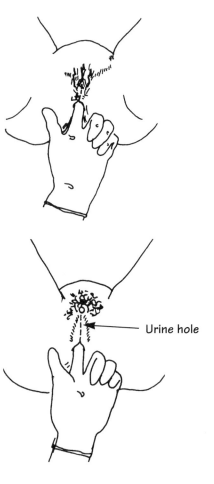

Urine hole

1. Put a finger under the band of scar tissue.

2. Inject local anesthesia, if you have it (see p. 400).

3. Cut the old scar open by snipping the bands of scar tissue until you can see the woman's urine hole. The vagina will probably now stretch to allow the baby to come out.

After the baby is born, talk to the woman about whether she wants to be circumcised again (recircumcised), or if she wants to be repaired.

To recircumcise the woman

1. Place local anesthesia on the 2 sides of the scar.

2. Stitch the cut edges of the scar together with interrupted stitches of 00 or 000 suture.

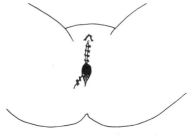

Recircumcision (option)

To repair the cut

1. Place local anesthesia on the 2 sides of the scar.

2. Loosely sew any raw surfaces together with a *blanket stitch* (a continuous locked stitch) of 000 chromic gut or Vicryl suture to stop any bleeding.

After any of these procedures, wash the area often and keep it as dry as possible.

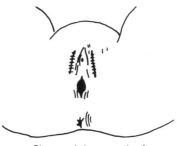

Circumcision repaired

7. Turning a breech or sideways baby

Turning a breech baby

Some midwives have been taught to massage the womb to try and turn a breech baby. If a breech baby does not turn head down by the time of birth, it is far safer for the mother to give birth in a maternity center or hospital than to try to turn the baby or give birth at home. Doctors in a hospital can use forceps (pulling instruments) if the baby gets stuck. Or they can do a cesarean section.

Caution! Massaging the womb to try and turn the baby is extremely dangerous! You should try to turn the baby **only** if you are sure that the baby is in a breech position, if you have been taught how to do it properly, and if you can get medical help. (If you are unsure if the baby is breech, get medical advice.)

Also, do not try and turn the baby if the mother's waters have broken or if the baby has settled down into her pelvic bones. Do not try to turn the baby if the mother has ever had vaginal bleeding, high blood pressure, or surgery on her womb or a cesarean section.

If you try to turn a breech baby, follow these steps:

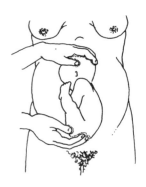

1. Remember that you must be absolutely sure of the baby's position. Also remember that the best time to turn the baby is 2 to 4 weeks before the due date.

2. Ask the mother to empty her bladder.

3. The mother should lie on her back with her knees bent.

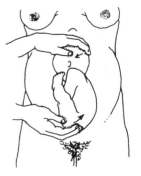

4. Check the baby's heartbeat to be sure it is OK. If you doubt the baby is healthy, do not try to turn it.

5. Be sure of the baby's position. Gently grasp the baby's head with one hand and push the baby from the bottom with your other hand. Push the baby up high to the top of the womb.

6. Try to move the baby in the direction it is facing. If it does not move easily, try the other direction. Be gentle. Hold the baby in place with one hand and push with the other. Try to keep the baby's position so its chin is on its chest.

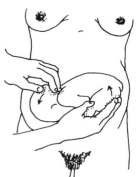

7. Each time you get the baby to move—even a little—stop and listen to its heartbeat. If the baby's heartbeat speeds up, STOP. If the heartbeat slows down a little but then quickly goes back to normal, it is OK. If it does not return to normal, STOP. Ask the woman to lie on her left side and take slow deep breaths. Recheck the baby's heart.

8. Keep gently turning until the baby is in a head down position.

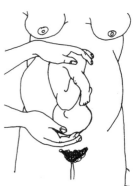

Caution! If you have to push hard or the mother is uncomfortable, STOP! You may be about to break the womb. (It is OK for the mother to feel pressure, but not pain.) **Never force the baby to turn.**

Turning a sideways baby

If at all possible, a sideways baby should be born by cesarean section in the hospital.

Some sideways babies will turn very easily, with just a gentle push. This is especially true if the mother has had other babies. But if this does not happen, the baby must be born in the hospital.

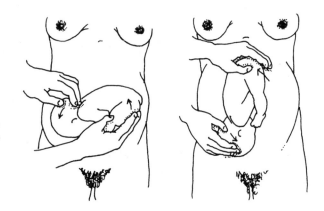

Caution! Pushing on the womb will tear it. Only turn the baby if it goes easily.

8. Giving fluids rectally

When a woman is in shock or is very dehydrated it is important to give her fluids as fast as possible. Sometimes this can be done by giving her fluids by IV. If you cannot give her fluids by IV, you can give the woman fluids rectally to treat shock or dehydration. If she is very dehydrated, she will absorb the fluids from her rectum.

1. Use the same equipment you would use to give an enema (see p. 174).

2. Ask the woman to lie on her left side. Put some oil on the tip of the rectal tube. Gently place the tube in the woman's rectum. Hold the container with the water (or the funnel) at the same level as the woman's hips, so that the water runs into the tube slowly. It will take about one hour for the water to go in.

3. When all the water is gone and the container is empty, slowly take the tube out of the woman's rectum. The woman will not feel like emptying her bowels (shitting). Her body will soak up the water. If the woman is still shows sign of dehydration or shock after two hours, you can give her another 500 cc (2 cups) of water the same way.

Special procedures inside the hospital

Chapter 25 contents

Special procedures inside the hospital

Building good relationships with hospital people before you need them

If you care for pregnant women and babies in the community, there will be times when an emergency or serious risk comes up. You will want to take or send a woman to the hospital or maternity center for special care. This will be much easier to do if you have already built a good relationship with hospital people in your area.

A good relationship is built when people can talk easily with one another, and when there is mutual respect and support. We encourage you to seek out medical and hospital people who recognize that midwives are important and who are willing to work with you to give women better care. Let them get to know you. Talk about the particular needs of women in your area. Ask them for what you need—more training, equipment, and so on. If hospital people in your area are not interested in getting to know midwives, try to talk with them anyway. If this does not work, you may need to approach them in a more organized way. For example, a group of midwives could get together with a local women's group and arrange a meeting with local hospital people. Or you might ask helpful medical people to speak to others for you.

When talking with hospital people, emphasize how a good relationship with community midwives will benefit everyone. Midwives will benefit by getting more training and equipment, and by knowing where to send women with complications. They will also be more willing to refer women with complications if they know medical people. Once a woman is in the hospital, midwives can give hospital people important information about the health history of each woman they refer, and help explain procedures to the mother so she will not be afraid.

Hospital people will benefit by getting important information about local health needs and about the local beliefs that affect health care. And if midwives refer women with complications more quickly, doctors will be able to give better care.

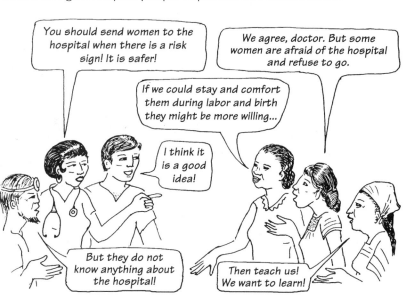

You should send women to the hospital when there is a risk sign! It is safer!

We agree, doctor. But some women are afraid of the hospital and refuse to go.

If we could stay and comfort them during labor and birth they might be more willing...

I think it is a good idea!

But they do not know anything about the hospital!

Then teach us! We want to learn!

At the hospital

A hospital is like another world. There are rules and procedures to follow, and doctors and nurses are often too busy to explain each one. So it is important for midwives to know about this world and how to work with hospital people. This section gives some general guidelines to follow. The rest of the chapter describes specific medical procedures that you will see in the hospital.

1. Talking with hospital people

When talking with hospital people, try to remember these things:

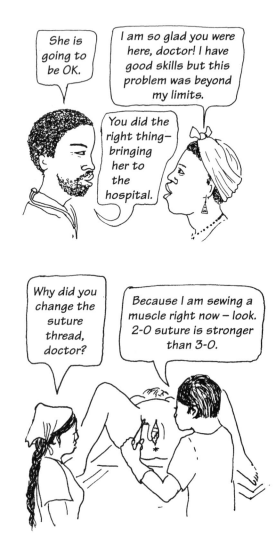

- Be tactful and respectful. Remember that doctors and nurses are not only busy but often very tired. They need to know that they are appreciated. Let them know that they are important, but do not forget that you have important skills, too.

  There may be times that you disagree with doctors or nurses. You will need to use your own judgment about whether or not to say anything. If you do decide to speak, there is a greater chance you will be heard if you speak with respect.

- Ask questions. Watching hospital people at work is a good opportunity to learn. If a doctor or nurse seems friendly, let them know you are eager to learn. They may be able to explain procedures to you, or to discuss things later when they are less busy.

2. Respecting new procedures

To respect hospital procedures:

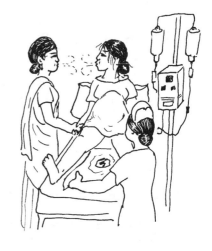

- Stay out of the way during procedures. Some hospital people fear that if they let midwives into the birth room, they will just have another person to take care of. Show them that this is not true. Look around the room and find a place to stand, away from any equipment. When in doubt, ask "Where would you like me to be?"

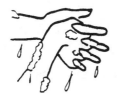

- Do not touch any instruments or sterile cloths unless a doctor or nurse says that it is OK. Always keep your hands very clean.

- Do not try to do any midwife procedures unless a doctor or nurse asks you to. For example: Do not massage the woman's genitals or give her water to drink unless someone tells you it is OK.

3. Making yourself useful

Even if you are not doing midwife procedures, you can be helpful in other ways. For example:

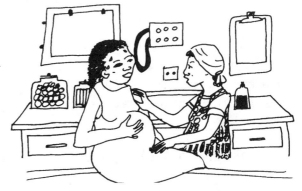

- Help the mother stay calm and relaxed. This is one of the most important things you can do. A calm, relaxed mother will usually have an easier, safer labor and be easier for the hospital staff to care for.

- Look for practical jobs to do that do not interfere with hospital routine. For example, you can ask the nurse: "Would you like me to change the pads on the bed?" or "Shall I bring the mother some water?" In many hospitals nurses are very busy and appreciate this kind of help.

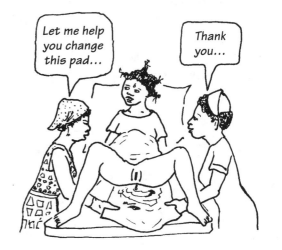

Let me help you change this pad...

Thank you...

4. Helping change hospital practices

As you get to know hospital people better, you may be able to help influence how they care for pregnant women. (But remember: It usually helps for hospital people to know you very well first.) Here are some of the most important practices to encourage:

- Describing any medical procedures in a clear, simple way so that women understand what is going to be done, why it is being done, and the choices they have.

- Allowing women to sit, stand, lie down, or walk around during labor.

- Allowing women to give birth in a sitting, squatting, kneeling, or standing position. They do not have to lie flat on their backs unless there is a medical emergency.

- Allowing women to touch and hold the new baby right away. They should be allowed and encouraged to breast feed within minutes after the baby is born.

- Letting babies stay with their mothers (rather than sending babies to a nursery) unless there is a medical emergency.

- Including the family in medical decisions and care.

Common hospital practices

In this section we will explain some of the most common hospital practices. We look at each of these practices in the same way that we looked at traditional and modern medicine—to see if it is helpful, harmless but useless, or harmful (see p. 23–28). We also explain what a midwife can do to help with each practice, if anything.

1. IV fluids (no drinking liquids by mouth)

IV stands for *intra venous* or *in the vein.* When a woman is given IV fluids, a needle is first put into her vein. Fluid flows from a bottle or bag through a tube and into the vein. Her body gets all the fluid it needs but her stomach stays empty.

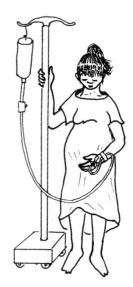

Some hospitals give every woman in labor an IV—even if the labor is normal and there are no risk signs. The benefits of an IV during labor are:

- An IV prevents dehydration. This is especially important if a woman is nauseated and cannot keep fluids in her stomach.

- The stomach stays empty. If an emergency operation is needed, the woman will not have fluid in her stomach. This is important because the medicine that puts people to sleep during an operation sometimes makes them vomit, and they may choke on it. If the stomach is empty, a person will not vomit.

- Emergency medicines can be given quickly—right in the vein.

The risks of an IV during labor are:

- An IV is uncomfortable for the woman and limits her movements during labor. This may make labor longer and more difficult. (A woman with an IV does not have to lie down. She can carry the IV on a pole that has wheels, but this is sometimes difficult.)

- A woman could get a serious infection of the blood from the IV. This is a small but serious risk.

Since there are risks in giving an IV, we recommend that an IV not be given unless there is a medical problem.

What you can do

When a woman has an IV and is told not to take liquids, her mouth may feel very dry. You can help by letting her suck on a wet cloth. This makes her mouth feel better without filling her stomach with liquids.

2. Sterile fields

A *sterile field* means an area where everything is free from germs (sterile). The sterile field helps prevent infection. When the time comes for the birth, hospital people will put sterile cloths on the woman's belly and thighs, so that only the genitals show. Sometimes those people attending the birth wear special clothes and masks over the nose and mouth. These masks are to keep people from breathing germs onto the mother and baby.

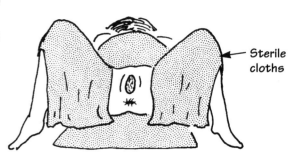

Sterile cloths

In a birth where there is an episiotomy or an operation, sterile fields are very important. But we do not believe that all the practices hospitals use to create sterile fields in normal births are necessary. For example: Some hospitals shave the woman's hair before washing the genitals with disinfectant soap. They are afraid that the woman's hairs may provide a place for harmful germs to hide—even after washing. In some places women keep their hair shaved off all the time, so there is no problem. But in places where shaving is not the custom a woman may find shaving uncomfortable, and there may be some itching when the hair grows back later. Also, shaving makes little cuts in the skin that could get infected later on.

What you can do

It is very important to not touch anything in a sterile field—unless you have scrubbed and are wearing sterile gloves. It is probably best to stay near the mother's shoulders, away from the sterile field, where you can help explain what is happening and help her relax.

3. Routine vaginal exams

In some hospitals, the nurse, midwife, or doctor put their hands in the woman's vagina to check the cervix. These vaginal exams can give the hospital people a lot of useful information about how much the cervix has opened and about the position of the baby. There is little harm in these exams as long as they are only done a few times, and if the person wears sterile gloves and makes sure everything around the vaginal opening is very clean. There is more risk of infection if the waters have broken.

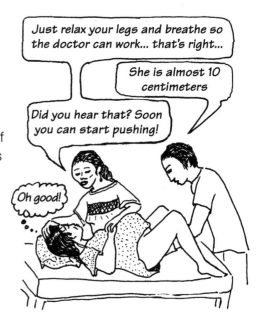

Just relax your legs and breathe so the doctor can work... that's right...

She is almost 10 centimeters

Did you hear that? Soon you can start pushing!

Oh good!

What you can do

If you live in an area where women are very modest about their bodies, explain to the mother that a male doctor's touch is medical, not sexual, and does not affect her virtue. It might be best to talk with women and their families about this during pregnancy, rather than waiting until they are in the hospital.

If a woman is afraid or tense during a vaginal exam, you can help by holding her hand gently but firmly, and encouraging her to relax her bottom and leg muscles. Help her breathe slowly and calmly. Reassure her. Explain what is happening.

4. The birth table and lying flat for the birth

Hospitals use different kinds of things to support a woman during birth. Some hospitals use ordinary beds. Some use **birth chairs** or "bean bag" chairs that support the mother in a sitting or squatting position. Some use **birth bars** so that the woman can stand while giving birth. Some use a **delivery table** where a woman lies flat on her back to give birth.

We believe that lying flat on the back for a normal birth is useless and sometimes harmful. It often makes it harder for the woman to push the baby out. To help, many hospitals now use a pillow on the delivery table, so that the woman can sit up part way during the birth. This is an easy, inexpensive way for hospitals to improve a mother's position during birth.

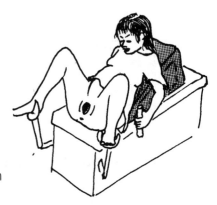

If there is a complication and the doctor needs to do a special procedure, it may be best for the woman to lie flat on her back.

What you can do

If the hospital uses a delivery table, you can suggest that a woman can push better if there are pillows helping her sit part way up.

5. Routine episiotomy

An episiotomy is a cut in the vaginal opening to make it larger. In some areas, doctors do episiotomies on all women or on all women who are having their first baby.

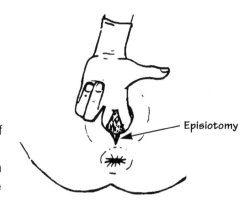

Episiotomy

An episiotomy can help a baby be born faster. It also helps the doctor get inside the mother to help the baby if there are problems. But there are also risks to doing routine episiotomies. They are often painful after the birth and heal more slowly than natural tears. They also cause bleeding and can become infected.

We believe that if the vaginal opening is normal, there is no need to do an episiotomy. The skin can stretch open during childbirth, and most tears can be prevented by controlling the birth of the head (see p. 187) and massaging the vaginal opening (see p. 186). However, an episiotomy is necessary when there are circumcision scars and in certain problem births.

Hospital procedures that deal with problems

The following procedures can be very useful, but they should only be done when there is a real problem.

1. X-rays and ultrasounds

X-rays and ultrasounds are ways to look inside a woman's body without cutting or hurting her. X-rays are used to look at the mother's bones and the baby's bones. X-rays are like a kind of light that cannot be seen. The x-ray machine sends this light through a woman's body, and then makes a picture on film (just like a camera makes a picture).

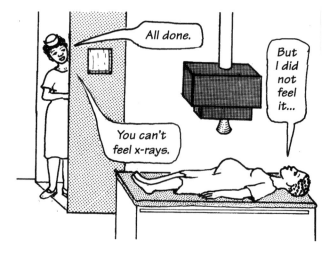

There are 2 kinds of ultrasounds used for pregnant women. *Sonograms* use a special kind of silent sound much like the x-ray machine uses light. The sonogram machine sends a silent sound through the woman's body, and then a picture appears on a television screen showing what is going on inside. A picture like a photo can be made from the TV screen.

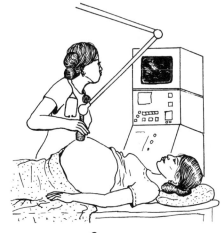

Sonogram

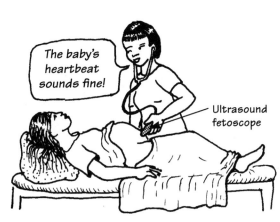

The baby's heartbeat sounds fine!

Ultrasound fetoscope

An *ultrasound fetoscope* makes the baby's heartbeat easy to hear, but it does not make a picture.

X-rays and sonograms can give a lot of useful information. They can show how old the baby is and the position of the placenta, if the baby is too big to fit through the mother's pelvic bones, or if there are twins. Ultrasound fetoscopes can often find the baby's heartbeat when a regular fetoscope cannot. This information can help the doctor make decisions which could save the life and health of the mother and baby.

What you can do

Explain to the mother that the x-ray machine or ultrasound machine will not hurt her. It is only going to make a picture or listen to the baby's heartbeat. Be sure she knows why an x-ray or ultrasound is being done.

2. Starting or strengthening a labor

Hospitals often use 2 methods for starting or strengthening a labor: *breaking the bag of waters* and *oxytocin drip*.

Breaking the bag of waters

When a woman has been in labor for a while but is not making good progress, a doctor or professional midwife may decide to break the water bag. He or she puts a special sterile instrument with a sharp tip into the vagina and pokes a hole in the bag.

Breaking the bag of waters may help bring the baby's head down harder against the cervix. Sometimes this causes better contractions. But it can also cause a greater chance of infection (especially if the labor is long) or make the cord prolapse (see p. 250). In a hospital, the benefits usually outweigh the risks, but this should not be done at home.

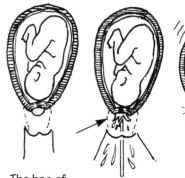

The bag of waters is not yet broken.

The bag of waters is broken.

The baby's head comes down harder on the cervix.

Oxytocin drip

When it is important to start or strengthen a labor, and other methods have not worked, the doctor may give a woman an oxytocin drip (oxytocin in an IV). Oxytocin is a chemical which is very much like the natural body chemical oxytocin—which causes stronger, longer, more useful contractions.

When oxytocin is used correctly, it can make a long, difficult labor shorter, and it can save lives. If oxytocin is given incorrectly (too much or too fast), it can cause contractions that are too strong and too close together. These contractions may cause brain damage to the baby, the placenta may separate early, or the womb may tear. These complications can damage or kill the baby and mother. For this reason, oxytocin should only be given by trained medical people. The baby's heartbeat should be checked often after giving oxytocin.

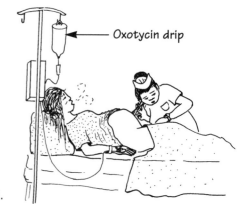

Oxotycin drip

> **Caution!** Oxytocin during labor should only be given IV, not by injection or by mouth. This way the doctor can control how much medicine the woman is getting and how fast it is going into her body.

What you can do

For both practices explained above, you can help by explaining to the mother what is happening and why it is happening.

3. Birth by instruments

Sometimes the cervix opens but the baby gets stuck going down the vagina. There are 2 main kinds of instruments that may be used to get the baby out: *forceps* and *vacuum extractor*.

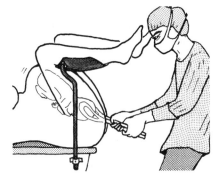

Forceps are special tools made to grab the baby's head while it is still inside the mother. The doctor puts the forceps inside the mother on either side of the baby's head. Sometimes it is only necessary to change the position of the baby's head, and then the doctor takes the forceps out and the mother pushes the baby out. At other times, the doctor will need to carefully pull the baby out through the vagina with the forceps. The doctor may need to do an episiotomy to make more room.

Forceps

A vacuum extractor is like a suction cup that is put on the baby's head to help pull the baby out.

One or both of these instruments may be useful when:

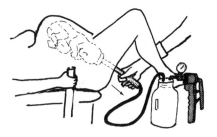

Vacuum extractor

- the baby is small enough to go through the mother's pelvic bones but is a very tight fit.

- the baby's head is at an unusual angle and needs to be straightened out inside.

- the baby is facing the mother's front and gets stuck.

- the baby is breech and the head comes too slowly.

- the baby is in some other danger and needs to be born quickly.

- the mother cannot push well because she has taken drugs for pain, or is very sick, or for some other reason.

Both these instruments can help save the lives and health of the mother and baby. They may prevent brain damage by helping the baby be born quickly. These instruments also have risks. For the baby, they can cause brain damage or the baby can be paralyzed. They may also cause the baby's head to be bruised or swollen, but this should go away in time. For the mother, these instruments can injure her insides, causing her more pain and a greater chance of infection after birth.

We recommend that these instruments not be used at normal births. But when there are problems like those listed above, it is worth the risk.

What you can do

If you are allowed to stay with the mother during a birth where the doctor uses forceps or a vacuum extractor, you can help by explaining what is happening and giving good labor support. Encourage the mother to relax her body and let the doctor work. If the doctor wants her to push, help her push correctly. Warn the mother that the baby's head may be bruised or swollen.

4. Birth by operation

Sometimes a baby cannot fit through the mother's pelvic bones. The baby may be too big, or it may be in a position that makes normal birth impossible. Or there may be a reason to believe that the mother or baby is in immediate danger. For example: slow fetal heartbeat, detached placenta, prolapsed cord. In these cases the doctor may decide to do an operation. He may do a ***cesarean section (C-section)*** or a ***symphisiotomy***, depending on what the problem is.

Cesarean section

A cesarean section is helpful when there is no other way to get the baby out, or when the mother or baby is in immediate danger. There are also risks. The mother may have a bad reaction to the medicine putting her to sleep, or she may have heavy bleeding or infection after the birth.

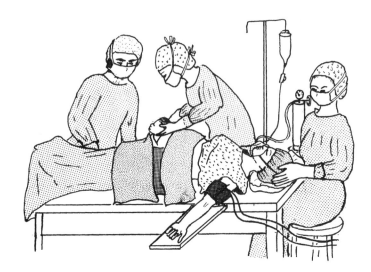

What you can do

Before the operation, you can help by telling the mother what to expect. Her belly will be painted with disinfectant and shaved. She may be put completely to sleep or the lower part of her body only may be asleep. If she is not completely asleep she will not feel any pain, but she may feel some tugging and pushing. After the operation, her belly will be sore and must be watched closely for signs of infection.

You may not be allowed in the operating room. However, you can be useful by giving support and comfort to the woman's husband or family. If the family is not there and you are allowed to watch the operation, you may learn a lot about how the body is made. Do not touch anything unless a doctor or nurse gives you permission. If the mother is awake, reassure her. Tell her when the baby is born, and whether it is a boy or a girl. Describe what the baby looks like.

Symphisiotomy

A symphisiotomy is an operation in which the middle of the mother's pubic bone (the softest part) is cut open. This makes the space between the mother's bones larger, so that it is easier for the baby to get out. This operation is only done in a few parts of the world.

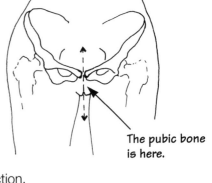

The pubic bone is here.

The benefits of an symphisiotomy are:

- It is easier to do than a cesarean section.

- It can be done with less equipment than a cesarean section.

- There is no scar left on the womb.

- When the pelvis heals, it may be larger for future births.

The risks of a symphisiotomy are:

- Healing may be very painful afterwards.

- Sometimes the bone does not heal well and the mother may be mildly disabled for life.

- The urine tube or bladder may be cut by accident.

What you can do

Before the operation, you can help by telling the mother what to expect. The woman's belly will be washed with disinfectant soap and she will be given an injection of local anesthesic (see p. 400) to numb the pubic bone. Either a doctor or nurse midwife will do the procedure, and they may ask you to hold the woman's legs so they stay apart. Once the pubic bone has been cut, the woman's legs must be pressed together. An episiotomy is also usually done at this time. After the baby is born, the woman's legs will be wrapped together at the knees. She will probably stay in the hospital for a week or more.

5. IV blood for hemorrhage

If a woman has bled too much during or after the birth (hemorrhage), she is in danger. She will be weak and vulnerable to infection, and it is sometimes necessary to give her blood in her vein. This is blood that another person has given to the hospital to save lives, or perhaps that her family has given for her at this birth.

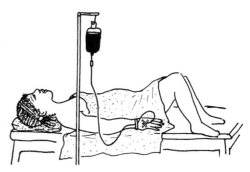

Blood should be given in an IV only when the mother is very weak. There is always a risk that the person giving the blood had a serious illness (like AIDS) and that the mother can get that illness, too.

6. IV antibiotics for infection

Antibiotics are usually given by injection or by mouth. But if the mother or baby has a serious infection, it is sometimes better to give the medicine in an IV. An IV puts the medicine right into the blood where it will do the most good and work most quickly. Also, some hospitals will give IV antibiotics to a mother whose bag of waters had broken more than a day and a night before the birth.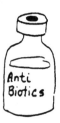

When a baby needs an IV, it is sometimes put in a vein in the cord, leg, or head. The nurse or doctor will use the vein that looks the strongest and is the easiest to reach.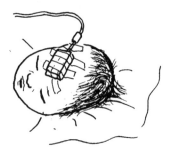

Antibiotics are very helpful if the mother or baby has an infection. But they should not be given without a good reason.

7. Sick or early babies

In areas where there are very few medical resources, sick babies may get very little medical attention. People may feel that it is better to let a sick baby die than to try and save it. They may prefer to spend their limited time and money trying to save older children and adults.

But some hospitals do have special equipment and medicines that can save many babies from both death and brain damage. This is some of the equipment that may be used:

- An *incubator* is a special box made to keep the baby warm. This way the baby can use its energy to get stronger rather than to make body heat.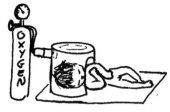

- An **oxygen tent** or **oxygen hood** gives the baby extra oxygen. This may help a baby if its lungs are not strong enough (or are too infected) to get all the oxygen it needs from plain air. Oxygen must be given correctly. Too much oxygen can make the baby blind.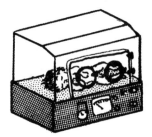

- A *respirator* is a special machine that helps a baby breathe. A tube is put into the baby's throat. Then the machine sends air in and out of the baby's lungs, until it is strong enough to breathe for itself.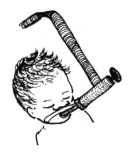

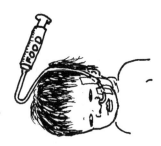

- A ***feeding tube*** is a tube put through the baby's mouth or nose all the way into its stomach. This is used when the baby is too weak to suck well. Since it is usually best for the baby to have breast milk, the mother can milk her breasts by hand or with a pump (see p. 337) to give the baby through the tube.

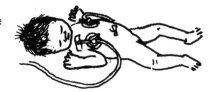

- Measuring devices may be put on the baby's chest to make sure the heart is beating well.

Sometimes it looks terrible to see a little baby with needles and tubes all over it. It is natural to think, "Why not let the poor baby die?" But it is also true that these methods can sometimes save a baby's life and health. He or she may get well and grow up to be a strong, healthy, happy person.

What you can do

Explain what is happening to the mother. If the mother can visit the baby, explain that she may be asked to wear a special, sterile robe. This is to protect the baby from infections. Sometimes the mother can hold the baby. If she cannot, she can stroke it, sing to it, and give it comfort. If possible, encourage the hospital to let the mother stay with the baby.

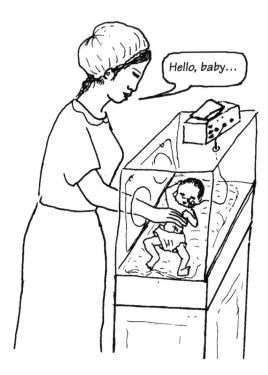

Hello, baby...

Appendix A: Homemade, low-cost equipment

Homemade timers

Sometimes midwives need to measure the number of heartbeats or breaths per minute, but they may not be able to afford or keep a clock or watch with a second hand. Instead, midwives can make simple instruments for measuring time.

When you first make a timer, be sure you have a watch to "set" the time. It is also a good idea to check your timer (especially the water timer) from time to time with someone's watch. If this is not possible, you can make 2 timers and check one against the other.

Here are some ideas that have been tried and work fairly well:

Water timers

Water timers are easy to make but less accurate than sand timers (see below).

Using a syringe

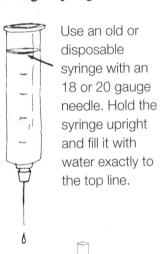

Use an old or disposable syringe with an 18 or 20 gauge needle. Hold the syringe upright and fill it with water exactly to the top line.

Using a watch with a second hand, measure how far the water level drops in exactly one minute.

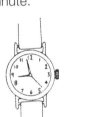

Check this a few times, and then mark the spot with ink, nail polish, or a piece of tape. If the water drips out too slowly, break off the needle to make it drip faster.

Using a glass or plastic tube

Instead of a syringe, you can use a glass or plastic tube. The longer and thinner the tube, the more accurate it will be as a timer.

To form a narrow hole in a glass tube, hold it over a hot flame, then stretch, cool, and break it (see p. 428).

Using an old intravenous (IV) kit

A fairly accurate timer can be made from an old IV kit. Open the wider tube at the top to serve as a funnel. Hold the tube in the air or have someone hold it for you. Fill the tube with water (be sure there is no air in the tube).

Using a watch with a second hand, mark the distance the water drops in one minute. Check it several times to be sure.

To help keep the tube straight, tie a weight at the lower end.

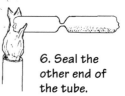

Start here →

One minute →

Rock or other weight →

23–25 gauge needle →

Sand timers

A sand timer consists of a tube of glass closed at both ends, with a narrow neck in the middle. It is partly filled with fine sand. The sand runs from the upper to the lower half in an exact period of time.

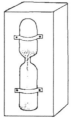
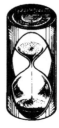

Egg timers, or 3-minute sand timers, can be purchased at low cost in some areas. To use one, count the number of pulses or breaths for 3 minutes, and then divide by 3 to know the number of pulses or breaths per minute. This can also be used to tell when contractions are 3 minutes apart.

1-minute sand timer

To make a 1-minute sand timer, follow these steps:

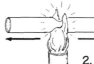

1. Heat the middle of a glass tube over a Bunsen burner or other small, very hot flame.

2. Stretch the tube to make a thin neck in the middle.

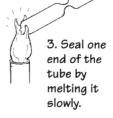

3. Seal one end of the tube by melting it slowly.

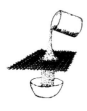

4. Wash some fine sand to remove the dirt. Dry it in the sun, and sift it through a very fine strainer. Then heat the sand to remove moisture.

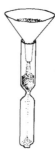

5. Put just enough sand in the tube so that it takes exactly one minute for all of it to run from one part to the other. (Use someone's watch with a second hand to check this.)

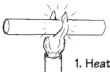

6. Seal the other end of the tube.

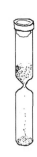

An easier method is to use a "soft glass" test tube, or a blood collection tube. Instead of melting the end, simply seal it with a cork or rubber stopper. This timer may be less accurate in a moist climate.

Do not be surprised if you have to make a sand timer several times before you get it just right. Try to make sure you have the right amount of sand before you seal the tube. If the sand sticks, try to find a smoother, finer sand, and be sure it is absolutely dry. Protect the timer by keeping it in a box with cotton, as it can break very easily at the neck.

Note: For both water timers and sand timers: Sometimes a timer will get partly clogged and give a false reading. So it is a good idea to check your timer from time to time.

Homemade stethoscopes

A stethoscope is a hollow tube that makes it easier to listen for sounds inside a person's chest or belly. It is a good tool for listening to the baby's heartbeat inside the womb.

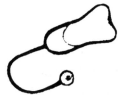

The best stethoscopes are made of metal and plastic, and can be expensive. But there several kinds of homemade stethoscopes you can make:

- Use a hollow tube of bamboo, wood, or clay.

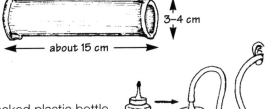

3–4 cm

about 15 cm

- Use the top of a narrow-necked plastic bottle and a piece of rubber tube.

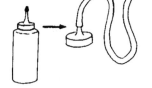

- Cut off the top of a rubber suction bulb.

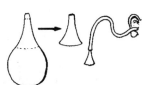

Homemade scales

These scales are less accurate and less easy to use than store-bought scales, but they are cheap and easy to make.

4 kinds of scales

Beam scale

This is the easiest kind to make and probably the most accurate. The beam can be made of dry wood or bamboo. The movable weight can be a bag, bottle, or tin filled with sand.

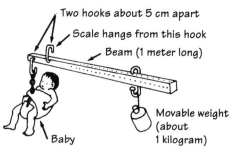

Two hooks about 5 cm apart

Scale hangs from this hook

Beam (1 meter long)

Baby

Movable weight (about 1 kilogram)

Folding scale

This scale is easy to carry from place to place. It works best if made of metal or plywood strips.

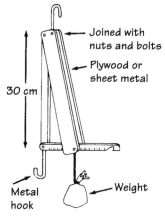

Joined with nuts and bolts

Plywood or sheet metal

30 cm

Metal hook

Weight

Quarter-circle scale

If this scale is made with plywood, use sheet metal to reinforce the upper corner. The weight should be between 1 and 2 kilograms. It can be made from scrap metal or a piece of heavy pipe.

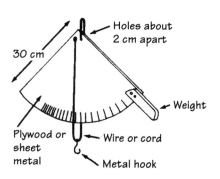

Holes about 2 cm apart

30 cm

Weight

Plywood or sheet metal

Wire or cord

Metal hook

Spring scale

This scale is made with a coil spring inside a bamboo tube. The spring should be about 30 centimeters long and squeeze to half its length with a weight of 15 kilograms.

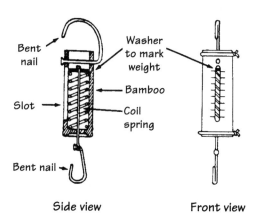

Bent nail

Washer to mark weight

Bamboo

Slot

Coil spring

Bent nail

Side view

Front view

How to make the scales accurate:

To do this, you will need some accurate standard weights. Perhaps you can...

- Borrow some weights from a merchant at the market.

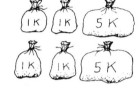

- Use a merchant's
scales to prepare
several sand weights.

- Borrow some 1-kilogram packages or cans of food.

To mark your scale:

1. Hang 1 kilogram on it.

2. Balance the movable weight.

3. Mark the spot with a small line and write a "1."

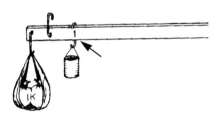

4. Now add 1 more kilogram at a time, making a mark each time,
until you have 5 marks on the scale.

Appendix B:
Teaching materials

Most people learn better when they can hear and see what they are learning about. In this section we describe how to make some materials for teaching about women's bodies, and about pregnancy and birth. These materials can be used when teaching other midwives, pregnant women and their families, or people in the community who want to learn about women's health.

At the end of this section there are 3 addresses for ordering teaching aids for midwives. For a list of places to get general teaching materials, see *Where There is No Doctor,* by David Werner. This book is available from the Hesperian Foundation (see p. 20).

1. 3 basic methods for making teaching materials

To use the materials on the following pages, you will need to use some of these methods:

Copying a pattern

Some teaching materials come with *patterns* for making models. To copy this pattern, put a thin sheet of paper over the pattern. If possible, tape it down lightly so it does not move around. Then trace the pattern onto the thin paper. Remove the thin paper and pin (or tape) it on the cloth or cardboard you are going to cut out.

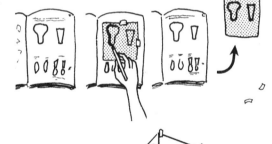

Making a slide into a poster

Put a large piece of paper or a large cloth on a wall. Then put a slide into a slide projector and shine the picture onto the piece of paper or cloth. Trace the picture exactly. Once you have the outline, color it in.

Making models out of paper mache

Paper mache is a good material for making models of parts of the body. For example, if you want to make a model of a baby's head, use a balloon or some dry, crumpled newspaper in a plastic bag. Then make a paste of flour and water. Dip strips of news-

paper or other paper in it, and layer the strips over the balloon or newspaper. Make several layers and let it dry (it dries best in the sun or in a low temperature oven). Paint the outside so it looks like a baby's head.

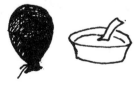
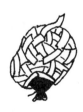
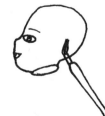

2. Making a model of a non-pregnant woman's body

It is good for women to know about their bodies before pregnancy and birth. These materials can help you teach them.

A paper pelvis

You can make a simple model of the pelvic bones by using a large piece of stiff paper.

1. Make a pattern by tracing this shape on thin paper:

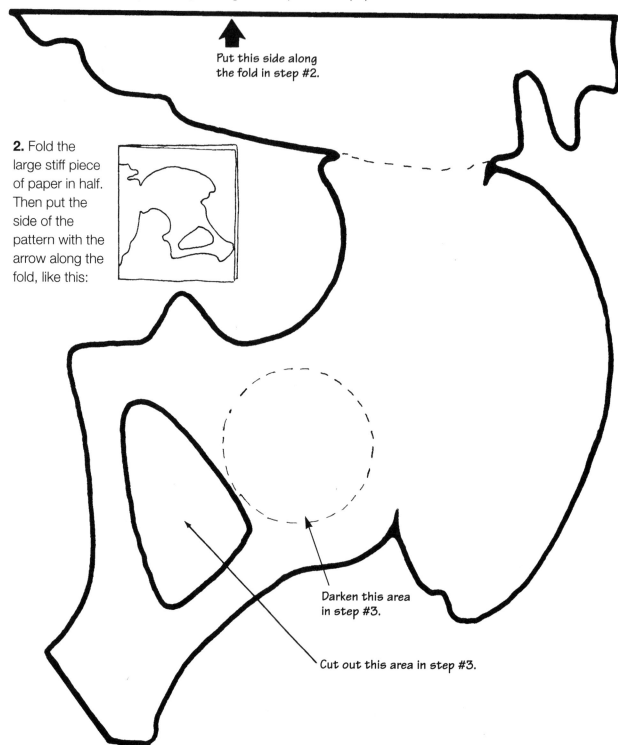

Put this side along the fold in step #2.

2. Fold the large stiff piece of paper in half. Then put the side of the pattern with the arrow along the fold, like this:

Darken this area in step #3.

Cut out this area in step #3.

3. Cut the paper along the edges of the pattern, and then unfold the paper. Draw a dark spot on each side to show where the leg bones go. Cut out the holes here.

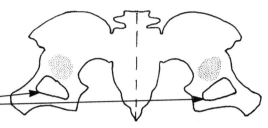

4. Bend the paper around and join the ends together to make a pubic bone in front. Be sure to keep the dark spots on the outside. To keep the front of the pelvis round, put a thin strip of cardboard across the inside of the pubic bone. Gently curl the hip bones (at the top on each side) back.

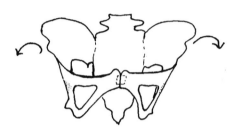

5. Bend the tail bone back.

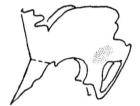

6. Then curl it forward.

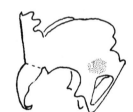

7. Fold the little tips so that they point inward.

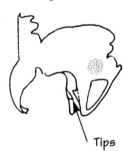

Tips

A womb and vagina made from cloth

The womb

1. To make the outside of the womb, cut 2 pieces of cloth this size. Stretchy material is best. (If you cannot get stretchy material, cut the material a little larger than this picture.) Purple is a good color, but use whatever you can get.

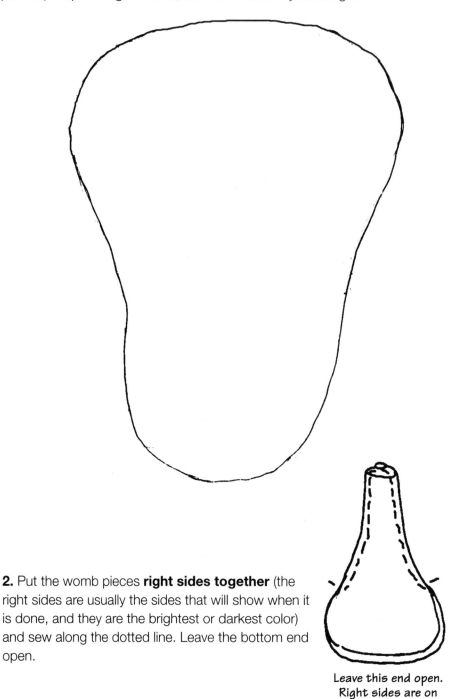

2. Put the womb pieces **right sides together** (the right sides are usually the sides that will show when it is done, and they are the brightest or darkest color) and sew along the dotted line. Leave the bottom end open.

Leave this end open.
Right sides are on
the inside.

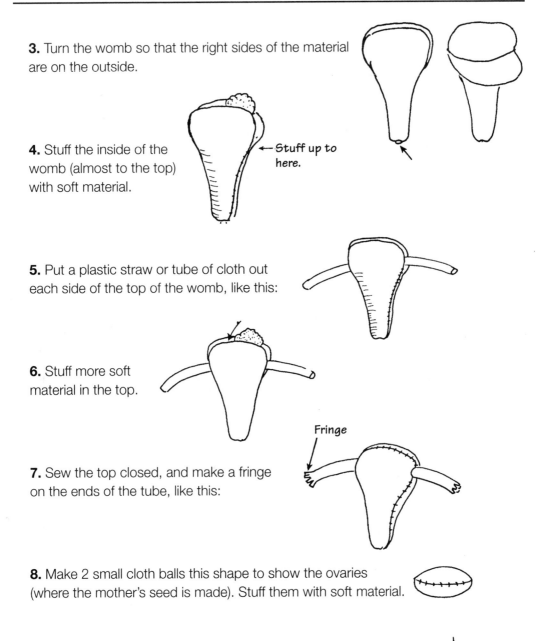

3. Turn the womb so that the right sides of the material are on the outside.

4. Stuff the inside of the womb (almost to the top) with soft material.

←Stuff up to here.

5. Put a plastic straw or tube of cloth out each side of the top of the womb, like this:

6. Stuff more soft material in the top.

7. Sew the top closed, and make a fringe on the ends of the tube, like this:

Fringe

8. Make 2 small cloth balls this shape to show the ovaries (where the mother's seed is made). Stuff them with soft material.

9. If you are using a plastic straw to show the tubes, sew a strong string to one ovary. Put the string through the straw and attach it to the other ovary. If you are using cloth tubes, sew one ovary to each end.

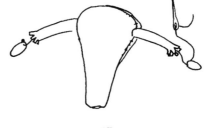

10. The finished womb should look like this:

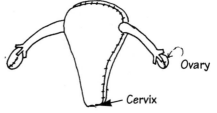

Ovary

Cervix

The vagina

1. Cut a piece of material this size and shape:

2. Sew a little soft wire or plastic along the flat edge of the **wrong side** of the material. The wrong side will be inside when it is done and is less dark or brightly colored.

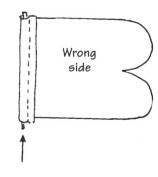

Wrong
side

Small opening

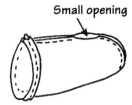

3. Fold the right sides of the material together (so you cannot see them) to make a tube. Sew, leaving a small opening.

4. Sew a piece of cloth here.

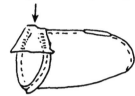

5. Turn the tube so the right sides face out. Make a knot here to show the clitoris. Make a dot or a hole to show the urine hole.

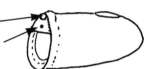

6. Attach the womb to the vagina by putting the bottom of the womb into the opening in the vagina.

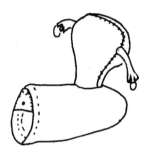

Using the model for teaching

Here are a few ways you can use this model in teaching:

1. Students can put their fingers into the vagina and feel the cervix.

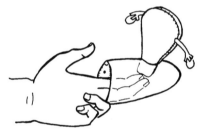

2. You can hold the womb in front of your belly so people understand where the womb is in the body.

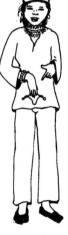

3. You can show how to stop a hemorrhage after birth (see p. 277). Fold the womb over a board or stick (the pubic bone) and apply pressure.

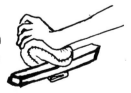

3. Making a model of pregnancy: the womb, placenta, cord, and baby

When teaching people about pregnancy and birth, the following models can be very helpful.

A womb made from a gourd

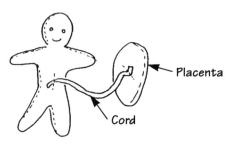

1. Look for a gourd shaped like this.

2. Make a hole in the bottom and open the top.

3. Make a simple doll from cloth. Make the doll small enough to fit inside the gourd. Use a small piece of rope or string for the cord, and a small pillow for the placenta. (For another way to make a doll, see the next section below.)

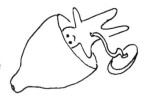

Placenta

Cord

4. Put the doll inside the gourd. You can glue the placenta to the inside wall of the gourd.

5. Make a vagina out of a tube of leather, cardboard, rubber, or some other material. Make a hole in the top. Leave one end open and sew the other end closed.

Leave this end open.   Make a hole here.

Sew this end closed.

6. Put the bottom of the womb into the hole in the top of the vagina. Perhaps you can find some way to prop it up.

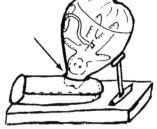

7. If you want to show an open cervix, make another gourd womb with an open bottom, like this:

A pregnant womb

1. Cut 2 pieces of material this shape. The material should be about 33 centimeters or 13 inches long. It should be about 27 centimeters or 10 ¹/₂ inches wide at the top, and about 15 centimeters or 6 inches wide at the bottom. Stretchy material is best. Purple or pink are good colors, but use whatever you can.

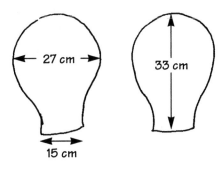

2. Cut a circle of red cloth the same size as the placenta (see below). Sew it to the wrong side of one of the womb pieces. This circle shows the spot where the placenta is attached.

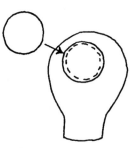

3. Put the right sides of the womb together and sew like this. Leave the bottom end open.

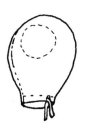

Leave this end open.

4. Turn up the open end and sew. Leave enough space for a drawstring to fit inside. This will be the cervix.

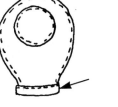

5. Turn the womb right side out. Put a drawstring or piece of elastic in the bottom.

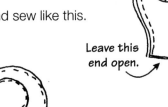

The placenta and membranes

1. To make the placenta, cut 2 pieces of cloth (red cloth is good) about the size of the big circle. It should be at least 22 centimeters or 8½ inches across. The circles do not have to be exactly round.

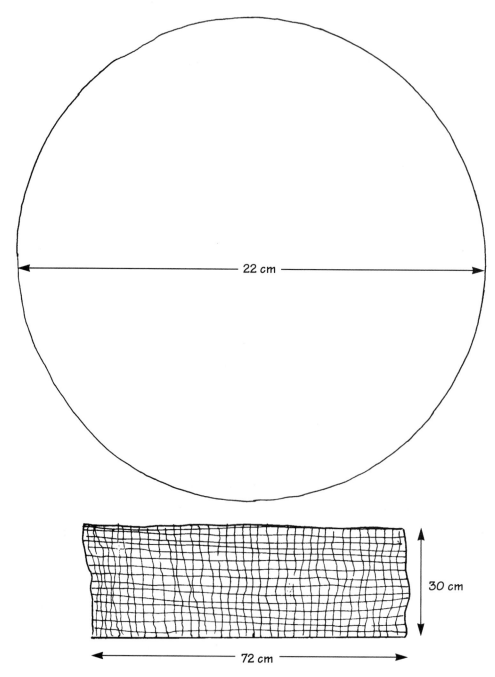

2. To make the membranes (the bag of waters), use thin material you can see through. White or light blue material is best. Cut the material about 30 centimeters or 12 inches wide, and about 72 centimeters or 8 inches long.

3. Lay one of the circles face down on the middle of the thin cloth. Sew the circle down, leaving a space around the edge.

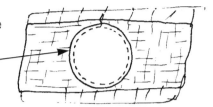

4. Turn the cloth over and fold the thin cloth carefully away from the edge of the circle and pin it down, so it is entirely contained in the circle. Leave the edge of the circle sticking out.

Opening

5. Put the other circle face down over the first circle and folded thin cloth. Sew almost all the way around, leaving a small opening.

6. Turn the circles so the right sides of the circles face out. Take out the pin, and the membranes will be on the outside. Stuff the placenta with some soft material like foam rubber, old rags, or even dried grass.

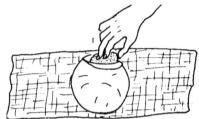

7. Stuff the placenta until it is this shape. Do not fill it too tight. Then sew the opening closed.

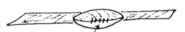

Sew it closed here.

8. Turn the placenta to the side that has no thin cloth over it. This is the bottom of the placenta—the side that is attached to the womb wall. If you like, quilt the bottom to show the segments in the placenta. Do not let the quilting go through to the top side of the placenta. The top should be smooth.

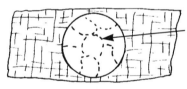

Quilt line on bottom

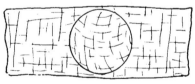

Smooth top

9. Let the thin material hang down and sew the sides together to make a tube.

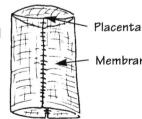

Placenta

Membranes

10. Turn up the bottom of the tube and sew it, leaving a space that a drawstring can fit through. Thread a drawstring through the bottom of the tube.

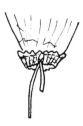

The cord

1. Cut a long piece of cloth about 52 centimeters or 20 inches long, and 8 centimeters or 3 inches wide. Blue is a good color to use, but use whatever you have.

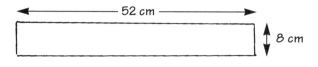

52 cm

8 cm

2. Fold the right side of the material together, lengthwise, and sew along the edge.

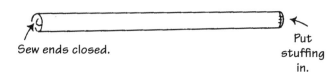

3. Turn the material so the right side is now on the outside. Stuff it with something soft, just as you stuffed the placenta.

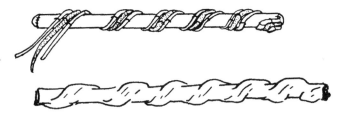

Sew ends closed.

Put stuffing in.

4. To show the arteries and vein in the cord, wind 3 thick strings or pieces of yarn around the cord and sew them down, so they do not get tangled. Two of the strings should be the same color. If possible, cover the cord with a piece of thin material like you used for the membranes, so it looks like this:

5. Sew one end of the cord onto the top side of the placenta (the side covered with thin material). Draw veins on this side of the placenta with an felt tip or ink pen.

6. Attach the other end of the cord to a doll (see next section). You can sew the cord to the doll or fasten it with a safety pin.

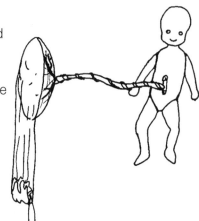

To demonstrate the baby inside the bag of waters, put the doll into the bag and close the drawstring. To demonstrate the bag breaking, open the drawstring.

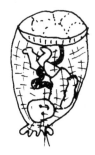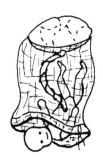

The baby

Although any doll can be used as a baby, the best kind of doll has a hard head and a soft body. If you are making a doll, follow these instructions:

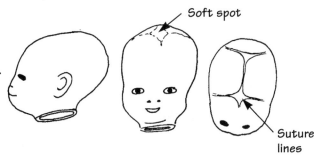

Soft spot

Suture lines

1. Make a hard head with a hollow center with paper mache (see p. 433). Paint a face on the head, and then paint on the soft spots or suture lines (see p. 216).

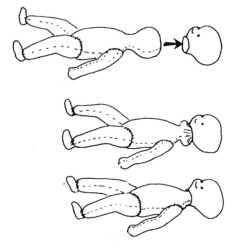

2. Sew a life-size body for the doll— with a round head a little smaller than the hard head you just made. Stuff the cloth with foam rubber, rags, or dried grass, so that it looks like a baby's body. Then stuff the cloth head into the hollow center of the hard head.

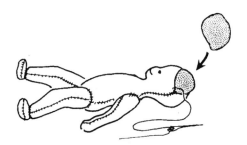

If paper mache is not easy to use, you can try this way of making a hard head. Stuff the body and face with soft material, then stuff the top of the head with one of these: a gourd; a hard ball; a smooth, round piece of wood; or a round stone.

Using the model for teaching

To demonstrate how the baby, placenta, and membranes are arranged inside the womb, put the baby inside the membranes with the placenta, then put the membrane bag into the womb. Put the bottom of the placenta up against the red circle inside the womb and pin it with a pin.

1. Pull the drawstring to close the cervix.

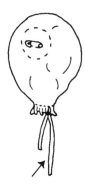

2. Then open the drawstring so the baby can be "born." (If you want to show that the waters have broken, open the drawstring on the membranes.)

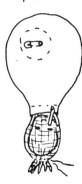 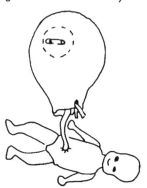

3. Take off the pin and squeeze the placenta out to show the birth of the placenta.

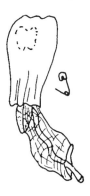

4. Explain that the red circle inside the womb is like an open wound that bleeds. Squeeze the womb to show how it must contract to stop the bleeding.

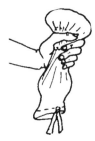

4. The *birth box* and *birth pants*

The birth box

To demonstrate birth, cut and paint a cardboard box to look like a woman's body. Make a hole that the doll can fit through. Make a belly out of the front flap of the box and breasts out of the back flap.

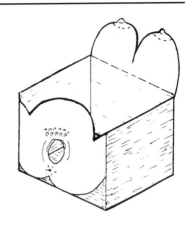

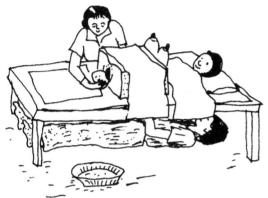

To make the box more real, you can put it on a cot under a cloth or blanket. Put a doll above the box on the cot so it looks like a woman, then have someone lie underneath the cot. This person can push up on the box to show contractions and make panting and moaning sounds as if giving birth.

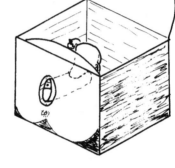

Or you can put the womb and vagina you made above (see p. 436–439) in the birth box to give people a better view.

The birth pants

Birth pants give a more real view of birth. Cut an old pair of pants with a hole for the vaginal opening. Then have a woman dress like and act like a woman in labor, and wear the birth pants over her clothes. The woman then pushes a doll hidden in her own clothing out through the hole in the birth pants.

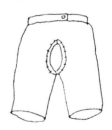

Addresses for teaching materials

ICEA Book Center
PO Box 20048
Minneapolis, MN 55420
USA
Fax: 512-854-8772
Telephone: 612-854-8660

Childbirth Graphics
PO Box 21207
Waco, TX 76702-6461
USA
Fax: 817-751-0221

Women's International
Network
187 Grant Street
Lexington, MA 02173
USA

The Green Pages: Table of medicines

Whenever possible, pregnant women should avoid using medicines. When a woman takes medicine, the medicine first gets into her blood and then gets into the baby's blood. Some of these medicines will not harm the baby, but other medicines can cause birth defects or serious problems.

In this book we recommend medicines only when needed. In this section we give more information about these medicines, their risks for the mother and unborn baby, and whether they are safe to use while breast feeding. Sometimes you will need to decide if the mother's health problems are serious enough to justify using a medicine that has some risks. Medicines with risks should be used only for serious problems or life-threatening illnesses.

> **Caution!** Whenever possible, avoid giving medicines to pregnant women.

How to use the Green Pages

Finding the medicine you want

The medicines in this section are grouped according to their uses. If you want to find a specific medicine, look it up in one of these lists: (1) the List of Medicines, which lists medicines according to their use, and begins on p.451, or (2) the Index of Medicines, which lists medicines alphabetically (beginning with "A," then "B," and so on), and begins on p. 452.

Medicines are listed according to their generic names (their scientific names) rather than their brand names (names given by the companies that make medicines). In a few cases, well-known brand names are given in bold italic in parentheses ( ) after the generic name. We list medicines according to their generic names because these names are similar everywhere, but brand names differ from place to place. Also, generic medicines are often cheaper.

Understanding how the information is arranged

Some medicines are part of larger groups of medicines. Since these medicines have many things in common, we often talk about them as a group first, and then give specific information about each medicine. It is important to read about both the group and the specific drug. For example:

Information about all cephalosporins

Cephalosporins

Cephalosporins are powerful antibiotics that kill many different kinds of bacteria. They are often expensive and not widely available. However, they generally have fewer risks and *side effects* than other antibiotics and can be useful in treating serious infections, such as infection of the womb, or certain sexually transmitted diseases. Cephalosporins are safer for pregnant and breast feeding women than other antibiotics.

Brand name
Generic name

Cefazolin *(Ancef)*

Information about one kind of cephalosporin

Often comes in: vials for injection with 250 milligrams (mg), 500 mg, and 1 gram

Dosage for infection of the womb

Inject 1 gram every 6 hours.

Under each medicine, we give 3 kinds of information: (1) the form the medicine often comes in (for example: tablets, vials, syrup); (2) the medicine's use (if this has not already been explained under a group description); and (3) the dosage for different uses. For example:

Note: The medicines and dosages listed here are those used by midwives in many places. But you should check with local health authorities for medicines and dosages used in your area.

Erythromycin

Form — Often comes in: tablets or capsules with 250 mg; syrups with 125 or 200 mg in 5 ml

Use — Erythromycin is a common antibiotic that is safe for pregnant and breast feeding women. It can be used to treat infection of the breast, and also some sexually transmitted diseases (syphilis in persons allergic to penicillin, chlamydia, and chancroid). Erythromycin sometimes works for gonorrhea (see Chapter 23).

Dosage — *Dosage of erythromycin for serious infections*

Give 4 times a day, preferably with food to avoid stomach upset.

For adults, give 500 mg in each dose.

For breast infection, take for 10 days.

For syphilis, take for 15 days.

For chlamydia, chancroid, and gonorrhea, take for 7 to 10 days.

More information on dosages

In these pages we have given dosages for adult women and babies. But it is even better to figure out the dosage according to a person's weight. If you have a scale, look for information about weight in parentheses. This is especially important when giving dangerous drugs, or giving medicines to babies.

For example, if you read:

(15 mg/kg/day)

This means that during a 24 hour period you would give 15 milligrams (mg) of the medicine for each kilogram (kg) the person weighs. So a 50 kg woman would receive 750 mg of this medicine in one day. This total amount should be divided up, depending on whether it is given 2, 3, 4, or 6 times each day. If the medicine is given 3 times a day, you would give 250 mg in the morning, 250 mg in the afternoon, and 250 mg in the evening.

Sometimes you will need to give part of a tablet of medicine. Dosages that are less than 1 whole tablet are written as **fractions**. For example:

1 tablet = one tablet =

$\frac{1}{2}$ tablet = half a tablet =

$1\frac{1}{2}$ tablets = one and a half tablets =

$\frac{1}{4}$ tablet = one quarter or one fourth of a tablet =

$\frac{1}{8}$ tablet = one eighth of a tablet
(dividing it into 8 equal pieces and taking 1 piece) =

CAUTION! Many of the medicines listed here are also used for illnesses not discussed in this book. But doses are often different for various health problems. Get advice from a health worker, or refer to a book such as *Where There Is No Doctor* before using these medicines for purposes other than specified here.

List of medicines in the Green Pages

Listed by use, in the order in which they appear.

Index of medicines in the Green Pages

Listed in this order: A B C D E F G H I J K L M N O P Q R S T U V W X Y Z

see page

Antibiotics

Use of Antibiotics

Antibiotics are medicines that fight infections caused by bacteria. Used correctly, they can save lives. But used incorrectly they can cause death or great harm.

Some antibiotics are generally safe for pregnant and breast feeding women. Others should be avoided during early or late pregnancy. Certain antibiotics have some risk of harming the growing baby, but may be needed in life-threatening infections. Sometimes it is necessary to compare the risks of the illness with the risks of the medicine and other available options (see p. 35). See the information given for each medicine for specific warnings for pregnant and breast feeding women.

Important guidelines for using antibiotics

1. As with all medicines, antibiotics should be used in pregnancy only when absolutely necessary. Antibiotics are not used to treat colds, coughs, diarrhea, or mild infections that will go away without medicine.

2. For mild to moderate infections, medicines given by mouth work as well and are safer than injections. For very severe infections, injections work faster and are sometimes necessary. Read p. 383–387 before injecting any medicine.

3. Before giving a medicine, always ask the woman if she has ever had an *allergic reaction* to that medicine (review p. 90 and 388). If she has ever had an allergic reaction, rash, fainting, or convulsions from the antibiotic, do not give her that medicine (or any other from the same group).

4. After giving the first dose of any antibiotic, either by mouth or by injection, stay with the woman for 20 to 30 minutes to see if she has a reaction to the medicine.

5. Be sure to give the full treatment. Incompletely treated infections may come back, and often these infections are more difficult to treat because bacteria sometimes become resistant to the antibiotic. Make sure she understands it is important to finish the full treatment, even if she feels better before taking all the medicine.

The Penicillins

Penicillin is one of the safest antibiotics for most people, including pregnant and breast feeding women, and babies. It can be useful for many different kinds of infections, including infection of the womb or breast, or blood infections in newborns. (For some life-threatening illnesses, an experienced health worker may need to give penicillin in addition to another antibiotic.)

There are several kinds of penicillins. This book mentions ordinary penicillin and 3 other members of the penicillin family: dicloxacillin, ampicillin, and amoxicillin. All these can be taken by mouth. But penicillin and ampicillin also come in injectable forms, which usually work faster and better for very serious infections. (If you are using a type of penicillin we have not listed here, be sure to get information about its correct use and dosage.)

Some bacteria have become resistant to penicillin, so it no longer works for certain diseases, such as gonorrhea. When treatment with penicillin fails, other medicines may be tried, or sometimes special forms of penicillin will work.

Guidelines, risks and precautions for all kinds of penicillin:

- Penicillin is measured in units (sometimes indicated with a "U") or milligrams (mg). Injectable penicillin is usually expressed in units, but penicillin by mouth is often written in milligrams. For penicillin G: 250 mg = 400,000 units.

- Penicillin is called short-acting, intermediate-acting, or long-acting, depending on how fast it works and how long it stays in the body.

- Too much penicillin does no harm. Too little will not completely stop the infection, and may make the bacteria more difficult to kill.

- In certain persons penicillin causes an allergic reaction. Mild allergic reactions include itchy raised spots or rashes. Often these come several hours or days after taking penicillin and may last for days. An antihistamine such as diphenhydramine or promethazine may help calm the itching.

- Rarely, penicillin causes a dangerous reaction called *allergic shock*. Soon after penicillin is injected (or swallowed), the person suddenly gets pale, has trouble breathing, and goes into shock (see p. 243). Epinephrine *(Adrenalin)* must be injected at once (see p. 388). Keep the person lying down.

- A person who has had any allergic reaction to penicillin should never be given any kind of penicillin (for example, ampicillin) again, either by mouth or by injection. This is because the next time the reaction would likely be far worse and might cause death.

Injectable penicillin

For very severe infections, injections of penicillin usually work faster and better than penicillin by mouth. However, there is more risk of allergic reaction from injections than from tablets.

Injectable penicillin comes in 3 main forms: Injectable **penicillin G** works quickly but does not last long in the body. **Procaine penicillin** and **benzathine penicillin** work more slowly but last longer. For most of the very severe infections discussed in this book (womb infection and blood infection in newborns) penicillin G injections are best. Procaine penicillin and benzathine penicillin are used for treating some sexually transmitted diseases, and for times when penicillin G is not available.

IMPORTANT: Before injecting penicillin, read the information and precautions for giving injections (see p. 383–387). Be sure to know the signs of allergic shock (pale skin, trouble breathing; weak or rapid pulse or heartbeat, loss of consciousness). **Always have epinephrine *(Adrenalin)* ready when you inject penicillin. See p. 388.**

Penicillin G injections (a short-acting penicillin)

Often comes in: vials of 1 million units (625 mg) or 5 million units (3125 mg)

Injectable penicillin G has many names, including crystalline penicillin, benzylpenicillin, aqueous penicillin, soluble penicillin, sodium penicillin, and potassium penicillin.

This kind of penicillin acts quickly but stays in the body a short time, so it must be injected several times in a day. It is usually the best choice for very severe infections when high doses are needed—such as infection of the womb, or infection of the blood or tetanus in the newborn.

Dosage for severe infections

For adults: Inject 2 million units every 4–6 hours.

For babies:

under 2 kg: inject 200,000 units every 12 hours.

2 to 4 kg: inject 300,000 units every 12 hours.

over 4 kg: inject 400,000 units 12 hours.

Procaine penicillin (intermediate-acting)

Often comes in: vials of 300,000 units, 400,000 units, and more

Procaine penicillin or **procaine penicillin aluminum monostearate (PAM)** works more slowly and lasts about a day in the body. It may be used for syphilis when benzathine penicillin is not available. In some areas, procaine penicillin still works to treat gonorrhea—get local advice. The dosage for procaine penicillin combined with a short-acting penicillin is the same as the procaine penicillin alone.

Dosage for syphilis

For adults: give 1 injection of 1,200,000 units a day for 10 days.

Dosage for gonorrhea that is not resistant to penicillin

Give 4,800,000 units. Inject half the dose in each buttock, and give 1 gram of **probenecid** by mouth at the same time. (Probenecid is a substance that makes penicillin more effective.)

Benzathine penicillin (long-acting)

Often comes in: vials of 1,200,000 or 2,400,000 units

Benzathine or **benethamine** penicillin or **bicillin** goes into the blood slowly and lasts up to a month. It often comes combined with faster-acting penicillins. Benzathine penicillin is mainly used to treat syphilis.

Dosage for syphilis

Inject 2,400,000 units one time only. (It is usually best to divide the dose and give 1,200,000 units in each buttock.)

Penicillin by mouth

Penicillin VK (penicillin V, phenoxymethyl penicillin, *Pen Vee K)*

Often comes in: tablets of 250 mg (400,000 units); syrups or powder to make syrup with 125 mg in 5 ml or 250 mg in 5 ml

Penicillin VK (penicillin by mouth) can be given for severe infections when injections are not available. They are also sometimes used to continue treatment after injections. To help the body make better use of the medicine, try to take penicillin VK on an empty stomach, an hour before or 2 hours after meals.

Dosage for severe infection

For adults: give 1000 mg 4 times a day.

Dicloxacillin

Often comes in: tablets of 250 or 500 mg

Dicloxacillin is a special form of penicillin that sometimes works against bacteria that have become resistant to ordinary penicillin. (Methicillin, nafcillin, oxacillin, cloxacillin are similar to dicloxacillin; get advice on uses and dosages if you have one of these.)

Dosage for breast infection

Give 500 mg by mouth 4 times a day for 10 days.

Ampicillin and Amoxicillin: wide-range (broad spectrum) penicillins

Ampicillin and amoxicillin are *broad spectrum* (wide-range) penicillins that kill many more kinds of bacteria than other penicillins. Like other penicillins, they are safe for pregnant and breast feeding women, and for babies, and very large doses can be given for serious infections.

Ampicillin can be taken by mouth or given by injection. Amoxicillin is only taken by mouth. They may be used for treatment of infections of the breast or womb, fever during labor, or blood infection in newborns. Ampicillin or amoxicillin by mouth is given to treat urinary tract infections.

Ampicillin

Often comes in: capsules, 250 mg; injections, 500 mg; solutions, 125 or 250 mg in 5 ml

Giving ampicillin by injection:

Dosage for fever during labor or infection of the womb

Inject 1 to 2 grams every 6 hours.

Dosage for infection of the blood in newborns

Inject 200 to 400 mg **twice** a day.

Giving ampicillin by mouth:

Dosage for urinary tract infection

Give 500 mg every 6 hours for 7 days.

Dosage for breast infection

Give 500 mg every 6 hours for 10 days.

Dosage for infection of the womb

Give 2000 mg every 6 hours.

Amoxicillin

Often comes in: capsules or tablets with 250 or 500 mg

Amoxicillin fights the same bacteria as ampicillin, but is taken 3 times a day instead of 4.

Dosage for urinary tract infection

Give 500 mg 3 times each day for 7 days.

Dosage for breast infection

Give 500 mg 3 times each day for 10 days.

Dosage for infection of the womb after childbirth

Give 1 gram 3 times each day.

Cephalosporins

Cephalosporins are powerful antibiotics that kill many different kinds of bacteria. They are often expensive and not widely available. However, they generally have fewer risks and **side effects** than other antibiotics and can be useful in treating serious infections, such as infection of the womb, or certain sexually transmitted diseases. Cephalosporins are safe for pregnant and breast feeding women.

There are many different types of cephalosporins, but in this book we have recommended 3 of the most common: cefazolin *(Ancef)*, cefoxitin *(Mefoxin)*, and ceftriaxone *(Rocephin)*. (Get advice before using cephalosporins other than those we have listed here.)

Cefazolin *(Ancef)*

Often comes in: vials for injection with 250 mg, 500 mg, and 1 gram

Dosage for infection of the womb

Inject 1 gram every 6 hours.

Cefoxitin *(Mefoxin)*

Often comes in: vials for injection with 1 or 2 grams

Dosage for infection of the womb

Inject 2 grams every 6 hours.

Ceftriaxone *(Rocephin)*

Often comes in: vials for injection with 250 mg, 500 mg, or 1 gram

Dosage for chancroid and gonorrhea in adults

Inject 250 mg one time only.

For gonorrhea, double this dosage (500 mg) may be needed.

Dosage for eye infection from gonorrhea in newborns

Inject 125 mg one time only.

Aminoglycosides

The aminoglycosides gentamicin and kanamycin are injectable antibiotics that should only be used by experienced health workers for very serious infections. It is important to give correct doses—too much of these medicines may cause permanent hearing loss or damage to the kidneys. Gentamicin generally has fewer side effects than kanamycin.

Gentamicin or kanamycin may be given for infection of the womb after childbirth, or infection of the blood in new babies. Spectinomycin is used only to treat gonorrhea and is safe to use during pregnancy.

Gentamicin *(Garamycin)*

Often comes in: vials for injection with 20 mg or 80 mg in 2 ml

Dosage of gentamicin (2 to 5 mg/kg/day)

For adults: inject 80 mg 2 times a day

For babies:

under 2 kg: inject 5 mg 2 times a day

2 to 4 kg: inject 7.5 mg 2 times a day

over 4 kg: inject 10 mg 2 times a day

(Sometimes smaller doses of gentamicin are given 3 times a day.)

WARNINGS:

- **Gentamicin should not be given to pregnant women except for life-threatening infections when safer medicines are not available;** this medicine may harm the growing baby.

- **Gentamicin should not be taken by people with kidney problems.** If ringing of the ears develops, see a health worker immediately.

Kanamycin *(Kantrex)*

Often comes in: vials for injection with 75 mg, 500 mg, or 1000 mg

Dosage of kanamycin (15 mg/kg/day)

For adults: inject 500 mg 2 times a day

For babies:

under 2 kg: inject 15 mg 2 times a day

2 to 4 kg: inject 24 mg 2 times a day

over 4 kg: inject 32 mg 2 times a day

WARNING: Kanamycin should not be given to pregnant women, or to people with kidney problems.

Spectinomycin *(Trobicin)*

Often comes in: vials for injection with 2 grams

Dosage for gonorrhea in adults

Give one injection of 2 grams one time only.

The sulfas or sulfonamides

The sulfas or sulfonamides are inexpensive medicines that fight many kinds of bacteria. But they are weaker than many antibiotics and more likely to cause allergic reactions (itching) and other problems.

Pregnant women should avoid taking sulfa or sulfonamide medicines in the last 3 months of pregnancy. These medicines are generally safe for breast feeding women, but mothers whose babies are ill, dehydrated, or premature may wish to milk their breasts and throw away the milk (see p. 337) while taking these medicines. Or these mothers can change to another medicine.

If you have a sulfa or sulfonamide medicine other than the ones mentioned here, get advice on its correct use and dosage.

WARNINGS:

- It is important to drink lots of water when taking sulfa or sulfonamides medicines, to prevent harm to the kidneys. Never give these drugs to a person who is dehydrated.

- Do not give to babies under 1 year old.

- If the medicine causes a rash, blisters, itching, joint pain, fever, lower back pain or blood in the urine, stop taking it and drink lots of water.

Co-trimoxazole (sulfamethoxazole with trimethoprim; SMZ-TMP)

(familiar brand names: ***Bactrim, Septra***)

Often comes in: tablets of 100 mg sulfamethoxazole with 20 mg trimethoprim; tablets of 400 mg sulfamethoxazole with 80 mg trimethoprim; syrup of 200 mg sulfamethoxazole with 40 mg trimethoprim in 5 ml

Note: This medicine also comes in double strength tablets *(Bactrim DS* and *Septra DS)* of 800 mg sulfamethoxazole with 160 mg trimethoprim. **Use half the number of tablets given below if the medicine you have is double strength.**

Co-trimoxazole is a combination medicine that fights a wide range of bacteria.

Dosage for urinary tract infections and chancroid

For adults: give 2 tablets of 400 mg sulfamethoxazole with 80 mg trimethoprim 2 times a day for 7 days.

Dosage for gonorrhea

For adults: give 10 tablets of 400 mg sulfamethoxazole with 80 mg trimethoprim each day for 3 days. Be sure the tablets are taken with lots of water!

Sulfafurazole

Often comes in: tablets of 250 or 500 mg

Dosage for urinary tract infections and chlamydia

Give 4 doses a day for 7 to 10 days.

For adults, give 500 mg in each dose.

Some other sulfa drugs, such as **sulfadimidine** or **sulfasoxazole**, can also be used. Give the same dose for the same length of time as for sulfafurazole.

Erythromycin

Often comes in: tablets or capsules with 250 mg; syrups with 125 or 200 mg in 5 ml.

Erythromycin is a common antibiotic that is safe for pregnant and breast feeding women. It can be used to treat infection of the breast, and also some sexually transmitted diseases (syphilis in persons allergic to penicillin, chlamydia, and chancroid). Erythromycin sometimes works for gonorrhea (see Chapter 23).

Dosage of erythromycin for serious infections

Give 4 times a day, preferably with food to avoid stomach upset.

For adults, give 500 mg in each dose.

For breast infection, take for 10 days.

For syphilis, take for 15 days.

For chlamydia, chancroid, and gonorrhea, take for 7 to 10 days.

Metronidazole *(Flagyl)*

Often comes in: tablets of 200, 250, or 500 mg

Metronidazole is used to treat vaginal infections caused by Trichomonas. It is also sometimes given together with other antibiotics to treat serious infections, such as severe infection of the womb after childbirth (see p. 298), or pelvic inflammatory disease (PID, see p. 363).

Pregnant women should avoid using metronidazole if possible, especially during the first 3 months of pregnancy; this medicine may cause birth defects. Some experts recommend that breast feeding women not give their babies breast milk for 24 hours after taking large doses of metronidazole.

Dosage for Trichomonas infections of the vagina

Give 500 mg 2 times a day for 7 days. Or, give 2 grams by mouth in one single dose.

Both the woman and the man should be treated at the same time for Trichomonas. The man should take medicine even if he has no signs of illness, or he will pass the infection back to the woman.

Dosage for infection of the womb after childbirth

Give 500 mg 3 times a day.

Dosage for pelvic inflammatory disease

Give 1 gram twice a day for 10 days.

WARNING: Do not drink alcoholic drinks when taking metronidazole. This causes severe nausea, and in pregnant women this may increase the possibility of harming the growing baby. People with liver problems should not use metronidazole.

Other medicines

For allergic reactions

Serious allergic reaction to penicillin injection is treated with injections of epinephrine and an antihistamine—usually promethazine or diphenhydramine. For allergic shock it is better to inject the antihistamine, rather than give it by mouth.

Epinephrine (adrenaline, *Adrenalin*)

Often comes in: ampules of 1 mg in 1 ml

Dosage for allergic shock

For adults, inject $1/2$ ml ($1/2$ mg) just under the skin or into the muscle.

If needed, a second dose can be given after 20–30 minutes, and a third dose in another 20–30 minutes. Do not give more than 3 doses, and do not give more than one dose in the same place. If the pulse goes up by more than 30 beats per minute after the first injection, do not give another dose.

WARNING: Be careful not to use more than the recommended amount of epinephrine.

Diphenhydramine *(Benadryl)*

Often comes in: capsules of 25 mg and 50 mg; injections—ampules with 10 mg or 50 mg in each ml

Dosage for allergic shock

Inject 25 to 50 mg. Repeat dose in 2 to 4 hours if necessary.

If injections are not available, give 25 to 50 mg by mouth.

WARNING: It is best not to use diphenhydramine in pregnancy except for emergency situations such as allergic shock.

Promethazine *(Phenergan)*

Often comes in tablets of 12.5 mg; injections—ampules of 25 mg in 1 ml; suppositories of 12.5 mg, 25, mg, and 50 mg

Dosage for allergic shock

Inject 25 to 50 mg. Dose may be repeated in 2 to 4 hours, if necessary.

When injections are not available, give 25 to 50 mg by mouth. Or, use a rectal suppository with 25 to 50 mg.

WARNING: Pregnant women should use promethazine only for emergency situations such as allergic shock.

For high blood pressure (antihypertensives)

Hydralazine and methyldopa *(Aldomet)* are medicines sometimes given to pregnant women to control dangerously high blood pressure, such as with pre-eclampsia (see p. 112).

Hydralazine *(Apresoline, Hydraline, Rozaline)*

Often comes in: tablets of 10, 25, 50 or 100 mg; ampules for injection of 20 mg/ml

Dosage

By mouth: Give 25 mg every 6 hours.

By intramuscular injection: Give 10 to 25 mg every 4 hours.

Stop giving hydralazine when the bottom number of the mother's blood pressure is 90 or below. Also, do not give more than 300 mg in 8 hours.

Methyldopa *(Aldomet)*

Often comes in: tablets of 125, 250, or 500 mg; syrup of 250 mg in 5 ml

Dosage

Give 250 mg by mouth every 3 to 4 hours.

For convulsions (anticonvulsants)

Magnesium sulfate is generally the best medicine to prevent convulsions in women with pre-eclampsia. But it should only be used when the mother's blood pressure is over 160/110. It is important to watch her blood pressure while giving this medicine (see p. 107–110). For this reason, it should only be used when equipment for measuring blood pressure is available.

When magnesium sulfate cannot be used, diazepam or phenobarbital may be given to prevent or control convulsions, although there is some chance these medicines will harm the growing baby. Sodium amytal may be given to control a convulsion.

WARNING: Too much of any of these medicines can slow down or stop breathing! Whenever possible they should be given in a hospital. Do not give too much, and be prepared to do rescue breathing if necessary.

Magnesium sulfate

Often comes in: Injections of 10 percent, 12.5 percent, 25 percent or 50 percent solution.

Dosage: Inject 5 grams in each hip. (Give 10 grams total—for example, 20 ml of a 50 percent solution.) Injecting this large amount requires a long needle and may cause discomfort; you may want to divide the dose again and give 2 smaller doses in each hip.

WARNING: Magnesium sulfate can be toxic to women with kidney problems. It is best for these women to be treated in a hospital where they can be very closely watched. Toxicity or overdose from magnesium sulfate may be treated with calcium gluconate.

Diazepam *(Valium)*

Often comes in: tablets of 5 mg or 10 mg; injections of 5 mg in 1 ml of liquid or 10 mg in 2 ml of liquid

Dosage to treat convulsions

Inject 10 mg intramuscularly.

With convulsions, this dose may be repeated every 3 hours.

See page 248 for instructions on how to give diazepam in the rectum during a convulsion.

WARNING: Pregnant or breast feeding women should only use diazepam for emergencies. Frequent or large doses during pregnancy can cause birth defects. Diazepam can be addicting (habit-forming) when taken too often.

Phenobarbital (phenobarbitone, *Luminal*)

Often comes in: ampules of 65 mg, 130 mg, or 200 mg in 1 ml

Dosage to treat convulsions

Inject 130 mg intramuscularly. Give only one injection—phenobarbital lasts a long time.

WARNING: Phenobarbital is used to treat epilepsy. Large amounts given over long periods of time may damage the growing baby. Pregnant epileptic women who use phenobarbital should take the lowest possible dose (get medical advice). However, possible harm to the baby from a convulsion is much greater than from the single dose of phenobarbital given here.

Sodium amytal (amobarbital sodium)

Often comes in: vials for injection with 250 or 500 mg

Dosage to stop a convulsion

Inject 250 mg intramuscularly to the mother during a convulsion.

For severe bleeding after birth (postpartum hemorrhage)

Oxytocics are medicines that contain ergonovine, ergometrine, or oxytocin. They cause contractions of the womb and its blood vessels, and are important medicines to control heavy bleeding after childbirth.

Ergometrine and ergonovine come in pills and intramuscular injections. Oxytocin is usually given by intramuscular injection, but for some emergency situations it may be given slowly in the vein—see sections of this book that explain specific complications.

Ergonovine *(Ergotrate)*, methylergonovine *(Methergine)*, or ergometrine maleate

Often comes in: injections of 0.2 mg, 0.25 and 0.5 in a 1 ml ampule; tablets of 0.2 mg

To prevent or control severe bleeding **after the placenta has come out**.

WARNING: Never inject ergonovine or ergometrine into the vein (IV). Never give these medicines before the baby is born or the placenta has come out! Do not give these medicines to a woman with high blood pressure.

Dosage of injectable ergonovine

Give 1 ampule (0.2 mg) by intramuscular injection. Dose may be repeated in $1/2$ hour to one hour.

Dosage of ergonovine or ergometrine by mouth

Give 0.2 mg (1 tablet). Repeat every 4 to 6 hours.

Dosage of injectable ergometrine

Give 0.5 mg by intramuscular injection. The medicine will take effect in about 6 or 7 minutes.

Oxytocin *(Pitocin, Syntocinon, Uteracon)*

Often comes in: ampules of 10 units in 1 ml

To help stop severe bleeding of the mother **after the baby is born**.

WARNING: The times when oxytocin is needed before the baby is born are very rare. For this purpose, it should only be given in the vein by a doctor or trained birth attendant. Using oxytocin to speed up labor or give strength to the mother in labor can be dangerous to both mother and child.

Dosage of oxytocin for the mother after the baby is born

Give 1 or 2 ampules (10 to 20 units) by intramuscular injection.

For pain and fever (analgesics)

For pregnant and breast feeding women, paracetamol (acetaminophen) is the best pain medicine. Aspirin should not be taken by pregnant women.

Paracetamol (acetaminophen)

Often comes in: tablets of 500 mg

Paracetamol is safe to use for short periods of time to relieve pain or to reduce fever.

Dosage

Give 500 mg every 3 to 4 hours.

Aspirin

Often comes in: tablets of 300 (5 grain) or 600 mg (10 grain)

Aspirin sometimes causes stomach pain. To avoid this, take it with milk or some food.

Dosage

Take 600 mg every 3 to 4 hours.

WARNING: Pregnant women should not take aspirin. Breast feeding women should avoid taking aspirin in large doses or for long periods of time, as there is a small risk it will harm the baby. Some experts believe these risks are greater in the first week of the baby's life.

For sewing tears (local anesthetic)

Lidocaine *(Xylocaine, Lignocaine)* 1 or 2 percent (without epinephrine)

Often comes in: ampules or bottles for injection

Lidocaine can be injected around the edges of a tear or episiotomy before sewing it, to make the area numb so it will not hurt. It is important to use lidocaine without epinephrine because epinephrine can stop the flow of blood and cause great damage. See p. 400 for how to inject lidocaine.

Nutritional supplements

Many pregnant women, especially those who are anemic or malnourished, need extra iron and folic acid. These can be obtained by eating dark green leafy foods, meat, and liver. In addition to eating nutritious foods, taking iron and folic acid tablets daily throughout pregnancy is very helpful to many women. Sometimes these nutrients come together in the same tablet.

Iron (ferrous sulfate, ferrous gluconate, or ferrous fumarate)

Often comes in: tablets of many different strengths, containing from 60 to 500 mg or more in each tablet

Iron sometimes upsets the stomach and is best taken with meals. Also, it can cause constipation, and it may make the stools look black. Fruits, vegetables, or a vitamin C tablet taken at the same time will help the body to use iron.

WARNING: Too much iron is poisonous. Keep tablets out of reach of children.

Dosage to prevent anemia in pregnancy

Take 60 mg (1 tablet) each day with meals.

Dosage to treat anemia

Women with severe anemia may need to take more: up to 325 mg of iron 3 times a day.

Folic acid (folate, folacin)

Often comes in: tablets of 1 mg or 5 mg

Dosage

Take 1 mg once each day by mouth.

Vitamin C

Often comes in: tablets of 500 mg

Dosage

Taking one tablet of vitamin C with iron and folic acid tablets will help the body to use these nutrients.

For acid indigestion and heartburn (antacids)

WARNING: Pregnant women should avoid using antacids that contain aluminum. Calcium carbonate can be taken for occasional indigestion or heartburn, but should not be used for long periods of time.

Calcium carbonate

Often comes in: tablets of 350 to 850 mg

Dosage

Chew one 850 mg tablet, or two 350 mg tablets when symptoms occur. Take another dose in two hours if necessary.

For yeast infections

Nystatin, clotrimazole, and gentian violet are used to treat yeast infections of the vagina. When possible, pregnant women should use nystatin or clotrimazole, as there is a slight risk of gentian violet harming the developing baby.

Nystatin

Often comes in: vaginal tablets with 100,000 international units; creams and ointments

Dosage to treat yeast infections of the vagina

Put 2 tablets high in the vagina each night for 14 nights.

Clotrimazole

Often comes in: vaginal tablets with 100 or 500 mg; creams with 50 mg in each application

Dosage for yeast infection of the vagina

Put one tablet of 500 mg high into the vagina for 1 night only. (Yeast infections are sometimes treated for 3 nights with 100 mg tablets, but this longer treatment does not work well for pregnant women.) Do not take this medicine by mouth.

Gentian violet (crystal violet)

Often comes in: dark blue crystals

This is a cheap and effective treatment for yeast infection of the vagina. But pregnant women should only use this when the above treatments are not available; there is some chance of gentian violet harming the growing baby.

Dosage for yeast infections of the vagina

> Dissolve a half a teaspoon of gentian violet in half a liter of water (this makes a 1% solution). Soak cotton balls with solution and put high in the vagina each night for 3 nights. Remove balls each morning.

WARNING: Do not use in the first 3 months of pregnancy.

To prevent health problems in newborn babies

Whenever possible, newborn babies are given two medicines at birth to prevent health problems: vitamin K to help prevent bleeding, and certain eye medications to prevent blindness from infection.

To prevent bleeding

Vitamin K (phytomenadione, phytonadione)

Often comes in: ampules of 0.5 or 1 mg

Newborn babies' blood cannot clot (harden to stop bleeding). An injection of vitamin K will help reduce the risk of bleeding.

Dosage

> Inject one ampule (1 mg) into the outer part of the newborn's thigh, one time only. Use a very small syringe and needle (tuberculin syringe).

To prevent eye infections

At birth, erythromycin eye ointment, tetracycline eye ointment or silver nitrate drops should be put in babies' eyes to prevent infection from chlamydia and especially gonorrhea, which causes blindness. Erythromycin is best, because it will prevent both these diseases. Tetracycline works against chlamydia and usually gonorrhea.

Silver nitrate drops work well against gonorrhea but not chlamydia. (See page 205.)

Antibiotic eye ointment—0.5 percent erythromycin *(Ilotycin)* or 1 percent tetracycline *(Latycin)*

Put a little ointment in the inner corner of each eye and do not wipe or rinse out.

Silver nitrate eye drops, 1 percent

Put a drop of 1 percent silver nitrate in each eye of the newborn to prevent blindness from gonorrhea.

WARNING: Do not use silver nitrate drops that may have become too concentrated because of evaporation—they can burn babies' eyes.

Family planning methods: birth control

In this section we give more details about different forms of birth control discussed in Chapter 22. Be sure to read the information in that chapter, too.

Condoms (see p. 347)

There are many different brands of condoms (also called rubbers, prophylactics, and sheaths). Some are lubricated, some come in different colors, and some have spermicide.

In addition to helping prevent pregnancy, **condoms can also help to prevent the spread of sexually transmitted diseases, including AIDS.** Spermicide is helpful in preventing these diseases, and so is lubrication, because a condom is less likely to break when it is moistened. However, do not use cooking oils or other "home methods," as they can weaken the condom. Pharmacies sometimes sell special lubricants that are safe to use with condoms.

Many people use condoms along with another form of birth control to make it more effective and to prevent disease.

Contraceptive foam *(Emko, Lempko, Delfen)*
(see p. 348)

These foams and jellies with spermicide are put in the vagina with a special applicator. They are fairly effective alone, and very effective when used together with a condom.

Contraceptive suppository *(Neo Sampoon)*
(see p. 348)

This is a tablet containing spermicide that a woman puts deep in her vagina near her cervix. The suppository should be put in 15 minutes before having sex. It is a fairly effective method of birth control alone, and very effective if the couple also uses a condom.

Diaphragm and Cervical cap (see p. 349)

Diaphragms and cervical caps are worn over the cervix. A trained health worker can fit the woman for the best size and teach her how to put it in and use it correctly. To be effective, spermicide cream or jelly should be put in the diaphragm or cap. They can be washed and used over and over.

Contraceptive sponge (see p. 349)

This is a special sponge with spermicide that goes deep in the vagina in front of a woman's cervix. It is fairly effective, but expensive, because the sponge must be thrown away after one use.

Intrauterine device (IUD) (see p. 350)

There are several different kinds: Copper T, Copper 7, Lippes Loop, and the Safety Coil. Another kind, called Progestasert, must be replaced more often than others. One kind of IUD, the Dalkon Shield, causes more problems than others and should not be used. A trained health worker must put the IUD in the womb.

Because infection and other problems can occur with IUDs, only women who live close to a health center should use them. The best time to have a IUD put in is while the woman is having her monthly bleeding.

Oral contraceptives (birth control pills)

Read about the use, risks, and precautions for birth control pills, pages 351 to 355. The following information is about choosing the best pill for individual women if there is a choice available.

Most birth control pills contain 2 chemicals, or hormones, similar to those produced in a woman's body to control her monthly bleeding. These hormones are called estrogen and progesterone. The pills come under many different brand names, with different strengths and combinations of the 2 hormones.

Generally, brands that contain a relatively small amount of both hormones are safest and work best for most women. Most women should start with pills from Group 1 or 2.

GROUP 1 (fairly low amounts of estrogen and progesterone)

Common brands:

> *Brevicon 1 + 35*
> *Neocon*
> *Norinyl 1 + 35, 1 + 50*
> *Norimin*
> *Ortho-Novum 1/35, 1/50*
> *Perle*
> *Noriday 1 + 50*
> *Ovysmen 1/35*

The amount of hormone in these brands changes during the month, so it is important to take the pills in order:

> *Logynon*
> *Synophase*
> *Trinordiol*
> *Trinovum*
> *Triquilar*
> *Triphasil*

To assure effectiveness and minimize small amounts of bleeding between monthly bleeding (spotting), take the pill at the same time each day, especially with pills that have low amounts of hormones.

If spotting of blood continues after 3 or 4 months, you can change to one of the brands in Group 2. If there is still spotting after 3 or more months, try a brand from Group 3.

As a rule, women who take birth control pills have less heavy monthly bleeding. This may be a benefit, especially for women who are anemic. But if a woman misses her monthly bleeding for months or is disturbed by the very light monthly bleeding, she can change to a brand with more estrogen, in Group 3.

For women who have very heavy monthly bleeding, or whose breasts become painful before their monthly bleeding begins, a brand low in estrogen but high in progesterone may be better. For example:

GROUP 2 (high in progesterone, low in estrogen)

Common brands:

Lo-Femenal
Lo-Ovral
Microgynon 30
Microvlar
Nordette

Brands from Group 2 are not recommended for women who have pimples, or a lot of hair on their arms or lip. High progesterone may make these conditions worse—or even cause them.

Women who continue to have missed periods or spotting after using a brand from Group 2, or who became pregnant previously while using another type of pill, can change to a pill that has a little more estrogen. For example:

GROUP 3 (a somewhat higher amount of estrogen, most with higher progesterone)

Common brands:

Minovlar
Norlestrin
Ovcon 50
Femenal
Eugynon
Nordiol
Ovral
Primovlar
Neogynon

The brands Ovulen and Demulen will often control spotting that continues even when taking pills from Group 3. But these are very strong in estrogen, and for this reason are rarely recommended. They are sometimes useful for women with severe acne.

Women who are disturbed by morning sickness or other side effects after 2 or 3 months of taking the pill, and women who have a higher risk for blood clots can use a birth control pill that is very low in both estrogen and progesterone. For example:

GROUP 4 (very low in both estrogen and progesterone)

Common brands:

Brevicon
Brevinor
Modicon
Ovcon
Ovysmen
Perle LD
Loestrin 1/20

The disadvantages of brands in Group 4 are that they often cause spotting between monthly bleeding, and that there is an increased chance of pregnancy if only one pill is forgotten.

Women who are breast feeding, or who should not use regular pills because of headaches, mild high blood pressure, or because they are over 40, may want to use a pill with only progesterone. This is also called the 'mini-pill'. For example:

GROUP 5 (progesterone only—the mini-pill)

Common brands:

Femulen
Micronor
Microlut
Micronovum
Nor-Q D
Ovrette

These pills should be taken at the same time every day, even during the period. Menstrual bleeding is often irregular. There is also an increased chance of pregnancy if a pill is forgotten.

Injectable contraceptive *(Depo-Provera, Net-En)* (see p. 355)

This is an injection of the hormone progesterone that is given to a woman every 2 or 3 months. It is a very effective form of birth control. Like the mini-pill and implants, injections may be a good choice for women who cannot take the regular pill because of medical risks or side effects (see page 354).

Monthly bleeding may be irregular, and often becomes very light or stops after the first year. This is not serious, but worries some women. Older women may mistake this for the menopause, stop getting more injections, and become pregnant. Seek medical advice if very heavy bleeding occurs.

Contraceptive implant *(Norplant)* (see p. 356)

Implants are a very convenient and highly effective form of birth control. Because they contain only progesterone, they can be used by women who should not use regular pills because of headaches, mild high blood pressure, or because they are over 40 years old.

Six small rubber tubes are put under the skin in a woman's upper arm by a specially trained health worker. They prevent pregnancy for about 5 years, but can be removed sooner if the woman wants to become pregnant. The tubes should be inserted 7 days after the woman starts her monthly bleeding.

Use this space to write information about other medicines or home remedies useful in your area.

Use this space to write information about other medicines or home remedies useful in your area.

Use this space to write information about other medicines or home remedies useful in your area.

Use this space to write information about other medicines or home remedies useful in your area.

Vocabulary

This vocabulary is listed in the order of the alphabet:

A B C D E F G H I J K L M N O P Q R S T U V W X Y Z

A

Abortion (Planned abortion, Induced abortion) A woman purposely ends a pregnancy before the baby can live on its own.

Abortion pill (RU486) A pill that ends a pregnancy before the baby can live on its own.

Abruption (Detached placenta) When the placenta comes off the wall of the womb before the baby is born. Abruption can happen during the last few months of pregnancy or during labor or birth. The baby can die and the mother will bleed very heavily.

Abscess A sack of pus caused by an infection.

Active labor When the labor contractions get longer, stronger, and closer together.

Acupressure A type of massage in which pressure is applied to certain parts of the body. The massage is based on an ancient method of Chinese healing.

Afterbirth see **Placenta**

After pains When the mother feels very strong contractions after the birth.

Agony Extreme pain.

AIDS (Acquired Immune Deficiency Syndrome) A disease caused by the HIV virus, which reduces a person's ability to fight infections and diseases.

Albusticks see **Uristicks**

Allergic shock A very severe reaction to a medication: a woman's skin becomes cool, moist, pale, or gray; she has difficulty breathing; she has a weak, rapid pulse or heartbeat; and she loses consciousness (see **Allergy**).

Allergy A reaction to a medicine that may cause a rash, swelling, or difficulty breathing. This can be very dangerous and even cause death if the person takes the medicine again at any time.

Allis forceps An instrument used to grasp the muscle around the anus in the repair of a third degree tear.

Ampule A small glass bottle that contains medicine for injections. The top is broken to get the medicine out.

Anemia When the blood is thin or pale because there aren't enough red blood cells. Anemia is usually caused by lack of iron in the diet and is very common in pregnant women.

Ante-natal exams see **Prenatal checkups**

Ante-partum exams see **Prenatal checkups**

Antibiotic A medicine that fights infections caused by bacteria.

Antibiotic cream A medicated cream that helps fight infection.

Anus The butt hole or shit hole.

Apex The top or tip of a tear.

Apprenticeship When a new midwife or student works with an experienced midwife to learn to do checkups and give care at births.

Arteries The tubes that carry oxygen and blood from the heart to the rest of the body.

Arthritis A disease of the joints. Arthritis cannot be passed from one person to another.

Asthma When people have difficulty breathing.

Auxiliary midwife A midwife who has had some medical training and may work in a hospital, maternity center, or in the community.

Average birth When the baby's head starts to show after $1/2$ hour of good pushing.

i

B

Bacteria Small germs that cause infection and cannot be seen.

Bag of waters The sack inside the womb that holds the baby, the placenta, and the waters (see **Membranes**).

Beam scale A scale made of dry wood or bamboo with a moveable weight–usually a bag, bottle, or tin filled with sand.

Benefit The good that something may cause.

Bilirubin A chemical in the blood that causes many babies to turn yellow after birth. This is probably OK if it happens 2 to 5 days after birth. It is very dangerous if it happens the first day, or after the 5th day, of a baby's life (see **Jaundice).**

Birth bar A bar that a woman can hold while standing to give birth.

Birth box A cardboard box cut and painted to look like a woman's body. This can be used to demonstrate birth.

Birth canal (Vagina) The path the baby follows from the mother's womb to the outside during birth.

Birth chair A chair that supports the mother in a sitting or squatting position while giving birth.

Birth control (Contraception) Any method of preventing pregnancy (see **Family Planning**).

Birth control pills When a woman takes pills that contain hormones; these pills make her body think she is already pregnant, so her eggs do not come down into her womb.

Birth defect When a child is born with physical or mental problems—such as a harelip, club foot, or an extra finger or toe.

Birthing positions The different positions in which a woman can give birth. Four common positions are the hands-and-knees, half-sitting, sitting, and squatting positions.

Birth pants A teaching tool to show people how the baby comes out of the woman's body.

Bladder The bag that stores the urine inside of the body. As it fills, it stretches and gets bigger.

Blanket stitch A continuous locked stitch.

Bleeding inside see **Hidden bleeding**

Blood clot When blood hardens into a semi-solid piece.

Blood infection A disease in which the baby seems very sleepy, has yellow skin or eyes, and vomits or has diarrhea. It is more common for babies who were born after long labors or when the mother's bag of waters broke a long time before birth.

Blood pressure The force or pressure of the blood upon the walls of the blood vessels (arteries and veins).

Blood pressure cuff An instrument used to check blood pressure.

Blunt-tipped scissors Scissors with blunt tips that are good to use for cutting the cord.

Body relaxation A method to release tension in the body.

Bottom of the placenta The side of the placenta that is attached to the wall of the womb and has many lumps (see **Top of the placenta**).

Bowels The end of the large intestine; stool (shit) passes through the bowels on the way to the anus.

Breaking the bag of waters When the bag of waters is broken by a trained person before it would have broken naturally. This is done in hospitals to start or strengthen labor.

Breast abscess A type of breast infection; there is a pocket of pus in the breast that feels like a hard, round ball.

Breast bone The bone in the center of the chest that protects the heart and lungs. The ribs are attached to the breast bone.

Breast feed When a mother feeds her baby with the milk in her breasts.

Breast infection (Mastitis) An infection inside the breast which can be very painful and make it difficult for the baby to suck the nipple. The signs of a breast infection are a hot, red, sore area or lump on the breast; fever and chills; and body aches and pains.

Breast pump A machine that the mother can use to remove milk from her breasts if she must be away from the baby. This will keep her breasts making milk.

Breath holding A method of breathing that helps the mother push during labor.

Breathing exercise A method that helps a woman relax and prepare for her labor.

Breech birth When a baby is born feet or butt first, instead of head first. This can be more dangerous for the baby.

Breech position (Complete breech, footling breech, frank breech) When the baby is butt first or butt down inside the mother. If the baby is breech at the end of pregnancy, the mother may need to deliver in a hospital (see **Head down position** and **Sideways position**).

Broad spectrum antibiotics Antibiotics that kill a wide range of bacteria.

Brown waters (Green waters, Meconium) When the baby has a bowel movement (passes meconium) before the birth, the waters are brown, green, or yellow. This is a risk sign for the baby.

Buboes Very swollen lymph nodes.

Bulb syringe (Ear syringe, Suction trap) An instrument used to clear a baby's nose or mouth which is clogged with fluid or mucus.

Bunsen burner A small lamp with a very hot flame.

Burp A mother can help a baby get rid of gas pains by patting the baby on its back, or laying the baby on its belly across the mother's knees and patting him on the back.

C

Calcium A mineral which helps make bones and teeth strong.

Calcium deposits Small white spots, like tiny rocks, which are found on the lumpy (bottom) side of the placenta of a baby who is born late.

Calibrate Marking the scale of a measuring instrument so that it is accurate.

Cancer A tumor or lump that grows and may keep growing until it finally causes death.

Candida see **Yeast Infection**

Candle breathing A method of slow breathing to help a woman relax and stay calm. The woman breathes in through her nose and out through her mouth gently enough to bend a candle flame, but not to blow it out.

Caput A swelling on the baby's head. This may happen when the head is pressed aginst the cervix during labor.

Castor oil drink A drink made of castor oil and fruit juice to help start or strengthen labor.

Catheter A rubber tube used to drain urine from the bladder to drain urine.

Catheterization Putting a catheter into the bladder to drain urine.

Centigrade (C) A unit of measurement for body temperature.

Cervical cap A method of birth control; a small, shallow cup fits over the woman's cervix and prevents sperm from entering the womb.

Cervix The opening of the womb at the back of the vagina.

Cesarean section A birth by operation.

Chancre A sore on the genitals, finger, or lip that can be the first sign of a sexually transmitted disease. It may look like a pimple, a blister, or an open sore.

Chromic gut One of the best kinds of thread to use when sewing tears and episitomies. The thread slowly dissolves (disappears) so it is not necessary to take out the stitches later.

Circumcision An operation to remove the skin around the tip of the penis. In some areas, women are also circumcised: the clitoris, some skin over the clitoris or the labia (lips) of the vagina are removed. (see **Pharonic circumcision** or **Infibulation**).

Circumcision scar The scar tissue surrounding the area where a woman was circumcised. These scars may not stretch enough for a baby's head to come out.

Cirrhosis A disease of the liver caused by drinking too much alcohol.

Cleft lip (Harelip) An opening or gap on a baby's upper lip, often connecting to the nostril.

Cleft palate A split or abnormal opening in the roof of the baby's mouth.

Club foot When a baby's foot turns inward and must be straightened by surgery or by wearing special shoes.

Cold sores A sore or blister on the lips or nose caused by germs that can be very dangerous and even kill a baby.

Colic Sharp pain in the baby's stomach caused by gas, spasms, or cramps.

Colostrum (First milk) A clear yellowish fluid which may leak out of the nipples during the last months of pregnancy. This liquid also comes out of the mother's breasts for the first few days after the baby is born. It is very rich in vitamins and will help protect the baby from disease.

Common complaints Things that many pregnant women complain about. These complaints are usually bothersome but not serious.

Complete breech When the baby is breech (or butt down) inside the mother. This position may be risky for the baby.

Complications Problems or things that go wrong.

Compress A folded cloth or pad that is put on a part of the body to ease the pain of a sore. The compress may be soaked in hot or cold water.

Condom (Rubber, Prophylactic) A narrow bag of thin rubber that the man wears on his penis while having sex. The bag traps the man's sperm so that it cannot get into the woman's womb. This helps prevent pregnancy and the spread of sexually transmitted diseases.

Constipation When a person has a hard time moving the bowels (passing waste, shitting stool). The stools may be hard or dry.

Contagious When a disease can spread easily from one person to another.

Contraceptive foam (Contraceptive jelly, Contraceptive cream) A method of birth control; a special foam, jelly, or cream (containing a chemical that kills sperm) is put inside the vagina.

Contraceptive jelly or **Contraceptive cream** see **Contraceptive foam**

Contraceptive sponge A method of birth control; a small sponge filled with contraceptive cream (or jelly or foam) fits over the woman's cervix. The contraceptive sponge prevents sperm from getting into the woman's cervix and also kills the sperm.

Contraception (Birth control) Any method of preventing pregnancy (see **Family Planning**).

Contract To squeeze tight or hard.

Contractions (Pains, Labor pains) When the womb squeezes up and becomes hard during the end of pregnancy. Contractions open the cervix and help push the baby out of the womb.

Convulsions An uncontrolled fit. A sudden jerking of part or all of a person's body. These convulsions may be caused by eclampsia. Babies sometimes have convulsions if they have a very high fever.

Cord (Umbilical cord) The cord that connects the baby at its navel to the placenta. The cord is fat and blue when the baby is born because the baby is still getting oxygen from its mother.

Cord guiding A method to remove the placenta from the mother's womb, if the placenta has not come out on its own one hour after birth.

Cord infection When the baby's cord stump becomes hot and red, smells bad, and drains pus.

Creativity The ability to make something new out of materials and information you already have.

Cretinism When a child is short and mentally slow, usually due to lack of iodine in the mother's diet.

Crowning When the baby's head stretches the vaginal opening during labor to about the size of the palm of the hand. The baby's head stays at the vaginal opening, even between contractions.

Curved needle A special type of needle which makes it easier to sew tears or wounds.

Cyst An abnormal, round sack of fluid which grows in the body.

D

D & C (Dilation and curettage) A kind of planned or induced abortion done by scraping the inside of the womb (see **Abortion**).

Deep slow breathing A method to calm and relax a woman in labor. A woman breathes in deep, slow breaths that expand her chest and belly.

Dehydration When the body loses more liquid than it takes in. Dehydration is especially dangerous in babies.

Delivery table A table a woman lies on to give birth.

Detached placenta see **Abruption**

Diabetes When a woman has too much sugar in her blood. If a pregnant woman has diabetes, it can cause the baby to be born early, to be very big, or to have breathing problems.

Diaphragm A method of birth control: a soft rubber cup filled with contraceptive jelly or cream is worn over the cervix during sex.

Diarrhea Frequent runny or liquid stools.

Dilation and curettage see **D & C**

Diluted A liquid that has been made weaker by adding water.

Direct entry midwife see **Traditional midwife**

Discharge The clear (or somewhat yellowish) wetness or fluid that comes out of the vagina.

Disinfectant solution A liquid that can be used to sterilize equipment, tools, and containers.

Disposable Things that are meant to be used once and then thrown away.

Downward traction Pulling or drawing the baby out and down during labor.

Due date The day the baby will probably be born.

E

Early baby (Premature, Preterm) A baby born before the 8th month of pregnancy.

Ear syringe see **Bulb syringe**

Eclampsia A disease of pregnancy caused by high blood pressure. It causes convulsions, and the baby may be born early, too small, or dead (see **Pre-eclampsia, Toxemia, Convulsions**).

Ectopic pregnancy A pregnancy in the wrong place; a fertilized egg attaches itself to the tubes instead of inside the womb.

Egg timer see **Timer**

Emotional pain Pain that is caused by thoughts or feelings.

Emotional relaxation Exercises that help calm the mind, and calm tension and fears.

Empowerment Helping others to make their own decisions and change their lives for the better. It gives people the courage to use their own abilities and take pride in their culture.

Enema A solution of water that is put up the anus to cause a bowel movement.

Engagement (Engaged) When the baby's head starts to settle down through the mother's pelvic bones in preparation for birth.

Engorged breasts When the breasts become very full and hard shortly after the baby is born, or if the mother does not get to nurse the baby as often as she usually does. An engorged breast can lead to a breast infection.

Epilepsy A disease that causes people to have seizures.

Episiotomy When the vaginal opening is cut to make it larger. This helps a baby be born faster.

Equipment Any tools, supplies, or instruments used by a midwife in her work.

Ergometrine (Methergine, Ergonovine) A medicine which can help stop heavy bleeding of the womb after a woman gives birth. This medicine should not be given to women with high blood pressure.

Express milk When a mother removes milk from her breasts by herself. She can feed the expressed milk to her baby with a spoon.

Eye Ointment (Ilotycin, Latycin) A medicated cream with 0.5% erythromycin or 1% tetracycline, which prevents blindness in newborn babies.

F

Face first When a baby is lying with its face against the cervix, instead of the top of its head. This type of birth may be very difficult or impossible.

Fahrenheit (F) A unit of measurement for body temperature.

Fallopian tubes (Tubes) The tubes that lead from the ovaries to the womb. The eggs move down these tubes to the womb.

Family planning Using birth control methods to plan how many children to have, and when (see **Birth control** and **Contraception**).

Fast birth When a baby is born more quickly than is usual; the head comes out after just 1 or 2 pushes.

Fats Foods which give the body energy. Fats are found in animal meat, nuts, eggs, seeds, vegetable oil, butter, ghee, and lard.

Fear A feeling of concern or fright.

Feeding tube A tube put through the baby's mouth or nose all the way into its stomach. This is used when the baby is too weak or ill to suck the mother's breast for feeding.

Fertile The time of a woman's monthly cycle when she is able to get pregnant.

Fetoscope A tool for listening to and counting the heartbeat of the baby inside the mother's womb.

Fever A body temperature higher than normal (37°C or 99°F).

First milk see **Colostrum**

Flare To get larger.

Float When a baby rests in the womb, above the mother's pelvic bones (see **Engagement**).

Folding scale A scale that is very easy to carry from place to place. It is usually made out of metal or plywood strips.

Fontanels see **Soft spots**

Footling breech A baby that is born legs first. This can be very dangerous because there is a much greater chance of a prolapsed cord.

Foot-reflex test A method to check for active reflexes when a woman's blood pressure is high during pregnancy or labor.

Forceps An instrument used to help pull the baby during birth.

Forehead first When a baby is lying with its forehead against the cervix. This type of birth may be very difficult or impossible.

Foreskin The skin around the tip of the penis. This is the skin removed in circumcision.

Formula A special drink for newborn and small babies who are not able to breast feed. It can be made from powder or made from local ingredients.

Frank breech When the baby is lying inside the mother with its head and legs up, and the butt comes out first. This type of birth can be dangerous for the baby.

G

Gas Air that gets into the a baby's stomach when it sucks or swallows.

Gauze A soft, loosely woven cloth used for bandages.

Genitals The organs of the reproductive system, especially the sex organs.

Genital bulge During labor a mother's genitals swell outwards as a sign that the baby is coming soon.

Genital ulcers Sores on the genitals. Genital ulcers are usually a sign of a sexually transmitted disease.

German measles (Rubella, 3-day measles) A contagious or infectious disease. If a pregnant woman gets this disease, especially in the early months of her pregnancy, it can make the baby blind or have other problems.

Germs Very small organisms that can grow in the body. Germs can cause some infectious diseases.

Glow foods Foods which contain vitamins and minerals. Glow foods help the body resist disease and recover after an illness or disease.

Go foods Foods which contain sugars and fats. Go foods give energy.

Goiter A swelling on the lower front of the neck (enlargement of the thyroid gland) caused by the lack of iodine in the diet.

Gonorrhea blindness When a baby is born blind because the mother had the sexually transmitted disease called gonorrhea during birth.

Green waters see **Brown waters**

Grimace When a baby makes a face when someone puts fingers in its mouth or suctions its mouth and nose. A grimace is a normal reaction.

Grow foods Foods which contain protein. This helps build strong muscles and bones.

Guard the labor When the midwife or labor partner protects the labor from interference.

Guide the labor When the midwife or labor partner helps keep the labor on a healthy path.

H

Harelip see **Cleft lip**

Head down position When babies are lying in the womb with their heads toward the vaginal opening. This is the safest and most common position for birth (see **Breech position** and **Sideways position**).

Healthy signs The signs in the woman's body or in the baby that things are going well.

Heartbeat The sound of the baby's heart. During pregnancy, the midwife hears the heartbeat by using a stethoscope or **fetoscope**, or by placing her ear on the mother's belly (near the end of pregnancy).

Heartburn see **Indigestion**

Heart massage A method to help start or strengthen a baby's heartbeat by gently rubbing the baby's breast bone. Sometimes it is also necessary to do **Rescue breathing**.

Hee breathing When a woman in labor makes a sound like a strong but soft hee, hee, hee.

Hematoma Bleeding under the skin.

Hemorrhage Severe or dangerous bleeding.

Hemorrhoids Small painful bumps or lumps at the edge of the anus or inside it. They are a type of swollen veins which may burn, hurt, or itch.

Hemostats Blunt clamping instruments. These are used for clamping the baby's cord, especially when the cord must be cut because it is wrapped tightly around the baby's neck.

Hepatitis A serious illness of the liver. This is a sexually transmitted disease, which a pregnant woman can pass on to her baby.

Hidden bleeding (Bleeding inside, Internal bleeding) When a mother bleeds inside her body, so it is difficult to know that she is bleeding. Hidden bleeding can be very dangerous. The woman can lose a lot of blood and go into shock.

High blood pressure When the force or pressure of the blood upon the walls of the arteries and veins is harder than normal. In pregnancy this can cause problems for both the mother and baby (see **Pre-eclampsia, Eclampsia**).

HIV (Human Immune-deficiency Virus) The virus which causes AIDS.

Hives Hard, thick, raised spots on the skin that itch severely. Hives are a kind of allergic reaction.

Hold-the-breath pushing When a woman in labor takes a deep breath and fills her chest completely, and then holds this breath while pushing as hard as she can.

Homemade sponge A method of birth control; a woman puts a sponge that is wet with water and vinegar (or lemon juice) in the vagina before having sex.

Home method see **Traditional medicine**

Hormones Chemicals which are made in a woman's body. Estrogen and progesterone are hormones that regulate a woman's monthly bleeding and her chance of becoming pregnant. These chemicals increase greatly during pregnancy, and cause many of the changes women notice when they are pregnant.

Hot water bottle A bottle filled with hot water and wrapped in a cloth to help keep the baby warm.

Hydrocephalus When a baby has water on the brain. This can cause serious problems for the baby.

I

Ilotycin see **Eye ointment**

Immunizations (Vaccinations) Shots or injections that are given to prevent some infectious diseases—like tetanus, tuberculosis, and measles. Babies should be given immunizations early.

Implant (Norplant) A method of birth control; a trained health worker puts 3 to 6 small, soft tubes of hormone under the skin of a woman's arm. The hormone prevents pregnancy for 2 to 5 years.

Incubator A special box, usually found in a hospital or maternity center, to keep a newborn baby warm.

Indigestion (Heartburn) A burning feeling or pain in the stomach or between the breasts, usually caused by the baby growing and crowding the mother's stomach. Indigestion is not dangerous and usually goes away after birth.

Induced abortion see **Abortion**

Infection A sickness caused by bacteria or other germs.

Infectious disease A disease that is easily spread or passed from one person to another (see **Contagious**).

Infertility When a woman is unable to become pregnant.

Infibulation (Pharonic circumcision) A type of female circumcision when all of the skin around a woman's vagina is removed. A tiny hole and a lot of scar tissue are all that remain.

Inflammation An area that is red, hot, and painful, often because of an infection.

Injectable medicine Medicine (either a liquid or a powder mixed with a liquid) that is given as a shot or injection.

Injections When medicine or other liquid is put into the body through a needle. One kind of birth control is done this way, when a woman is given a shot of hormones every 2 or 3 months to keep her from getting pregnant.

Interference When someone or something gets in the way.

Internal bleeding see **Hidden bleeding**

Internal exam When a midwife or other trained health worker feels inside the woman's vagina to check the cervix or the position of the baby.

Interrupted stitch A single stitch that is tied in a 3-layered knot and then clipped on both sides. An interrupted stitch is recommended for sewing most tears and episiotomies.

Intestines The tubes that connect the stomach to the anus. Stool moves through the intestines on its way out of the body.

Intoxicated To be drunk from too much alcohol.

Intramuscular injection An injection given into a person's muscle.

Intrauterine device (IUD) A plastic birth control device placed in a woman's womb by a trained health worker. The IUD will help stop pregnancy until it is taken out by a trained health worker.

Intravenous fluids (IV fluids) Fluids given through tubes placed into a person's veins. IV fluids are often given for shock.

Intravenous injection (IV) A medicine or other liquid that is injected in the vein through a needle.

Intuition The knowledge that comes through feelings. This knowledge is important, but it is not always right.

Inverted nipples When the nipples sink into the breast instead of sticking out.

Iron A mineral which helps make the blood healthy. Iron is found in most animal foods, but in pregnancy some women need to take iron pills (in addition to eating animal foods) to stay healthy.

J

Jaundice Yellow color of the eyes and skin. It can be a sign of diseases such as hepatitis or newborn jaundice.

K

Kit A container which holds all of a midwife's equipment and supplies used in prenatal, birth, and after birth care.

Knee-chest position When the mother gets on her hands and knees and then bends her arms so that her head is lower than her hips. This helps increase the flow of blood to the baby inside the womb.

Knot The way a thread is tied to fasten the stitches. We recommend tying a **3-layered knot**, which won't come undone.

L

Labia The outer folds of skin in the vagina.

Labor The work that a woman's body must do to move the baby from inside her womb to the world outside.

Labor contractions The contractions which open the cervix. They are usually felt low in the belly or back and usually get longer, stronger, and closer together as labor progresses.

Labor partner A person who gives a mother support during the labor and birth.

Labor positions Different positions a woman can try to be more comfortable during labor. Some positions are sitting, standing, side-lying, or hands-and-knees. A woman may want to try many positions during her labor.

Labsticks see **Uristicks**

Last monthly bleeding The last time a woman had her monthly bleeding before she became pregnant. If a woman knows this date, the midwife can tell when the baby will be born.

Late labor When labor contractions last up to 1 and $1/2$ minutes, with only 2 or 3 minutes between them. The mother may shake, and feel like she wants to vomit and can't go on.

Latycin see **Eye ointment**

Ligaments Tough cords inside the body that hold the womb in place.

Light labor When labor contractions are short and come every 15 or 20 minutes. The contractions may be mild and felt low in the belly, either in front or in the lower back.

Light panting When a woman takes quick shallow breaths into the chest, not into the belly.

Local anesthetic Medicine given by injection to numb a small area around a wound or tear that needs stitching.

Lockjaw see **Tetanus**

Loss of elasticity When the skin loses its normal stretchiness.

Low-back exercise (Angry cat) An exercise a woman can do between contractions to help move the baby into a better birth position. Low-back exercise can also be done during pregnancy to relax the back muscles.

Lymph nodes Small lumps under the skin in different parts of the body. These lumps are traps for germs and can become painful and swollen if they get infected.

M

Main foods Foods that provide a healthy source of energy.

Malaria An infection in the blood that causes chills and high fever. Malaria can be worse in pregnancy, and can cause the mother to have a still birth or early baby. Malaria is spread by mosquitoes.

Malnutrition When a woman does not get enough food or the right kinds of food.

Mask of pregnancy The dark colored areas that appear on the faces of some pregnant women. They are not harmful and usually go away after pregnancy.

Massaging the womb When the womb is rubbed to make it hard and to stop bleeding after the baby is born.

Mastitis see **Breast infection**

Meconium The blackish-brown or green, sticky substance on the inside of the baby's intestines. If there is meconium in the mother's waters it may be a sign of a problem (see **Brown waters**).

Median cut (Median episiotomy) When the cut for an episiotomy goes straight down towards the anus. The median cut should not go into the anus (see **Episiotomy**).

Medicine given by mouth When medicine is given to a person as pills or a liquid. Medicine given by mouth does not usually work as fast as medicine given by injection.

Mediolateral cut (Mediolateral episiotomy) When the cut for an episiotomy goes to the side, not straight down towards the anus (see **Episiotomy**).

Membranes The thin layers that hold the bag of waters (see **Bag of waters**).

Meningitis A brain infection which causes a baby to have a stiff neck, a bulging soft spot (fontanel), and to lie with its head and neck bent back.

Menopause When a woman's monthly bleeding stops forever and she can no longer get pregnant.

Methergine A medicine which can help stop heavy bleeding from the womb after a woman gives birth. This medicine should not be given to women with high blood pressure (see **Ergometrine**).

Migraine headaches A severe, throbbing headache, often on one side of the head. A person who has a migraine may see spots and feel nauseated.

Minerals Substances that are found in certain foods. Minerals help the body fight disease and help it get better after a sickness or an injury (see **Glow foods**).

Miscarriage (Spontaneous abortion) When a baby is born before the woman is 6 months pregnant and before the baby can live outside the mother.

Moan or growl pushing When a mother works to push the baby out by taking a deep breath and letting it out, then taking another deep breath and pushing. While pushing, she lets her mouth go loose and moans or growls.

Modern medicine Medicine based on the knowledge of the body learned through Western science. Modern medicine can be helpful, useless, or harmful depending on how it is used.

Molar pregnancy When a tumor grows inside the womb instead of a baby. This can cause bleeding during pregnancy.

Molding When a baby's skull bones overlap during birth so its head can fit through the vagina.

Morning sickness see **Nausea**

Moro reflex When a baby opens its arms and hands widely when it is moved suddenly, dropped gently backward, or hears a loud noise. The Moro reflex is a normal reaction.

Mucous membrane see **Vaginal mucosa**

Mucous method A method of birth control; a woman looks at the mucus from inside her vagina to tell when she is fertile.

Mucous plug Mucus that covers the opening of the cervix. At the end of pregnancy or at the beginning of labor, this mucus will come out as the cervix starts to open.

Mucous show A pink or blood tinged mucus which is discharged 2 to 3 days before labor begins and also at the beginning of labor.

Mucus A thick, slippery liquid that moistens and protects the lining of the vagina. Mucus is also found in the nose, throat, stomach, and intestines (guts).

N

Narcotic drugs Drugs like heroin, opium, and morphine. If a mother takes these drugs during labor, it can be dangerous for the baby.

Nausea When a woman feels like she wants to vomit.

Navel The belly button; the place in the middle of the belly where the cord was attached.

Needle The instrument used for sewing tears. Another kind of needle is used to give injections or start an IV.

Needle holder An instrument which makes it easier to hold the needle when sewing tears or wounds.

Neonatal conjunctivitis An infection in a newborn baby's eyes. This happens when a mother who has gonorrhea or chlamydia passes the disease to the baby as it comes through the vagina.

Networking Finding other people–individuals, local groups, national groups, or even international groups–who can help you in your work.

Nipple stimulation Rubbing or sucking on the nipples to help start a labor or to make the labor stronger.

Nitrazine papers A method to check if the mother's waters have broken by testing any wetness on her genitals or pad. If the papers stay orange when put into the wetness, the wetness is only urine. If the papers turn blue or purple, the wetness is waters.

Normal saline A liquid that is just as salty as blood and is given by IV to people who have lost a lot of blood or are dehyrated. Normal saline comes in sterile bags or bottles.

Norplant see **Implant**

Nurse see **Breast feed**

Nurse midwife see **Professional midwife**

Nutrients Substances found in foods that make the body healthy and strong.

Nutrition A woman has good nutrition when she eats enough food and the right kind of food.

O

Oral contraceptives see **Birth control pills**

Oresal see **Rehydration drink**

Organizing the community Getting the members of the community to work together for change.

Ovaries Small sacks in a woman's belly next to her womb. Ovaries produce a woman's eggs.

Oxygen bag A bag that holds oxygen for a person who needs help breathing.

Oxygen mask A device attached to an oxygen tank which is put over a baby's mouth and nose to help it breathe. Oxygen can also be given to a woman who is bleeding or in shock.

Oxygen tank A special storage container that holds oxygen.

Oxygen tent (Oxygen hood) A machine that gives the baby extra oxygen.

Oxytocin A medicine which helps the womb contract (stay hard) after the baby is born. Oxytocin will stop or slow down bleeding. It should never be used to start or speed up labor.

Oxytocin drip A method used in hospitals to give oxytocin. This medicine should only be given by IV in a hospital. It should **never** be given by injection or by mouth.

P

Pacifier Something the baby sucks on, usually made of soft rubber. A pacifier is also called a dummy.

Packing (a baby) Holding a baby against the mother's body to keep the baby warm.

Pains see **Contractions**

Pant-and-blow (Pant breathing) When a woman takes shallow, quick breaths into her chest and then blows out.

Pant pushing When the mother pants like she would in pant breathing and then pushes whenever she wants to. Pant pushing helps push the baby out.

Paper mache A mixture of water, flour, and paper used to make dolls and models for teaching.

Pap smear A medical test to check a woman for cancer of the cervix.

Parasites Worms and tiny animals that live in or on another animal or person and cause disease. You cannot always see parasites.

Patterns Models for making teaching materials.

Pelvic bones The bones inside a woman's belly that the baby must fit through to be born.

Pelvic Inflammatory Disease (PID) An infection which often starts as a sexually transmitted disease and then travels up the vagina into the womb, ovaries, and fallopian tubes.

Penis The male sex organ.

Pharonic circumcision see **Infibulation**

Physical signs Signals from the body that tell you what is happening. Some physical signs are the pulse, the blood pressure, and the temperature.

The pill see **Birth control pills**

Pitocin (Syntocinon) An oxytocin medicine that may be given as an injection or a pill after the birth of the baby to help the womb contract and stop bleeding.

Pitting edema Severe swelling of the lower legs and ankles. A pit or hole forms in the skin when you push your finger against the swelling.

Placenta (Afterbirth) The organ that gives the baby food and air (oxygen) during pregnancy. The baby is connected to the placenta by the cord. After the baby is born the placenta also comes out of the womb.

Placental site The place where the placenta was attached to the wall of the womb.

Placenta previa When the placenta is too low in the womb and lies over the cervix. There is a high risk of dangerous bleeding as the cervix starts to open. If a woman is bleeding late in pregnancy she should go to a hospital at once. A midwife should never do an internal exam on a woman bleeding in late pregnancy.

Planned abortion see **Abortion**

Pneumonia A lung infection. A baby who is grunting, sucking in the skin between its ribs, flaring its nose, and taking more than 50 breaths a minute may have pneumonia. This baby needs medical attention.

Postpartum The time after the baby is born.

Postpartum exam When a midwife visits a mother after the baby is born to check on her health and the baby's health.

Postpartum hemorrhage Heavy bleeding from the womb after the baby is born.

Post-term birth (Post dates) When a baby is born more than 3 weeks after the due date.

Practice contractions Contractions which happen throughout the pregnancy. Practice contractions are usually irregular and mild, and are felt high in the belly.

Pre-eclampsia (Toxemia) A condition of pregnancy with high blood pressure, swelling of the face and fingers, and protein in the urine. Women with pre-eclampsia should get medical help because they will probably need to give birth in the hospital.

Premature baby see **Early baby**

Prenatal The time between when a woman gets pregnant and when she gives birth.

Prenatal day A day when many pregnant women come to see a midwife for their regular checkups (see **Prenatal checkup**).

Prenatal checkup (Ante-natal checkup, ante-partum checkup) When a midwife visits a pregnant woman to check on her health and make sure the pregnancy is going well.

Preterm baby see **Early baby**

Procedure The steps a midwife follows to get things done. For example, she follows a procedure to cut the baby's cord, or put medicine in the baby's eyes.

Professional midwife A midwife who has a lot of medical training or nursing training, and works in the hospital, maternity center, or in the community.

Prolapsed cervix When the cervix has dropped down to the vaginal opening.

Prolapsed cord When the baby's cord comes out of the vagina before the baby or lies across the opening of the cervix below the baby's head. This can be very dangerous for the baby.

Prolapsed uterus A fallen womb.

Prophylactic see **Condom**

Protein A substance found in certain foods. Protein helps the muscles and bones grow strong (see **Grow foods**).

Pubic bone The front part of the pelvic bones.

Pulse The number of times a person's heart beats in one minute. The pulse can be taken (counted) on a person's wrist or neck, or by listening to the chest.

Pupil The dark spot in the center of the eye that lets the light in. It gets smaller in bright light and larger in the dark.

Pus White or yellow fluid filled with germs. Pus may be found inside a tear or wound.

Push When the mother helps the baby come out of the womb. The mother should hold her bottom down and keep her thighs relaxed and open while pushing.

Pushing positions The different positions that make it easier for a woman in labor to push the baby out. Some common pushing positions are on hands-and-knees, squatting, lying on the side, and standing.

Push-moan When the woman takes a deep breath and gives a long, hard push, while relaxing her mouth and making a moaning sound.

Q

Quarter-circle scale A scale that can be made at home out of plywood.

R

Rectal fluids Fluids put into the rectum to treat dehydration or shock (when the woman cannot drink and the midwife cannot start an IV).

Rectal sphincter The round muscle around the anus.

Rectal tube The tube put into the anus when giving an enema or rectal fluids (see **Enema** and **Rectal fluids**).

Rectum The end of the large intestine. The part that is near the anus.

Reflexes The body's natural and unthinking reactions to things. Good reflexes are a sign that the brain and nerves are working well together.

Rehydration drink A drink that prevents or stops dehydration. It can be made with boiled water, salt, and sugar. Rehydration drinks can also be purchased in pre-made packets such as Oresal.

Rescue breathing When a midwife helps a baby start breathing by gently blowing puffs of air into the baby's mouth.

Resistant A bacteria is resistant when it is not killed by an antibiotic.

Respirator A special machine that helps a baby breathe.

Rhythm A method of birth control; a woman counts the days from the beginning of her last monthly bleeding to find out when she is most fertile. She avoids having sex during her fertile period if she doesn't want to get pregnant.

Ringer's lactate A commonly used IV fluid.

Risk The harm, injury, or loss that something could cause.

Risk signs The signs that show that something may be wrong.

Rooting reflex When the baby turns its head toward a hand that is stroking its cheek. This is a normal reaction.

RU486 see **Abortion pill**

Rubber see **Condom**

Running stitch A continuous unlocked stitch.

S

Saliva A person's spit.

Scope of practice The activities that a midwife is allowed to perform, depending on national or local rules or laws. Midwives from different parts of the world have different scopes of practice.

Scrotum The bag between a male's legs that holds the testicles or balls.

Scrub Washing the hands very carefully to kill germs.

Semen A man's sperm or seed.

Sexually transmitted diseases (STDs) Diseases of the genitals that are passed from one person to another through sexual contact. Sexually transmitted diseases used to be called venereal diseases.

Shock When a person has severe weakness, unconsciousness, dizziness, cold sweat, low blood pressure, and a fast or weak pulse. This is a dangerous condition. It can be caused by heavy bleeding, an injury, or severe illness.

Show see **Mucous show**

Side effects Problems caused by taking a medicine.

Sideways position When the baby lies across the womb horizontally. A baby in a sideways position can only be born by cesarean section (see **Cesarean section, Head down position,** and **Breech position**).

Signs The things a midwife looks for when she examines a woman.

Signs of dehydration Signs that show that a person is not getting enough liquids. When a woman in labor (or a baby) is dehydrated she does not pee often, has a dry mouth, sunken eyes, and her skin feels tight. A dehydrated baby also has a sagging soft spot on its head. Watch for these signs if a baby is not breast feeding very much, if the baby has diarrhea, or if it is very hot or has a fever.

Signs of separation The signs that show that the placenta is no longer attached to the womb and is ready to come out. The signs are a small gush of blood, the cord seems longer, and the womb rises a little.

Signs of shock The signs that show that a person may be going into shock. The signs are a fast, weak pulse; low blood pressure; cold sweat; dizziness; weakness; and unconsciousness.

Silver nitrate A type of medicine used in some areas to treat a baby's eyes right after the baby is born. This medicine will stop gonorrhea blindness, but not other types of blindness.

Sitting squat A position a mother may try when she is in labor, to help the baby move down into the vagina.

Sitting straight A labor position to help the baby move down into the vagina.

Soft spots (Fontanels) The spots on top of a baby's head where the bones have not yet come together. These spots help the baby's head change shape so it can move through the mother's vagina. The soft spot on the top of the new baby's head may sink in if the baby is dehydrated, or it may bulge up if the baby has meningitis.

Soft womb A womb that will not contract or tighten. This is often a cause of serious bleeding after the birth.

Sonogram A way to look inside a woman's body. A machine sends a silent sound through her body and shows a picture of the inside of her body on a special television screen (see **Ultrasound**).

Special procedures Procedures that a midwife might use if medical help is far away and the birth is complicated. These procedures would usually be done in a hospital or health center. A midwife should be taught these special procedures by a skilled person.

Spermicide A chemical that kills the man's sperm and helps prevent pregnancy (see **Contraceptive foam**).

Spiders Small purple spots that come from groups of veins under the skin. They are usually caused by swollen blood vessels. They are not harmful and usually go away after pregnancy.

Spit up When a baby vomits a small amount.

Spontaneous abortion see **Miscarriage**

Spotting When a woman has light bleeding between monthly bleedings or during pregnancy.

Spring scale A scale made with a spring inside a bamboo tube.

Squat When a mother bends her knees and puts most of her weight on the balls of her feet to try to help the baby move into the vagina.

Standing A position a mother may try to help the baby move down into the vagina.

STD see **Sexually transmitted disease**

Sterile Completely clean and free from germs (see **Germs**).

Sterile field An area where everything is sterile (free from germs).

Sterile gloves Disposable gloves from a sealed package or re-usable gloves that have been sterilized to prevent the spread of diseases. Sterile gloves should be used during all internal exams.

Sterile lubricant A sterile cream or jelly that is used to help make things slide smoothly inside the body.

Sterile packets Equipment that comes packaged in a sterile wrapping. This equipment can be used directly out of the package.

Sterile saline (Normal saline) A sterile salty liquid that is given IV to help replace fluids in the body. It is often used when a person goes into shock or has lost a lot of blood.

Sterilization 1) The process of making things sterile. 2) A method of making a man or woman permanently unable to have children (sterility).

Sterilizing by chemicals When tools and equipment are made sterile by soaking them in a strong disinfectant that kills germs.

Sterilizing by dry heat When tools and equipment are made sterile by baking them in a hot oven.

Sterilizing by wet heat When tools and equipment are made sterile by boiling them in water.

Stethoscope An instrument used to listen to sounds inside the body, such as the heartbeat.

Still birth When a baby is born dead.

Stools Shit or bowel movement.

Stroke A sudden loss of consciousness, loss of feeling, or loss of the ability to move. Strokes are caused by bleeding or a blood clot inside the brain (see **Blood clot**).

Strong blowing When a woman blows out hard and fast during labor.

Suction trap see **Bulb syringe**

Suffocate When a person does not get enough oxygen. This can cause serious brain damage or death.

Sugar A substance which gives energy. Sugars are found in sweet foods like fruits, white sugar, brown sugar, raw sugar, and honey.

Suppositories A bullet shaped tablet of medicine which is put up in the vagina or anus.

Suture Special thread that is used to sew tears or episiotomies.

Sutures (Suture lines) The lines that mark the edges of the bones on the top of a baby's head. The bones move in order to help the baby's head fit through the mother's vagina.

Symphisiotomy When the middle of the mother's pubic bone is cut open. This makes the space between the mother's bones larger and it is easier for the baby to get out during birth.

Syntocinon see **Pitocin**

Syringe An instrument with a tube that holds medicine and a needle on the end. A syringe is used when giving medicine by injection.

T

Tail bone The bone at the bottom of the back bone (the end of the spine).

Testicle The part of the male sex organ (inside of the scrotum) which makes the sperm.

Tetanus (Lockjaw) When a germ that lives in stools of animals or people enters the body through a wound and causes disease. Tetanus is a common infection in newborns if the instrument used to cut the cord is not clean, if the cord is left too long, or if dirt or dung are put on the cord.

The 3 cleans When a midwife has clean hands, a clean birth area, and practices clean cord cutting. The 3 cleans help the midwife prevent the spread of germs.

Thrush A yeast infection in a baby's mouth. The baby can get thrush during birth, when it comes through the vagina of a woman who has a yeast infection.

Thyroid The lump in the front of the throat.

Timer (Egg timer) An instrument used to count (measure) the number of heartbeats or breaths per minute.

Top of the placenta The side of the placenta where the cord goes in. The top of the placenta is smooth and shiny (see **Bottom of the placenta**).

Torn cervix When there is a small tear in the cervix that may cause bleeding during the birth. A cervix can tear when a mother begins pushing before the cervix is completely open.

Torn womb A very dangerous condition that is more common in long labors or when the baby is lying sideways or is too big to be born. If the womb tears, the mother will feel constant pain, the contractions may stop, the baby will have no heartbeat, and sometimes the baby can be felt outside the womb.

Toxemia see **Pre-eclampsia**

Traditional birth attendant (TBA) see **Traditional midwife**

Traditional medicine Medicine based on beliefs that have been passed down from midwife to midwife and from parent to child for many years. This type of medicine is based on a knowledge of the body and mind, contact with the spirit world, and knowledge of plant medicines.

Traditional midwife (Traditional birth attendant) A midwife who has learned her skills by experience, or from other traditional midwives, and works in the community.

Transfusion When blood is given to a person by IV.

Trickle A small or light flow of blood.

Tubal ligation An operation that cuts or ties the tubes inside a woman that carry the egg to the womb. A woman who has a tubal ligation cannot get pregnant.

Tubal pregnancy (Ectopic pregnancy) When a baby begins to grow inside a woman's fallopian tubes instead of inside her womb. The baby will become too big after about 10 weeks and the tube will break.

Tuberculosis A contagious lung disease.

Tubes see **Fallopian tubes**

Twin births When there are two babies inside the mother's womb.

Two handed pressure with hands outside A method to help stop heavy bleeding after the baby is born. The midwife massages the outside of the woman's womb with two hands.

Two handed pressure with one hand inside A method to help stop heavy bleeding after the baby is born. The midwife massages the woman's womb with one gloved hand inside the womb and one hand outside on the belly.

U

Ultrasound A method of looking at the inside of a woman's body without cutting or hurting her. An ultrasound machine uses sound to take a picture of the inside of the body in order to understand what is happening (see **Sonogram** and **Ultrasound fetoscope**).

Ultrasound fetoscope An instrument which makes the baby's heartbeat easy to hear.

Umbilical cord see **Cord**

Umbilical hernia When the baby's belly wall is not fully formed and some of the baby's insides push the skin out in the area around the cord.

Unconscious When a sick or injured person seems to be asleep and cannot be awakened.

Uristicks (Albusticks, Labsticks) Small plastic strips that are used to check urine for protein.

V

Vaccinations (Immunizations) Shots or injections that are given to prevent certain infectious diseases, like tetanus, tuberculosis, and measles. Babies should be given vaccinations early.

Vaccination schedule The list of the times when a baby should receive vaccinations.

Vacuum extractor An instrument that is like a suction cup. It is put on the baby's head to help pull the baby out during birth.

Vagina (Birth canal) The tube or canal made of muscle that goes from the opening of the woman's sex organs to the entrance of her womb (the cervix).

Vaginal mucosa The tissue that makes up the inside of the vagina.

Varicose veins Abnormally swollen, blue veins that sometimes appear in the legs or genitals of pregnant women. Varicise veins are often lumpy and winding.

Vasectomy An operation that cuts the tube that carries the man's sperm. When a man has a vasectomy, he cannot get a woman pregnant.

Vein A blood vessel that carries blood from the body back to the heart.

Very slow birth When the genitals do not bulge more and more after $1/2$ hour of strong pushing.

Virus A germ that is smaller than bacteria and causes some infectious diseases. AIDS is caused by a virus.

Visualization exercise A method to help calm a woman's mind and ease her tensions.

Vitamins Substances that are found in certain foods. Vitamins help the body fight disease and get better after a sickness or injury (see **Glow foods**).

W

Washing Cleaning things with soap and water.

Wear the baby When a person helps keep a baby warm by putting the baby next to her skin, wrapping it securely, and putting her regular clothes on over the baby.

Wet nurse A woman who breast feeds and cares for another woman's baby if the mother is sick or unable to breast feed.

Withdrawal A method of birth control; the man pulls his penis out of the woman before his sperm comes.

Womb The sack of strong muscle inside a woman's belly where a baby grows. The womb also holds the placenta, cord, and bag of waters.

Womb infection A sickness of the womb. A womb infection usually happens after the baby is born, but sometimes during a long labor or when the waters have been broken for a long time. The mother may have a tender or sore womb, she may have a fever and feel ill, or the blood coming out of the vagina may smell bad. A womb infection is very dangerous for the mother.

X

X-rays A machine using a special type of light to look at the bones inside of a woman's body, without cutting or hurting her.

Y

Yeast infection (Candida) A vaginal infection with white and lumpy discharge, itching, and burning. Yeast infections are common during pregnancy. They are uncomfortable, but not dangerous. A baby may get a yeast infection from its mother during the birth (see **Thrush**).

Yellow jaundice see **Jaundice**

Index

Ergotrate (ergonovine), 285, 460
Erythromycin, 334, 373, 374, 458
    eye ointment, 205, 462
Ethanol, 152, 156
Examinations *(See Checkups)*
Example, setting, 10
Exercise, 25, 57
Exercises
    angry cat, 69, 240
    breathing, 318–319
    lifted-hips (for breech baby), 130
    relaxation, 313–316
Exhaustion during labor, 241–242, 255
Eyelids pale inside, 110
Eye ointment, 149, 205
Eyes
    acupressure, 380
    blurred vision, 97, 112, 113, 115, 355
    changes in vision during labor, 246
    checking newborn baby's, 217
    double vision, 112
    flashing lights, 355
    gonorrhea blindness, 205, 363
    infected (baby's), 363
    medicine for newborn baby's, 205, 462
    no tears (baby), 305
    pus, swelling or redness in baby's, 205
    sunken, 171, 305
    yellow, 217, 370–371

F
Face
    grimace reflex, 203
    swollen, 97, 112, 246
Face first position (baby), 240, 255
Factory chemicals, 61
Faintness, 210, 243
Family
    alone time after birth, 212
    caring for new mother, 227
    feeding first, 54
    labor partner, 313–324
    special problems or needs, 92–93
    teaching people about birth, 310–327
    (Also see Community; People)
Family planning, 340–359, 463–465
    abortion, 358
    choosing a method, 342
    effectiveness chart, 342
    methods that often work well, 347–357
    methods that sometimes work, 343–346
    useless methods, 28
Fast birth, 185, 325
Fast breathing
    baby, 290, 292, 305
    mother, 110, 171

Fast heartbeat (baby's), 129, 203, 214, 235, 250, 259, 292
Fast pulse
    baby, 305
    mother, 106–107, 110, 171, 235, 248, 287
Fat mother, 88, 103–104
Fats (food), 49, 50
Fear
    after birth, 301
    during labor, 176, 242, 254
    during pregnancy, 63
    fast pulse from, 107
Feeding tube, 425
Feelings *(See Emotions; Intuition; Tension; Tiredness)*
Feet
    acupressure, 379–380
    baby's pale or blue, 283
    checking newborn baby's, 221
    itchy rash, 366
    numb or burning, 111
    reflex test, 115
    swollen, 70
Ferrous fumarate, 461
Ferrous gluconate, 461
Ferrous sulfate, 52, 461
Fertility awareness, 344–346
Fetoscope, 127
Fever, 86, 107, 115
    after birth, 287, 298–299
    in baby, 306
    breast infection, 333–335
    and dehydration, 171, 305
    during stage 1 of labor, 235
    frequent fevers, 87
    from malaria, 87
    medicines for, 461
    in past pregnancies, 85
    and sexually transmitted diseases (STDs), 362, 363, 370
    taking the temperature, 105
    (Also see Temperature)
Fingernails white, 110
First 2 to 6 hours after birth, 206–222
    complications, 231, 284–295
    overview, 135, 145
    signs (healthy and risk), 207–208
    signs (risk for baby), 290–295
    signs (risk for mother), 284–289
    what to do for the baby, 213–222
    what to do for the mother, 209–212
First 2 weeks after birth, 224–229
    complications, 231, 296–308
    overview, 135, 145
    signs (healthy and risk), 225–226
    signs (risk for baby), 302–308

Oxytocin, 176, 210, 274, 276, 278, 285, 382, 460–461
  drip (hurrying labor), 420
  Pitocin, 28, 176, 274, 382, 460–461
  Syntocinon, 176, 274, 460–461

P
Packing baby, 293
Pain
  after birth, 287, 298–300
  baby kicking, 68
  back, 69, 101
  belly, 67, 68, 101–102, 115, 363, 370, 373
  between contractions, 244–245
  between ribs, 246
  breasts, 300, 333–335
  during sex, 362
  gas pains (colic), 335
  headaches, 72, 97, 112, 113, 115, 246, 355
  joints, 69
  legs, 101–102, 354, 355
  medicines for, 461
  stomach, 67, 115, 461
  urination, 72, 362, 365
  in waist area, 235
Pains during pregnancy
  in belly, back, or legs, 101–102
  common complaints, 68–73
  constant pain and bleeding, 100, 257
  in lower front or back, 115
Pains, labor *(See Contractions)*
Palate, cleft, 295
Pale color
  baby, 283, 291
  cord, 144, 191
  gums, 110
  inside eyelids, 110
  skin, 243
  (Also see White color)
Panting exercises, 319
Pant pushing, 184, 321
Paper models
  paper mache, 433, 445
  pelvis, 434–435
Pap smear, 354
Paracetamol, 59, 72, 333, 461
Parasites, 98–99
Partner, labor, 313–324
Patterns
  cloth vagina, 438
  cloth womb, 436
  copying, 433
  paper pelvis, 434
  (Also see Models)
Patterns of labor, 141
Peas and other legumes, 49, 50, 56
Pee hole (urethra), 43

Peeing *(See Urinating)*
Pelvic bones
  baby too big to fit through, 238–239, 255, 391
  feeling baby's position, 124, 166
  illustrated, 43
  paper model, 434–435
  symphisiotomy, 423
Pelvic inflammatory disease (PID), 363–364
Penicillins, 235, 299, 307, 374, 453–455
Penis (baby's), 219
  (Also see Circumcision [male])
People
  hospital people, 411–412
  illiterate, 19
  labor partner, 313–324
  preparing to attend birth, 158–160
  teaching about birth, 310–327
  (Also see Community; Family)
Personal problems, 14
Pesticides, 61
Pharmaceutical drugs *(See Medicines)*
Phenergan, 459
Phenobarbital, 246, 460
Phenobarbitone (phenobarbital), 246, 460
Philippine birth care practices, 26
Phisohex, 161
Physical complaints during pregnancy, 68–73
Physical needs, 91–92
Physicians, 40
  (Also see Hospital; Medical help)
Phytomenadione (vitamin K), 205, 462
Phytonadione (vitamin K), 205, 462
Pictures in this book, 16–17
PID (pelvic inflammatory disease), 363–364
Piercing ears, 6
Piles (hemorrhoids), 71
Pills *(See Medicines)*
Pill, the, 351–355, 463–465
Pimples all over, 366
Pitocin, 28, 176, 274, 382, 460–461
  (Also see Oxytocin)
Pitting edema, 113
Placenta
  bleeding after it comes out, 276–279
  bleeding before it comes out, 270–274
  checking after birth, 200
  delivering, 197–199, 270–274, 275
  detached (abruption), 101, 244
  illustrated, 45
  membranes, 200
  missing piece(s) after birth, 200, 278–279
  model for teaching, 442–443
  not coming out, 275
  previa, 101, 244
  problems in past pregnancies, 85
  pushing out after birth, 144

List of references used for this book

Anderson, M. (1975). *Principles of Wound Healing in the Repair of the Episiotomy.* Hawthorn, New York: Margaret Anderson.

Anderson, R.M. and R. F. Romfh. "Knot Tying," *Technique in the Use of Surgical Tools.* New York: Appleton-Century-Crofts.

Abbatt, F.R. (1992). *Teaching for Better Learning: A Guide for Teachers of Primary Health Care Staff.* Geneva: World Health Organization.

Baker, C.A., G. J. Vill and L. B. Curet (1993). "Female Circumcision: Obstetric Issues," *American Journal of Obstetrics and Gynecology,* 269: 1616–1618.

Chow, M., B. Durand, M. Feldman, and M. Mills (1979). *Handbook of Pediatric Primary Care.* New York: John Wiley and Sons.

Davis, E. (1981). *A Guide to Midwifery: Heart and Hands.* Santa Fe, New Mexico: John Muir Publications.

Department of Health/MCHS/Philippines (in press). *Midwifery Manual of Maternal Child Health Care.* Manila: Department of Health.

Douglas, R.G. and W.D. Stromme (1965). *Operative Obstetrics.* NY: Appleton-Century-Crofts.

Eloesser, L., E. J. Galt and I. Hemingway (1973). *Pregnancy, Childbirth and the Newborn: A Manual for Rural Midwives.* Mexico: Instituto Indigenista Interamericano.

Frye, A. (1991). *Healing Passage: A Suturing Manual for Midwives.* Chelsa, Michigan: Labrys Press.

Gaber, I. A. (1985). "Medical Protocol for Delivery of Infibulated Women in Sudan," *American Journal of Nursing,* 85 (6): 687.

Gaskin, I. M. (1977). *Spiritual Midwifery.* Summertown, Tennessee: The Book Publishing Company.

Garrey, M. et al (1980). *Obstetrics Illustrated.* New York: Churchill Livingstone.

Gordon, G. (1990). *Training Manual for Traditional Birth Attendants.* London: Macmillan Education Ltd.

Kozier, B. and G. Erb (1989). *Techniques in Clinical Nursing.* Redwood City, California: Addison-Wesley.

Kwast, B., S. Miller and C. Conroy (1993). *Management of Life-Threatening Obstetrical Emergencies: Protocols and Flow diagrams for Use By Registered/Licensed Nurse-Midwives or Midwives in Health Centers and Private or Government Services.* Arlington, Virginia: MotherCare.

Lettenmaier, C. and M.E. Gallen (1987). "Counseling Guide," *Population Reports,* Series J, No. 36. Baltimore, Maryland: Johns Hopkins University, Population Information Program.

Lettenmaier, C. and M.E. Gallen (1987). "Counseling Makes a Difference." *Population Reports,* Series J. No. 35. Baltimore, Maryland: Johns Hopkins University, Population Information Program.

Lightfoot-Klein, H. L. and E. Shawn (1991). "Special Needs of Ritually circumcised Women Patients," *Journal of Gynecologic, Obstetric, and Neonatal Nursing,* 20(2): 102–107.

Marshall, M.A. and S.T. Buffington (1991). *Life-Saving Skills Manual for Midwives.* Washington, D.C.: American College of Nurse-Midwives.

Miller, S. (1993). *Technical Assistance to the Philippines: April 1, 1993–July 22, 1993.* Report to ACNM/MotherCare/USAID.

Ministry of Health, Ghana (1933). *A Manual for the Training of Traditional Birth Attendants in Ghana.* Ghana: Ministry of Health, UNICEF, and USAID.

MotherCare/Nigeria (1993). *MotherCare Counseling Training Module.* Washington, D.C./Nigeria: JSI/MotherCare.

Myles, M. (1981). *Textbook for Midwives.* New York: Churchill Livingstone.

Parke-Davis. *Female Reproductive Organs in Health and in Illness.* Morris Plains, New Jersey: Parke-Davis.

Pritchard, J.A. and P.C. MacDonald. *Williams Obstetrics,* 15th and 16th eds. New York: Appleton-Century-Crofts.

Oxorn, H. and W. Foote (1980). *Human Labor and Birth.* New York: Appleton-Century-Crofts.

Shearer, C., A.S. Kauffman, M.H. Shearer and P. Shrock (1987). *Directory of Instructional Materials in Perinatal Education.* Boston, Massachusetts: Blackwell Scientific Publications.

Sundeen, S. J., G. W. Stuart, E.D. Rankin and S.A. Cohen (1985). *Nurse-Client Interaction: Implementing the Nursing Process.* St. Louis, Missouri: C.V. Mosby.

Ross Laboratories. *Obstetrical Presentation and Position.* Columbus, Ohio: Ross Laboratories.

Varney, H. (1987). *Nurse-Midwifery.* Boston, Massachusetts: Blackwell Scientific Publications.

Werner, D. and B. Bower (1987). *Helping Health Workers Learn.* Palo Alto, California: Hesperian Foundation.

Werner, D. (1992). *Where There is No Doctor,* Revised Edition. Palo Alto, California: Hesperian Foundation.

Wind, G.G. and N.M. Rich (1987). "Surgical Knots and Suture Material," *Principles of Surgical Technique: The Art of Surgery,* Baltimore/Munich: Urban and Schwarzenberg, 41–52.

World Health Organization (1992). *Clean Delivery: A Complimentary Strategy in the Elimination of Neonatal Tetanus.* Jakarta: Expanded Program on Immunization Global Advisory Group, World Health Organization.

Other Books from the Hesperian Foundation

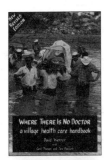

Where There Is No Doctor, by David Werner with Carol Thuman and Jane Maxwell, is perhaps the most widely used health care manual in developing countries today. The book provides vital, easily understood information on how to diagnose, treat, and prevent common diseases. Special importance is placed on ways to prevent health problems, including cleanliness, a healthy diet, and vaccinations. The authors also emphasize the active role villagers must take in their own health care. 512 pages. Available in English and Spanish.

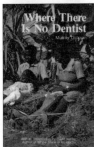

Where There Is No Dentist, by Murray Dickson, shows people how to care for their own teeth and gums, and how to prevent tooth and gum problems. Emphasis is placed on sharing this knowledge in the home, community, and school. The author also gives detailed and well-illustrated information on using dental equipment, placing fillings, taking out teeth, and suggests ways to teach dental hygiene and nutrition. 208 pages.

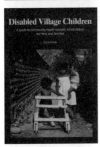

Disabled Village Children, by David Werner, contains a wealth of information about most common disabilities of children, including polio, cerebral palsy, juvenile arthritis, blindness, and deafness. The author gives suggestions for simplified rehabilitation at the village level and explains how to make a variety of appropriate low-cost aids. Emphasis is placed on how to help disabled children find a role and be accepted in the community. 672 pages. Available in English and Spanish.

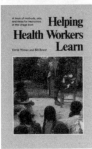

Helping Health Workers Learn, by David Werner and Bill Bower, is an indispensable resource for anyone involved in teaching about health. This heavily illustrated book shows how to make health education fun and effective. It includes activities for mothers and children; pointers for using theater, flannel-boards, and other techniques; and many ideas for producing low-cost teaching aids. Emphasizing a people-centered approach to health care, it presents strategies for effective community involvement through participatory education. 640 pages. Available in English and Spanish.

The Hesperian Foundation also distributes other books on health, rehabilitation, and development, as well as slide shows, videos, and writings on the politics of health. Please write us for a brochure describing all our materials, with prices and ordering information.

The Hesperian Foundation
P.O. Box 1692
Palo Alto, California 94302
U.S.A.

NOTES

NOTES

NOTES

NOTES

INFORMATION ON PHYSICAL SIGNS

Temperature

There are two kinds of thermometer scales: centigrade (C) and Fahrenheit (F). Either can be used to measure a person's temperature. Here is how they compare:

Centigrade

This thermometer reads 40°C (forty degrees centigrade).

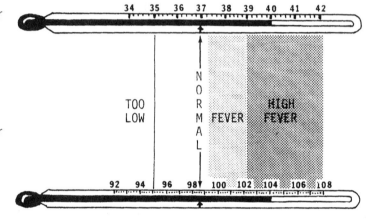

Fahrenheit

This thermometer reads 104°F (one hundred and four degrees Fahrenheit).

Pulse or heartbeat

For a person at rest

ADULTS... 60–80 beats per minute is normal.

NEWBORN BABIES... 120–160 beats per minute is normal.

For each degree centigrade of fever, the adult heartbeat usually increases about 20 beats per minute.

Blood pressure

(This is included for midwives who have the equipment to measure blood pressure.)

For a person at rest 120/80 is normal, but this varies a lot.

If the bottom number (when the sound disappears) is over 90, this is a danger sign of high blood pressure (see pages 107–110).